CATHERINE SAXELBY'S COMPLETE FOOD AND NUTRITION COMPANION

THE ULTIMATE A–Z GUIDE

To my mother Anne,

who first taught me to cook

and whose motto with all manner of

diets and food trends was always

'everything in moderation'.

CATHERINE SAXELBY'S COMPLETE FOOD AND NUTRITION COMPANION

THE ULTIMATE A–Z GUIDE

hardie grant books
MELBOURNE • LONDON

Published in 2012 by Hardie Grant Books

Hardie Grant Books (Australia)
Ground Floor, Building 1
658 Church Street
Richmond, Victoria 3121
www.hardiegrant.com.au

Hardie Grant Books (UK)
Dudley House, North Suite
34–35 Southampton Street
London WC2E 7HF
www.hardiegrant.co.uk

Cataloguing-in-Publication data is available from the National Library of Australia.
Catherine Saxelby's Complete Food and Nutrition Companion : the ultimate A–Z guide
ISBN 978 1 74066 841 5

Design and layout by Peter Dyson at desertpony
Author photo by Michael Cheetham
Typeset in Adobe Caslon Pro 10/12pt
Colour reproduction by Splitting Image Colour Studio
Printed in China by 1010 Printing International Limited

Contents

A note about trademarks

The following brands that appear in this book are trademarked products ™ or registered trademarks ®:

Actimel
Alcodol
Alka-Seltzer
All-Bran
Anlene
Aspro
Beano
Berocca
Betty Baxter
Biggest Loser
Burgen Soy-Lin
Cadbury Lite
Calfix
CalciPlus
Calcium Plus
Calrose
Cambridge Diet
Caro
Celebrity Slim
Chaser
Cirtavescent
Cordarone X
Corn Flakes
De-Gas
Doongara
Dymatize 12 hour meal
Ecco
Eno
Equal
Evian
Fairtrade
Farmers Best
Felodur
Fernwood
Fibyrax
Forbiotic
Fybogel
Gastrolyte
Gatorade
Hairy Lemon
Hangover Stopper
Heart Active
Heart Foundation Tick
Helga
Herbalife
Hi-Lo
Hi-Maize
HOWARU
Hungry Jacks
Hydralyte
Isowhey
Jenny Craig
Just Right
KFC
Kickstart
Lipex
Lipitor
Lite Start
Lite White
Logicol
Marmite
Maxim
McDonalds
Metamucil
Musashi
Natural Confectionery Company
Natvia
No Doze
Normacol
Normafibre
Nucolox
Nutella
Nutrasweet
Onedose
Optifast
Optislim
Panadol
Pero
Perrier
Physical
Pizza Hut
Plendil
Pro-activ
Pura Boost
Pura Heart Active
Pura Tone
Pure Blond Super Dry
Purevia
Quorn
Rebound
Red Bull
Rev
Rice Bubbles
RU-21
Russia Party
Shape
Skimmer
Skinny Milk
Slim Fast
Sob're-K
So-Good
Splenda
SteviaSweet
Subway
Sultana Bran
Sunola
Tabasco
Tony Ferguson
Trim
Ural
V
Vegemite
Vichy
Vita-Brits
Vitasoy
VSL#3
Weet-Bix
Weight Watchers
Xantrax
Yakult
Zimstat
Zocor
Zymil

Measurements and abbreviations used in this book

WEIGHT
ug = microgram
mg = milligram
g = gram
kg = kilogram
1000 g = 1 kg

VOLUME
ml = millilitre
L = litre
1000 ml = 1L

DISTANCE
mm = millimetre
cm = centimetre
m = metre
10 mm = 1 cm
100 cm = 1 m

KILOJOULES AND CALORIES

All energy values in this book are given in kilojoules, which are the metric unit of energy measurement. Kilojoules are approximately four times the value of calories. One calorie equals 4.186 kilojoules (4.2 or simply 4 is close enough for a quick conversion). For example, one slice of bread supplies 290 kilojoules or (290 divided by 4) 70 calories.

Food measures are based on level metric cup and spoon measures:
1 cup holds 250 ml
1 tablespoon holds 20 ml
1 teaspoon holds 5 ml

Preface

IF YOU'VE EVER WONDERED what's the difference between low-fat yoghurt and diet yoghurt, or how to eat to beat diabetes or high cholesterol, or simply to stay healthy and have more energy in your day, then this book is for you.

My passion is to provide you with the latest information about food, nutrition, diet and health. I want to cut through all the fads about food and misconceptions about healthy eating and prove that healthy eating doesn't have to be hard work. Yes, it can and should taste delicious.

I hope this book will teach and inspire you. Keep it close to hand as a reference for regular use as you make the best choices for you and your family's wellbeing. I want to help you live a long, happy and healthy life with energy and passion, and enjoy good food along the way.

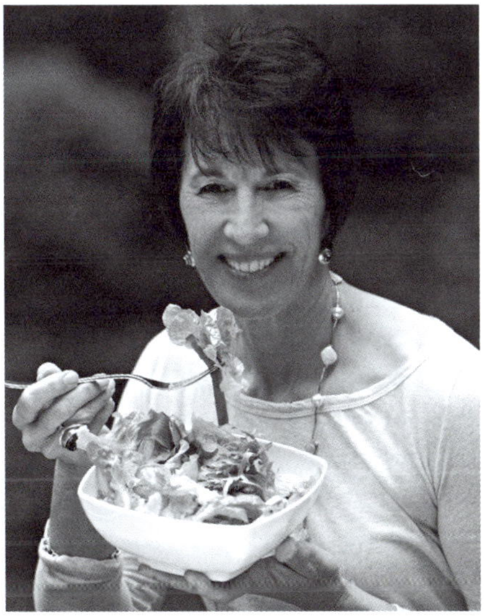

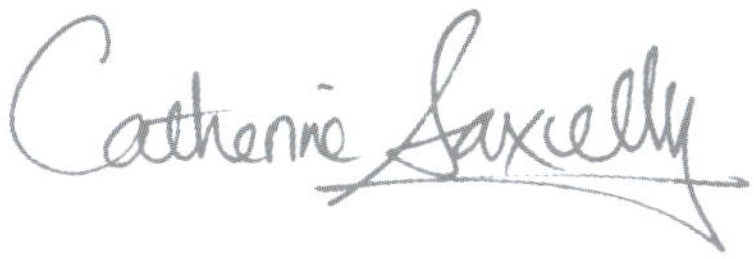

HOW TO USE THIS BOOK

Like all A to Z guides, you don't need to read this book from cover to cover. Just dip in or use the index to direct you to information that is relevant to your interest and needs today. All the latest facts and figures are here at your fingertips. It's like having your own personal food and nutrition coach on hand to answer any query!

ABOUT THE AUTHOR

Catherine Saxelby is an accredited dietitian and nutritionist who is passionate about helping people eat tasty, healthy, seasonal food. She is well known to readers and media for her easy-to-read articles and her invaluable Foodwatch website. In 2000, she received an award for Innovation in Nutrition Communication from the Dietitians Association of Australia for her books and blogs. This book is her eleventh book on food and nutrition and draws together a lifetime of professional experience.

You'll find a comprehensive glossary and reference list for this book on the Foodwatch website at **www.foodwatch.com.au**, where you can also access exclusive articles, video clips, recipes, information and all the latest nutrition news.

Acknowledgements

In a project as big as this, there are always many people to say thanks to. I've always valued the collective wisdom from their input.

First and foremost I'd like to thank the many members of my Foodwatch website who sent me queries, emails and comments, all of which help me write in a way that's clear and easy to read. I hope I've answered your curly questions.

Secondly, my thanks to all the experts who sent me their reference papers or who read a section of this book and gave me helpful feedback:

- Dr Trevor Beard, Founder of Salt Skip, now deceased
- Professor Jennie Brand-Miller, Professor of Human Nutrition at the University of Sydney
- Dr Louise Burke, dietitian at the Australian Institute of Sport
- Glenn Cardwell, dietitian; consultant Australian Mushroom Growers' Association
- Phil Daffy, Blackmores Australia
- Ian Hemphill, co-owner Herbies Spices and author
- Peter Howard, chef and author
- Professor Neil Mann, Head of Food Science, RMIT
- David Panasiak, food technologist and principal of Food Liaison
- Nicole Senior, dietitian and sustainability expert
- Greg Seymour, General Manager, Australian Mushroom Growers' Association
- Professor Andrew Sinclair, Professor of Nutrition Science at Deakin University
- Penny Stone, specialist early childhood dietitian
- Dr Anne Swain and the dietitians at the RPAH Allergy Unit in Sydney
- Holly Viner, organic food expert
- Lisa Yates, dietitian, consultant at Nuts for Life

Thirdly, to my dietitians who have conducted research and analysis for me over the years—in particular Karen Kingham, Airlie Lacey, Josephine Mollica, Anne Gregory, Caitlin Reid and Jess Hodgkinson.

To Munaiba Khan who has edited lots of posts, reviews and new ideas for the website and book (and never pushed her own opinions on what's healthy and what's not).

Not forgetting the team at Hardie Grant Books, particularly editors Sharon Mullins and Brooke Clark and designer Peter Dyson for his attractive design. A big thanks also to Sandy Grant, Julie Pinkham and Fran Berry for taking a big chance with this new book.

To my patient husband Dave, for putting up with the long time editing ('Is that still that book?') and to my darling kids, Guy and Georgia, for being guinea pigs along the way and taste-testing all those weird and wonderful creations from the kitchen. I know you both enjoy and strive to eat good food. Well, mostly.

Lastly to Philippa Sandall, publishing consultant and dear friend, without whom this book would never have seen the light of day.

A

Acai

Acai [ah-sigh-ee] is the fruit of the acai palm (*Euterpe oleracea*), native to South America's Amazon region. Although you may see it called 'acai berry', it's not actually a berry; it is a deep purple drupe (from the same family as plums), about the size of a large blueberry with a stone or seed that takes up about 80 per cent of the fruit, so there's not much flesh. It is highly perishable and is immediately processed after picking (frozen or freeze-dried). It is used in beverages, health products (bars, powders, capsules) and weight-loss supplements.

Around 2004, acai was 'discovered' and marketed to the world with amazing claims. Acai was a 'fountain of youth', 'the most nutritious and powerful food in the world', and an all–in–one multivitamin that could boost energy, improve sexual function, lower cholesterol, produce better sleep, strengthen your immune system and detox your body all at the same time. None of these claims have been proven by large, independent clinical trials published in peer-reviewed scientific journals.

MY TAKE *Time will tell if it's just another over-hyped (and in this case over-priced) fad like oat bran, lecithin, pine bark extract and wheat grass, which all came and went as wonder foods.*

NUTRITIONAL VALUE

Like all fruit, acai is nutritious. It has a high concentration of anthocyanins like other purplish-blue coloured fruits and berries. It's also rich in fibre and vitamin E and contains some minerals including a little calcium and iron. What is unusual for a fruit is its high proportion of essential fatty acids. I can't give you a nutritional analysis for acai because what you get depends on which acai product you buy (juice, bar or freeze-dried pulp), so check out the information in the nutrition panel. It is not very sweet, so has to be mixed with other juices or sugar to taste any good.

Acidity Regulators

See also **Food Acids.**

These are food additives that are used to hold the acid-alkali balance of a liquid at a constant level, like the gluconolactone (575) added to energy drinks.

Acidophilus

See also **Probiotics; Yoghurt.**

Acidophilus (*Lactobacillus acidophilus*) is the bacteria used in making yoghurt.

Acne and Diet

Acne has a huge impact on self-esteem and quality of life, no matter what your age. It's not just an adolescent affliction; some people suffer with pimples well into their twenties and beyond. Until recently, teens were told that food played no role in causing acne—not even those longtime villains like chocolate and greasy food. It was merely a case of hormones gone mad.

But recent Australian research shows that eating junk food *can* make acne worse, while eating less-processed foods with a low GI can help clear it up. Dietary modification is now considered when treating milder forms of acne, in place of the many skin treatments prescribed for pimple control. Researchers from RMIT University and the Royal Children's and Royal Melbourne hospitals in Victoria carried out a clinical trial with two groups of young men aged 15–25 years, comparing a typical Western diet high in processed and refined foods with a more natural diet based on wholegrains, low-GI carbohydrates, lean protein, fresh fruit and vegetables. After 12 weeks, eating the healthy, more natural low-GI and higher-protein diet had a dramatic effect, improving acne by over 50 per cent when compared to the diet high in processed and refined foods.

Foods eliminated from the low-GI and higher-protein diet were those we know aren't that nutritious such as high-GI white bread and rice, plus junk food like crisps, corn chips and fizzy drinks. Potatoes were also eliminated in this study as most have a high GI rating. The researchers believe that the diet worked by controlling some of the hormonal imbalances associated with acne, particularly an over-production of insulin and testosterone.

The five key features of the *Anti-acne Diet* include:

1. Lean, protein-rich foods—fish twice a week, red meat three to four times a week, three daily serves of low-fat dairy foods and lean protein at lunchtime
2. Low GI or wholegrain carbohydrate foods at every meal
3. Plenty of fresh fruit and vegetables (two serves of fruit and five serves of vegetables daily)
4. Good fats from olive and canola oils and spreads
5. Limiting highly processed foods such as sugary breakfast cereals, soft drinks, takeaway foods, ready-to-eat snacks, cakes and biscuits packed with refined starches.

DID YOU KNOW?

US researchers have observed that acne is rare or non-existent in the hunter-gatherer societies of Papua New Guinea and Paraguay where processed food is limited. In contrast, it's estimated that acne impacts between 79 and 95 per cent of adolescents and between 40 and 54 per cent of individuals older than 25 years in developed countries like Australia.

HORMONES AND INHERITANCE

Don't forget the key contributors to skin problems are still hormonal changes during adolescence and pregnancy, and stress. Acne also runs in families and may override even the healthiest diets. In their teens, my husband, his sister and all their cousins had terrible acne. It was clearly something that ran in that family and at the time there were none of the modern acne treatments available. Despite eating nothing fried, or any chocolate for most of his teen years, my husband's skin never really cleared up until his late twenties.

WHAT YOU CAN DO

You don't need to put up with acne. Mild acne usually responds to an improved diet and a regular cleansing routine using an oil-free moisturiser and special lotions that contain benzoyl peroxide, salicylic acid, retinoic acids or alpha-hydroxy acids.

Severe acne, where nothing seems to work, needs to be seen by a doctor or dermatologist, who can prescribe low-dose antibiotic therapy or oral retinoids.

Addiction, Food

Can you be 'addicted' to food in the same way as the nicotine in cigarettes? People regularly report suffering mood swings, the shakes, headaches and cravings when they cut refined flour and sugary foods from their diet. Although it may seem to make sense, there is circumstantial—not scientific—evidence for this, as there may be other contributing factors.

Researchers from the University of Auckland have suggested that food addiction could be an important factor in the obesity epidemic. They hypothesise that foods with a high GI cause blood glucose levels to spike, and this rush stimulates the same areas of the brain associated with addiction to nicotine and other drugs. The theory is based on evidence showing that people who binged on high-GI carbohydrate foods experienced loss of control and a compulsion to keep taking higher amounts to get the same 'buzz', and suffered withdrawal if they went 'cold turkey', which is why they find it hard to quit. If high-GI foods like corn flakes or white bread are the villains, then they suggest low-GI equivalents may be the saviour.

I asked GI expert Professor Jennie Brand-Miller about this food addiction hypothesis. 'It's a novel idea that draws on strong evidence that glucose consumption influences levels of the feel-good chemical serotonin in the brain,' she says. 'Although all foods take about 30 minutes to peak, and the overall shape of the post-meal glycaemia curve is similar for high-, medium- and low-GI foods, high-GI foods peak and fall at substantially greater levels. To control high blood glucose after meals, carbohydrate quality (its GI) and carbohydrate quantity (the amount you eat), both matter.' So her general message is stay 'low GI' with carb-rich foods, and keep portion sizes moderate.

See also **Cravings; Glycemic Index.**

Additives

Supermarket shelves are crammed full of food products that claim to be free of artificial colours and flavourings, or contain no preservatives. The increasing popularity to include the words 'natural', 'organic' or 'nothing artificial' on products are testimony to the image additives have as modern-day villains in our food supply. The growing interest in farmers' markets and genuine organic food further confirms this view.

Like everyone else, I want to avoid as many additives as possible in the foods I buy. But I also recognise that I choose to live in a large city away from the farms where my food is grown, and I also don't have the time to cook from scratch using only fresh produce each and every day. Without additives, I would face a restricted food choice and many foods would not be available all year round. For example, if I can't get fresh basil, my choices are to use dried basil, basil herb paste (made with the help of an emulsifier, thickeners, natural colour and a preservative), or no basil at all. So I know I need to accept some additives, such as the thickeners in my low-fat yoghurt or an emulsifier in a chilled soup; the ones that are unlikely to cause problems. But for me, the fewer additives in my food, the better.

DEFINITION

Food additives are substances added to food by manufacturers, in relatively small quantities, to improve the colour, appearance, flavour, texture, stability or storage life of food.

There are more than 300 additives permitted for use in food and drinks by Food Standards Australia New Zealand (FSANZ), and the maximum amount that can be used and type of food to which they can be added is clearly specified.

There are 18 major classes of food additives, each used for a different purpose. They have code numbers, and that's what you find on the food labels, although if you're travelling and shopping overseas, the numbers for their food additives will be different. For example, in the US additives are classified as GRAS meaning 'Generally Regarded As Safe' and additives listed as this can be used in any food.

THE 18 CLASSES OF ADDITIVES

COLOURS

Colourings are regarded by many as an unnecessary, cosmetic addition to food, added for eye appeal only. Whether they have a valid use (to make food appealing and enjoyable) is a debated issue. Fortunately, the list of permitted colours in Australia and New Zealand is more restricted than overseas. Colours can be divided into three groups:

1. Natural colours extracted from plants or animals such as caramels (150a–d), which are the most widely used food colours, carotene (160a), curcumin (100), carmine (120), beet red (162), anthocyanins (163) and annatto (160b).
2. Synthetic colours that are chemically identical to the natural colours and thus have the same code number.
3. Synthetic colours such as the yellow hues tartrazine (102) and Sunset Yellow FCF (110) or blue shades of indigotine (132) and Brilliant Blue FCF (133), which are not found in nature. A small number of people are sensitive to these azo dyes and coal tar dyes, and should check the ingredient labels for them. Tartrazine may cause an allergy-like reaction in a very small number of people.

PRESERVATIVES

Preservatives slow the growth of moulds, yeasts and bacteria, lessening food spoilage and waste. Some act as antioxidants to prevent food from oxidising or going rancid. The most commonly used are the sorbates (200–203) used in juice, cordial, jams and soft drinks; benzoates (210–213) used in acidic products like wine, cider and soft drinks; sulphur dioxide and sulphites (220–228) used in dried apricots and apples to keep their colour; nitrates (249–252) used in sausages to preserve sausage mince; and propionates (280–283) used in bread to inhibit moulds.

Each type of preservative acts against certain microorganisms in certain foods—no single one works in all conditions. Preservatives are only used where necessary. Remember that frozen, canned and pasteurised foods do not contain preservatives because the actual processes of freezing and heating act to preserve the food. Many household ingredients such as sugar (in jam, biscuits, confectionery), salt (in cheese, salami, olives) and vinegar (in pickled cucumbers, salad dressings) also function to preserve food. Foods made with high levels of these do not need preservatives.

COMMON ADDITIVES

- MSG (621)—flavour enhancer
- Citric acid (330)—food acid and antioxidant
- Caramel (150a)—colour
- Xanthan gum (415)—thickener, stabiliser
- Calcium propionate (282)—bread mould inhibitor/preservative
- Acetylated distarch adipate (1422)—thickener.

BENZOATES

Benzoates are naturally occurring food acids from fruit, vegetables, herbs and honey. Their salt, sodium benzoate (210), is a preservative used in some sauces and pickled vegetables. Both naturally occurring benzoates and the food additive forms can cause sensitivity reactions in susceptible people.

FOOD ACIDS

Food acids are added to give food a sharp or sour taste, which produces the correct flavour balance and ensures a consistent acidity level. They are identical to those that occur naturally like citric acid (330) in citrus fruit, malic acid (296) in green apples, tartaric acid (334) in grapes and acetic acid (260) in vinegar.

ANTIOXIDANTS

Antioxidants slow down oxidation reactions and so prevent fats turning rancid and food going brown. Vitamin E (tocopherols, 306–309) is a natural antioxidant which keeps oils and margarines from turning rancid. Another is vitamin C (ascorbic acid, 300), which keeps wine and cider from discolouring. As sodium ascorbate (301), it is used in cured meats, fruit salad and vinegars.

Butylated hydroxyanisole (BHA, 320) is one of the most widely used antioxidants in fats and oils, and in foods made with them such as snack foods, instant mashed potato, walnuts, pecans, crisps, cookies and muesli bars. It is often used in conjunction with a gallate, like propyl gallate (310).

MINERAL SALTS

Mineral salts improve the texture of foods such as ham, corned beef and deli meats, which are likely to lose meat juices. Various phosphates, chlorides and carbonates such as sodium carbonate (500) or potassium chloride (508) are examples.

VEGETABLE GUMS

Vegetable gums thicken and gel foods like ice-cream, desserts, dressings, sauces, mayonnaise and diet foods. Alginates (400–405), agar (406) and carrageenan (407) are extracted from seaweeds, while pectin (440), guar gum (412) and xanthan gum (415) come from plants. Others are produced from cellulose like carboxymethyl cellulose (466).

THICKENERS

Thickeners are added to foods such as soups, pasta sauces, toppings and custard to thicken them or give a smooth, uniform texture. Similar in function to cornflour or arrowroot used at home, they are based on a number of starches (1400–1405) and modified starches like acetylated distarch adipate (1422).

HUMECTANTS

Humectants include polydextrose (1200), sorbitol (420), mannitol (421) and glycerin (422) and are used in icings, cakes, soft tortillas, dried fruit and muesli bars to help maintain moistness and to prevent foods drying out.

EMULSIFIERS/STABILISERS

These are oily substances that stabilise mixtures and prevent oil and water from separating. Lecithin (322), a substance occurring in soy beans and egg yolk, is an emulsifier frequently used in margarine, chocolate, cake mixes, pastry and ice-cream. Others include sorbitan monostearate (491) and mono- and di-glycerides of fatty acids (471). Emulsifiers are closely related to fats and are digested the same way, so can be considered quite safe.

FLAVOUR ENHANCERS

Flavour enhancers bring out the flavour or aroma of a food but contribute no flavour of their own. Monosodium glutamate or MSG (621) is the most well-known example; others include disodium guanylate (627) and disodium inosinate (631). They are used in many savoury foods ranging from cracker biscuits to gravy powders, stock powders, sauce mixes and instant noodle sachets.

SWEETENING SUBSTANCES

Sweeteners are used to replace sugar in diet products such as soft drink, yoghurts, sugar-free jellies, chewing gum, peppermints and chocolate. Some can only be used in beverages and cold applications like aspartame (951) and xylitol (967), while others such as acesulphame potassium (950) and sucralose (955) are heat-stable and good for baked muesli bars. Often two sweeteners are used together—one as an intense sweetener, the other as a bulking agent.

ANTI-CAKING AGENTS

Anti-caking agents help foods such as salt, coffee whiteners or flavour sachets flow freely when poured and stop particles clumping together. Examples are sodium aluminosilicate (554) and magnesium carbonate (504).

COLOUR RETENTION AGENTS

Colour retention agents retain or intensify the colour of foods.

ACIDITY REGULATORS

Acidity regulators hold the acid-alkali balance of a liquid at a constant level, like the gluconolactone (575) in energy drinks.

GLAZING AGENTS

Glazing agents give a shiny appearance or a protective coating to foods and include beeswax (901) and shellac (904).

FLOUR TREATMENT AGENTS

Flour treatment compounds are added to flour to improve the action of the yeast during bread making, and to modify the gluten during baking.

PROPELLANTS

Propellants are gases used in aerosol sprays to expel the contents when the button is pressed, like isobutane (943b).

ANTI-FOAMING AGENTS

Anti-foaming agents stop excessive frothing on boiling or reduce the formation of scum. Examples are polydimethylsiloxane (900a), which is added to commercial frying oils, and polyethylene glycol (1521).

FLAVOURS

Like colours, flavours fall into three groups—natural, synthetic but 'nature-identical', and synthetic with no counterpart in nature. They are complex mixtures of many components, making them impossible to define as a single substance; hence they carry no code numbers. Many flavours have been extracted from herbs or spices, or the compounds responsible for the herb's flavour have been synthesised. The body isn't able to distinguish between them. Foods must list the word 'flavour' on the ingredients list, even if the flavour is a natural one. Flavours make food more palatable, maintain uniformity and restore what's lost during processing.

ADDITIVE SAFETY

All food additives in commercial use in Australia and New Zealand have been rigorously researched before being accepted as safe by Food Standards Australia New Zealand (FSANZ). For example, it must be demonstrated that a satisfactory product cannot be made without using an already approved additive or another method of manufacture.

Each food and additive is considered separately. If the additive is not specifically listed for that food, then it cannot be added to it.

READ THE LABEL

All additives are listed alongside other ingredients by their class name, followed by their chemical name or their code number. For example, the yellow colour tartrazine could appear on packs as COLOUR (TARTRAZINE) or simply as COLOUR (102).

WHITE BREAD

- ✔ Emulsifiers—481 sodium stearoyl lactylate and 471 mono- and di-glycerides of fatty acids ensure all ingredients in the dough stay mixed.
- ✔ Preservative—282 calcium propionate stops the loaf from developing mould in humid weather.

UNBLEACHED BAKER'S FLOUR, WATER, YEAST, GLUTEN, VEGETABLE OIL, IODISED SALT, SESAME SEEDS, SOYA FLOUR, EMULSIFIERS (481, 471), PRESERVATIVE (282), VITAMINS (FOLATE & THIAMIN).

SALAD DRESSING

- ✔ Food acid—330 citric acid gives the dressing a pleasant tang (like lemon juice).
- ✔ Vegetable gum—415 xanthan gum makes the dressing a little thicker.
- ✔ Colour—102 tartrazine imparts a golden hue.
- ✔ Antioxidant—320 butylated hydroxy anisole prevents the oil from turning rancid.

WATER, VEGETABLE OIL, SUGAR, VINEGAR, SALT, FOOD ACID (330), VEGETABLE GUM (415), SPICE, GARLIC, COLOUR (102), ANTIOXIDANT (320).

MUSTARD

- ✔ Food acid—330 citric acid imparts a pleasant tang.
- ✔ Emulsifier—322 lecithin keeps all ingredients blended.
- ✔ Colour—160a Beta-carotene imparts a rich golden colour; converted to vitamin A in the body.

WATER, MUSTARD, SALT, VEGETABLE OIL, SPICES, FOOD ACID (330), EMULSIFIER (322), NATURAL COLOUR (160A).

If the print on the label is hard to read, check out the manufacturer's website. Many major food companies post this product information there.

READING BETWEEN THE LINES OF ADDITIVE CLAIMS

NO MSG

This is misleading, as there are many sources of natural glutamates that may be present in many foods, especially protein foods. 'No added MSG' would be more realistic (and some food companies do say this), but it still does not solve the problem of how to avoid glutamates if you need to. Mushrooms, cheese, tomatoes and meat are all rich in natural glutamates, which contribute to flavour.

NO ARTIFICIAL COLOURS OR FLAVOURS

This is a key selling point with many consumers, but it is sometimes misused on foods when it is not permitted in a whole class of food. For example, breads and breakfast

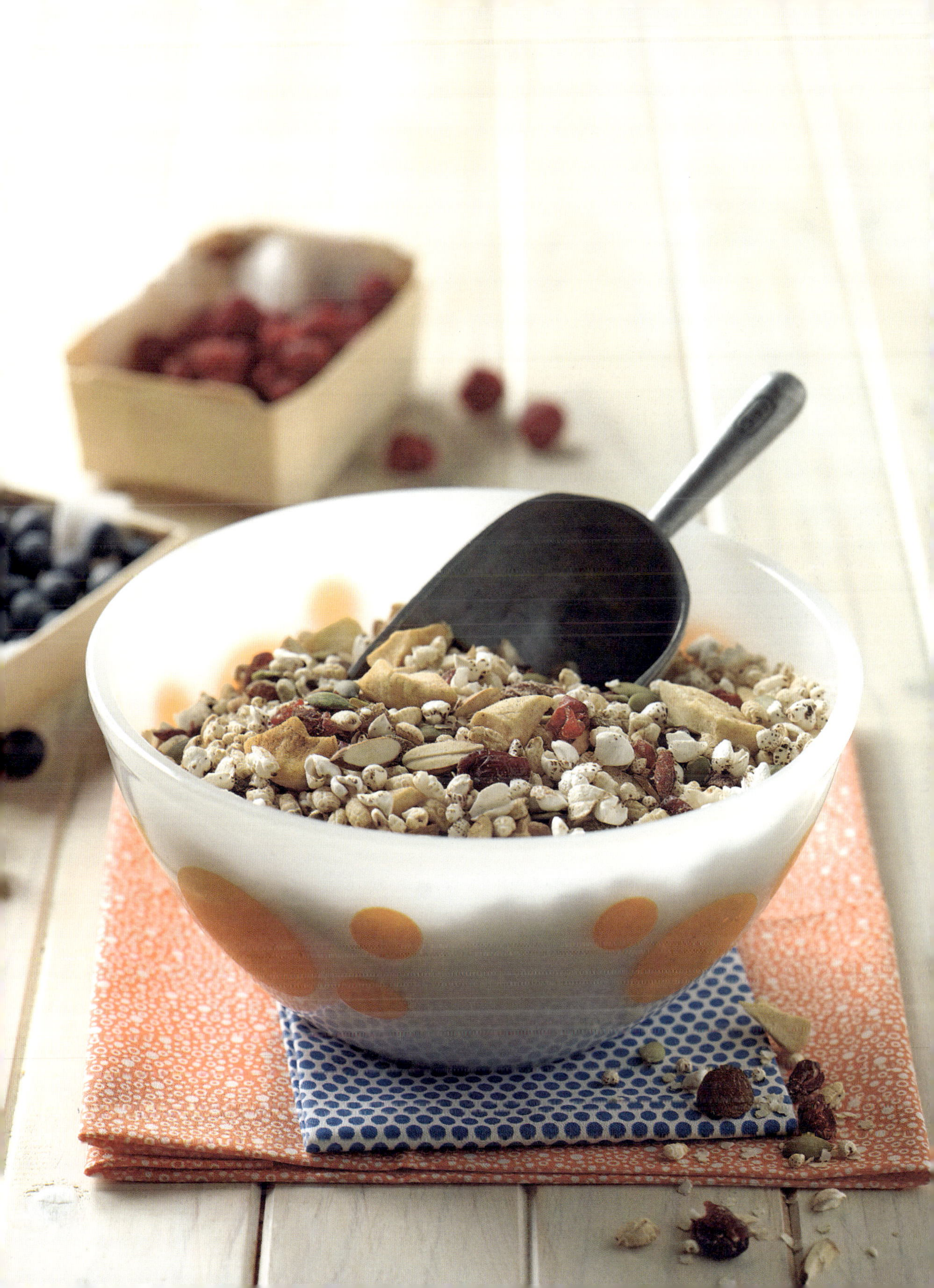

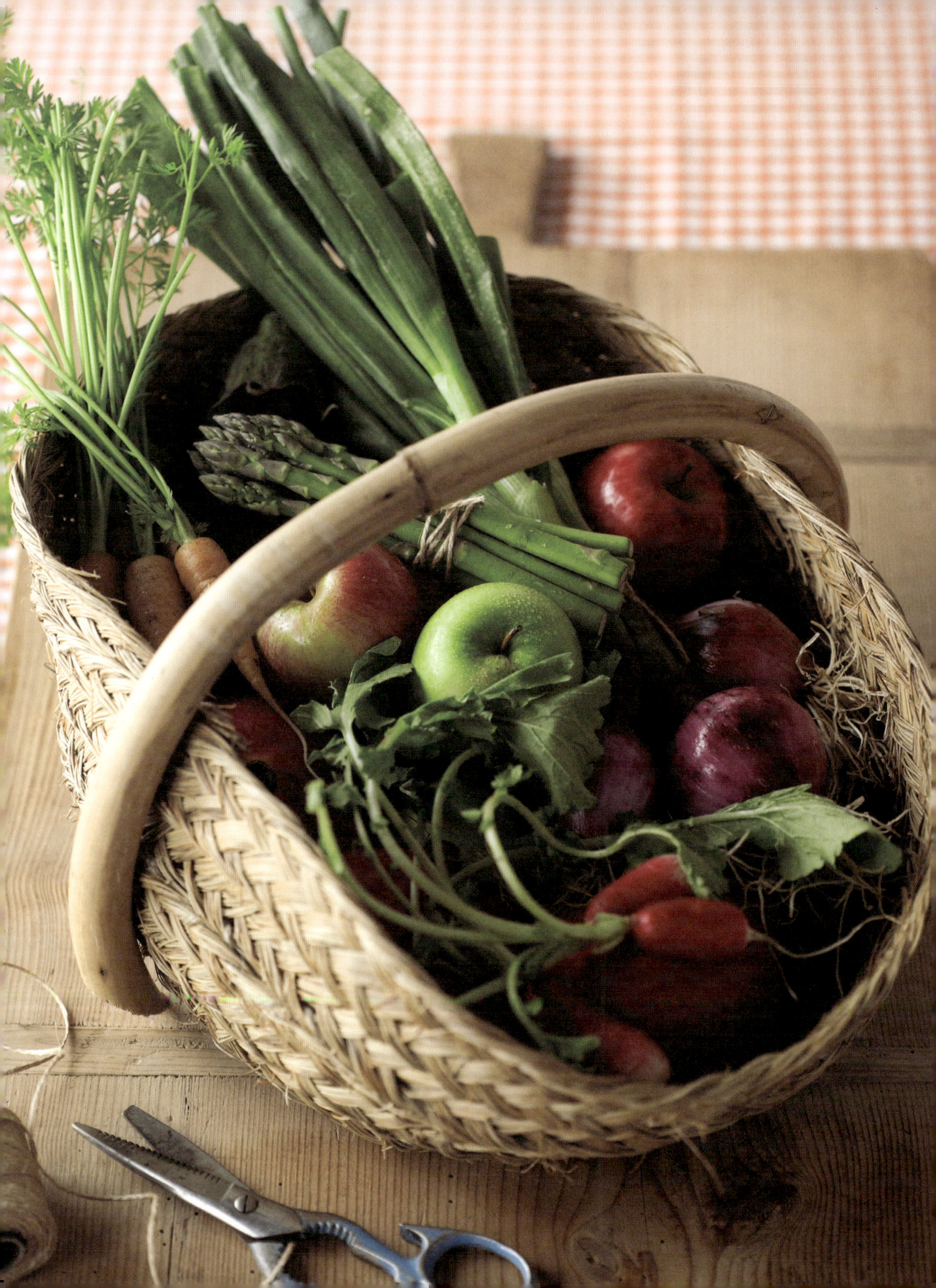

cereals are not permitted to contain artificial colours and flavours. However, they can still contain natural colours (like beta-carotene or caramel) or flavours and these will be stated on the ingredient list.

NO PRESERVATIVES

This is another key selling point. It generally lets you know that no chemical preservatives are present, although other methods of preservation like pasteurisation or vacuum packaging may have been used for the product. Because consumers are so fearful of additives, this term often appears on food packs as reassurance, even if preservatives are not actually permitted in that class of foods anyway.

NO ADDED CHEMICALS

This is a meaningless term as all food is composed of chemicals. Translated, it probably means 'No artificial colours, flavours or preservatives'.

AVOIDING ADDITIVES

- ✔ Avoid buying coloured, flavoured food in packets such as cordial, soft drinks, chips, soup mixes, simmer sauces, coloured lollies, biscuits with icing, cake mixes and instant puddings.
- ✔ Cook from scratch using meat, fish, fresh vegetables, fresh or pure dried herbs, homemade stock and flour or cream for thickening. For example, I can make my mum's beef stroganoff using beef, oil, onion, mushrooms, tomato paste, homemade stock and sour cream.
- ✔ Read the ingredient list for additives, not the claims on the front. Get familiar with the code numbers of the ones that are a problem for you. All FSANZ-approved additives and their code numbers are listed on my website.
- ✔ Compare two products side by side and buy the one with the least additives on the label. It's usually the plain version. Here's a comparison of two popular snack foods:

Original Grain Waves: 7 ingredients

WHOLEGRAIN CEREALS (66%) (CORN, WHEAT, OATS), VEGETABLE OIL, RICE, SUGAR, SALT

Sweet Chilli Grain Waves: 25 ingredients

WHOLEGRAIN CEREALS (61%) (CORN, WHEAT, OATS), VEGETABLE OIL, RICE, SUGAR, WHEY POWDER, SALT, FOOD ACIDS (262, 330), MALTODEXTRIN (TAPIOCA, WHEAT), FLAVOUR ENHANCERS (621, 627, 631, 955), SPICES (CHILLI, PAPRIKA), ONION POWDER, CORN STARCH, GARLIC POWDER, TOMATO POWDER, NATURAL FLAVOURS, NATURAL COLOURS (PAPRIKA EXTRACT, COCHINEAL, CARAMEL ANNATTO)

See also **Allergies, Intolerances and Diet; Sweeteners.**

Adolescents and Diet

13–18 years

Adolescents need a lot of calcium for their growing bones. This is the time to maximise their intake of calcium, magnesium and potassium so that strong, dense bones are laid down now, helping to prevent osteoporosis in later life.

Girls who start to menstruate need to increase their iron intake as their needs nearly double when periods start. However, healthy eating often gets railroaded during the teen years due to fast food and diet fads, which are common, particularly with girls.

Recommended daily intake for children
Ranges from 8900 kJ for a sedentary, inactive girl, to 15,600 kJ for a sporty, active boy.

GIRLS

Everything from 'going vegetarian' to the latest detox diet is embarked on and experimented with by many girls at this age. As a parent, take it in your stride but keep an eye on your daughter's health and watch for complaints of fatigue and feeling sick.

Many girls go vegetarian because they think it will lead to weight loss. While removing meat does remove kilojoules, going vegetarian can be a smokescreen for an eating disorder like anorexia. Australian research has found an unusually high incidence of vegetarianism among people with eating disorders. Vegetarianism doesn't cause eating disorders, but in the context of obsessive dieting and kilojoule counting, it can point to a problem.

You should discourage extreme weight loss diets as best you can. They can trigger an ongoing merry-go-round of unsustainable dieting followed by binge eating. Studies show that the more diets a teenage girl attempts, the more likely she is to binge eat. Explain to your child that fad diets don't work because they can make you so hungry that you eventually break out and binge on everything in sight. The ultimate aim is to build teens' resilience to negative body image pressures rampant in the fashion and advertising industries.

Try to be consistent and offer sensible, basic meals with extra salads, fruit and vegetables so they can choose healthier, lighter fare without following a rigid diet.

BOYS

In contrast to girls, boys have high kilojoule requirements due to the rapid growth spurts that occur during these years and the active, sporty lifestyle many teen boys have. They're hungry and they need food! I often hear stories from parents of teen boys recounting how their hungry son could consume twelve wheat biscuits or half a loaf of bread in one sitting after school.

Recommended daily intake for adults
This is wide and varied depending on your age, body weight and physical activity levels. It can be as low as 7400 kJ for an older woman over 70 years who is fairly inactive or housebound, to a high 13,500 kJ for a hard-working younger man doing labour-intensive work or strenuous sport.

Adults and Diet

18 + years

In general, the younger and more active you are, the more kilojoules you require from food. These needs decline as we get older, which explains the gradual weight creep that occurs with age.

PREGNANCY AND BREASTFEEDING

Requirements for most nutrients increase during pregnancy, but a boost in folate, iodine, iron, vitamin C and zinc is particularly important. Apart from a folate supplement, it is best to obtain nutrients from a healthy diet. Multivitamins not designed specifically for pregnancy should be taken with care, as there are dangers associated with excessive doses of nutrients such as vitamins A, D and B_6.

Kilojoule requirements vary greatly but on average a moderately active woman needs around 9700 kilojoules in her second trimester, rising to 10 000 kilojoules in the third. The average daily energy requirements for breastfeeding mothers are 2000 kilojoules per day more than that of a non-breastfeeding woman's needs. These energy requirements are based on full breastfeeding in the first 6 months, and partial breastfeeding after that time. Nutrient requirements also increase, particularly protein, folate, iodine, zinc, vitamin A and vitamin B_6.

The level of alcohol in breast milk is almost the same as a mother's blood alcohol level. An occasional drink is not harmful, but it's wise to stick to minimal amounts of alcohol when breastfeeding. Both pregnant and lactating women should also increase their fluid intake, mainly through water.

RECOMMENDED DAILY SERVINGS OF EACH FOOD GROUP

These are the minimum number of serves I recommend you eat for health and energy. If you're active, you'll need to eat more; if you want to lose weight without dieting, stick to these amounts and avoid any extras i.e. treats.

FOOD AND SERVINGS		AGE 1–3	AGE 4–7	AGE 8–11	AGE 12–18	ADULTS	PREGNANT WOMEN	BREASTFEEDING WOMEN
Vegetables	½ cup cooked vegetables or 1 cup salad leaves	1–2	2	3	4	5	5	5
Wholegrains	1 slice bread or ½ cup brown rice	3	3	3	3–4	4	4	4–6
Fruit	1 medium piece or ½ cup fruit salad	1	1	1	2–3	2	3	3–4
Dairy, low-fat	200 g tub yoghurt or 250 ml glass milk	3	3	3	3–5	2	3–4	3–4
Legumes	¼ cup, cooked	½	1	1	1	1	1	1
Lean meat, fish, chicken and eggs	100 g (cooked weight) or 3 eggs	½	½	1	1	2	2–3	2–3
Oils and spreads	2 tablespoons	1	1	2	3–5	2	2	2
Nuts and seeds	30–50 g handful	½	½	1	1	1	1	2
Water	1 glass	3–5	3–5	4–6	6–8	6–8	6–8	6–8

Aflatoxin

This is a poisonous compound produced by moulds growing on peanuts, wheat, corn and peas when they are grown or harvested in damp conditions. It causes liver cancer in animals, and has been correlated with liver cancer in Africa and South-East Asia where aflatoxin exposure occurs. Much has been done in Australia and New Zealand to minimise aflatoxin contamination in peanuts. The maximum allowable level of 0.015 milligrams per kilogram is enforced—when contamination has occurred, they have been withdrawn from sale.

Alcohol

Alcoholic drinks have been consumed for thousands of years and, in moderate quantities, they can be good for your heart. But there are good and bad side effects, so it pays to be restrained in the quantity you imbibe.

Alcohol (ethanol) is absorbed directly from the stomach and intestine and so enters the bloodstream within minutes of drinking—much faster than food. The rate of alcohol absorption varies from person to person depending on your individual sensitivity to alcohol, how often you drink, the type and concentration of what you drink, your genetic background and your body weight—the lower your weight, the greater its effect (which is why women are usually affected more quickly than men).

Alcohol is metabolised mainly by the liver, where it is converted to acetaldehyde and enters the body's biochemical pathways. A small proportion of alcohol is removed in the kidneys, sweat and breath (which explains why alcohol can be detected by breathalysers).

Alcohol and pregnancy

If you're pregnant, planning to fall pregnant or breastfeeding, it's best not to drink at all according to the NHMRC. This is particularly important during the first 3 months, when the risk of miscarriage, low birth weight and birth defects is highest. Once your pregnancy is past the first trimester, an occasional glass of champagne and orange is not something to worry about as long as it's just now and then. The real issue is becoming intoxicated or binge drinking.

THE GOOD NEWS

Although excess consumption is detrimental, studies show that people who drink modestly are less likely to suffer heart attacks, and more likely to live longer than total abstainers or those who consume three or more drinks a day. Alcohol appears to work by raising HDL cholesterol, the type that protects against heart disease, and by 'thinning' the blood and keeping it free-flowing.

The evidence is strongest for red wine, due to its protective grape antioxidants such as polyphenols and resveratrol—a fact that hasn't escaped wine lovers! In fact, red wine is held responsible for the 'French Paradox'; the moderate, regular consumption of wine by the French is thought to explain why they have one of the lowest rates of heart disease of any nation. But the research is far from conclusive as alcohol itself, whether from wine, beer or spirits, can also give similar benefits.

THE BAD NEWS

The positive effects of alcohol should not be taken as permission to over-indulge. Too much alcohol can inflame the lining of the stomach, intestine and pancreas, deplete the body of B vitamins, notably thiamin (vitamin B_1), zinc and magnesium, lead to cirrhosis of the liver (although not all heavy drinkers develop this disease), produce Wernicke-Korsakoff's syndrome (a disturbance in mental functioning caused by lack of thiamin), increase the risk of the common cancers (breast and colon) and some of the rarer forms (oral, oesophagus and stomach), lower the level of male sex hormones, causing loss of libido and decreased sperm production, and contribute to weight gain—pure alcohol is a concentrated source of kilojoules, having almost twice that of carbohydrate or protein. A glass of wine has 420 kilojoules, which is equivalent to one thick slice of bread (before you add any spread) or a large banana.

Binge drinking is particularly harmful and can lead to arrhythmia (disturbances in the heart rhythm) and platelet-rebound effect (a surge in blood clotting that results in stroke or sudden death) after alcohol withdrawal. The trend to binge drink among young people needs to be discouraged.

THE LATEST GUIDELINES FROM AUSTRALIA'S NATIONAL HEALTH AND MEDICAL RESEARCH COUNCIL (NHMRC) (2009)

- ✔ Women and men should limit their alcohol intake to just two drinks a day
- ✔ Women and men should consume no more than four drinks in total on any single occasion as the risk of injury from car accidents or assault jumps dramatically after this
- ✔ Children under 18 shouldn't drink at all.

SIDE EFFECTS

Hangovers aside, alcoholic drinks cause a fair share of side effects for certain individuals. Some people find that red wine produces more headaches than white because of its higher content of tannins and histamines. Asthma sufferers may find themselves unknowingly affected by white wines, which generally have more sulphur dioxide (additive number 220), a compound used since ancient times to delay oxidation. Wheeziness, sniffles or sinus problems can also be traced back to the sulphur. Sufferers of yeast allergies may also react to wine or beer.

And there is a long list of medications whose actions are antagonised or increased by alcohol. Anyone taking sedatives, anti-depressants, certain painkillers and flu tablets should check with a doctor or pharmacist before drinking alcohol. Often the medication pack carries a warning and it is essential to heed it, especially if driving or operating machinery.

ALCOHOL AND OBESITY

Given the growth in the quantity of alcohol consumed over the past 10 years, it's my belief that alcohol is the real problem behind many people's weight gain. Because it's a liquid, many people don't realise it's packed with kilojoules. Gram for gram, alcohol slogs you with 29 kilojoules per gram, second to fat at 37 kilojoules. A glass of dry white wine (the real-world 150 millilitre size, not the tiny 'standard' 100 millilitre glass that the government brochures talk about) has 500 kilojoules, while a trendy 275 millilitre bottle of alcopop such as Breezer or Cruiser adds a huge 730 kilojoules—almost as much as two thick slices of plain bread.

Alcohol also stimulates the appetite and loosens your inhibitions so you eat things you normally wouldn't (and possibly say things you normally wouldn't, too!). After a couple of drinks, foods like greasy chips, party pies, cocktail frankfurts and pizza start to look very appealing. Worst of all, research shows alcohol slows the burning of fat, as the body turns all its resources to eliminating the 'toxin' you've just drunk.

If you do sip, don't forget you can always dilute wine or spirits with ice and mineral water. Or ask for light beer rather than full-strength, or intersperse a juice or sparkling mineral water between regular drinks.

ALCOHOL CONTENT OF COMMON DRINKS

Different drinks have substantially different amounts of alcohol. Makers of alcoholic drinks must state on the label the percentage of alcohol, the number of standard drinks in the can or bottle and the presence of preservatives (such as sulphur) or colours.

ALCOHOL AND DRIVING

Alcohol is involved in around half of all serious car accidents in Australia and New Zealand. It takes the body about an hour to eliminate the alcohol from a single glass of wine or spirits, and about 12 hours to eliminate half a bottle of

KILOJOULE CONTENT OF COMMON DRINKS		
Wine, dry	1 glass, 150 ml	425 kJ
Wine, sweet	1 glass, 150 ml	415 kJ
Wine cooler	1 glass, 250 ml	550 kJ
Champagne	1 flute, 150 ml	405 kJ
Sherry, dry	1 small glass, 50 ml	235 kJ
Sherry, sweet	1 small glass, 50 ml	330 kJ
Spirits (brandy, whiskey, gin, vodka, bourbon)	1 nip, 30 ml	260 kJ
Beer, standard	1 can, 375 ml	565 kJ
Beer, light	1 can, 375 ml	395 kJ
Cider, dry	1 glass, 200 ml	290 kJ
Cider, non-alcoholic	I glass, 200 ml	350 kJ
Port	1 small glass, 50 ml	340 kJ
Liqueur	1 tiny glass, 30 ml	375 kJ

DRINK	% ALCOHOL BY VOLUME
Beer—extra light	less than 1
Beer—low alcohol	2–3
Beer—regular, low carb	4–5
Pre-mixed drinks or alcopops (Breezer, Cruiser)	5
Cider	4–5
Wine	10–13
Champagne	12
Sherry, vermouth, madeira	16–18
Port, muscat	18–20
Spirits (brandy, rum, whisky, gin, vodka, bourbon)	32–40
Liqueurs (Grand Marnier, Cointreau, Creme de Menthe, Drambuie, Kahlua)	30–40

Alcopops
Ready-to-drink alcopops (e.g. Breezers, Cruisers and Ruskis) are a cause for concern. Based on vodka, bourbon or rum, their sweetness and convenience make them effortless to drink. Relatively cheap and packaged in soft pastel colours, they are marketed squarely at young women. Research links alcopops with the rise in binge drinking in girls as young as 13 or 14—they are an easy transition from sweet soft drinks. One 275 millilitre bottle is a standard drink of 10 grams of alcohol but it also loads you up with some 20 grams of sugar and around 800 kiloJoules.

See also **Hangovers.**

spirits. If you plan to drink and drive, count your drinks so you stay under the blood alcohol limit of 0.05 grams per 100 millilitres of blood. For men this means two standard drinks in the first hour and then one drink every hour after that. For women this means one standard drink each hour.

After a night of heavy drinking, it is quite possible to be over 0.05 per cent the next morning. The only thing that will clear the alcohol from your blood is time. Coffee, fructose (fruit sugar), cold showers or exercise will not reduce your blood alcohol level.

Red wine is held responsible for the 'French Paradox'; the moderate, regular consumption of wine by the French is thought to explain why they have one of the lowest rates of heart disease of any nation.

Given the growth in the quantity of alcohol consumed over the past 10 years, it's my belief that alcohol is the real problem behind many people's weight gain.

FIVE TIPS TO DRINK LESS

- Quench your thirst with a non-alcoholic drink first.
- Have something to eat before and while you drink, to slow the absorption of alcohol into your bloodstream, especially something with fat or protein such as cheese, nuts, dip or milk. Avoid salty snacks as they only make you thirsty and so drink more.
- Beware of sparkling wines and carbonated mixer drinks. Their bubbles increase the rate of absorption of alcohol on an empty stomach.
- Lower the amount of alcohol in your drinks by diluting wine and spirits with soda or ice, or opting for light beer.
- Intersperse water or a non-alcoholic drink between regular drinks. Try a non-alcoholic apple cider, Clayton's and soda, tomato juice (refreshing in hot weather), lime, soda and bitters, grapefruit juice with mineral water, non-alcoholic wine, brewed soft drinks (they taste like beer but have no alcohol), diet soft drinks, ginger beer or iced tea.

WHERE TO GO FOR HELP

For information, counselling or other assistance to help moderate your alcohol intake, contact the Alcohol and Drug Information Service in your state or territory (or the Alcohol Drug Association in New Zealand). These centres are bound by confidentiality and you don't have to give your name if you don't want to.

Allergies, Intolerances and Diet

Sensitivity or allergy to certain foods is hard to live with—for some people even a tiny amount of a particular food can prove disastrous. If you wonder if food may be responsible for your skin rash, migraine or tummy troubles, read on.

ALLERGY

A true food allergy provokes the body's immune system, producing antibodies to specific food proteins. It occurs within minutes of consumption, mainly in infants and young children, and involves only a relatively small number of foods, notably eggs, milk, peanuts, fish and nuts. Blood or skin prick tests for detecting food antibodies are available.

One of the most severe forms of allergy is anaphylaxis, where the mouth, lips or throat swell, causing breathing difficulties and a potentially fatal collapse. Peanuts are the food most likely to cause death from anaphylactic shock, but tree nuts, fish, seafood or egg can also trigger it. Peanut allergy is on the rise for reasons researchers don't fully understand.

Allergy affects an estimated 5 per cent of infants, but only 1–2 per cent of young children and less than 1 per cent of the adult population. Most children grow out of milk and egg allergies by the age of four or five. Allergies to peanuts and seafood generally last for life.

INTOLERANCE OR SENSITIVITY

Food intolerance is often hard to recognise as the reactions do not always occur immediately after eating, and can be triggered by many different compounds, both natural and artificial. Food intolerance is more common than allergy (affecting 5–10 per of the adult population), but tends to run in families who may already suffer asthma, hay fever or eczema.

It is generally related to the dose consumed, whereby the body only reacts when its threshold has been crossed after a number of chemicals have been ingested. Don't forget that anything with a strong fragrance—pollens, perfumes, deodorisers, sprays, flowers and petrol—also spell trouble for the super-sensitive.

COMMON SYMPTOMS

- ✔ Digestive upsets (nausea, abdominal pain, diarrhoea or loose motions, wind)
- ✔ Swelling of the lips, mouth, tongue or throat (anaphylaxis)
- ✔ Hives (urticaria)
- ✔ Rash or redness (eczema)
- ✔ Hay fever
- ✔ Chronic runny nose (rhinitis)
- ✔ Coughing or wheezing
- ✔ Asthma
- ✔ Migraine, headaches
- ✔ Irritability, bad moods.

Correct diagnosis of allergy or intolerance is essential because their symptoms appear similar and may also have other causes. For example, stomach pains and diarrhoea could also be due to a gastric infection or to food poisoning, coeliac disease, lactose intolerance or excessive fibre.

If you suspect you have an allergy or intolerance to certain foods, do not self-diagnose. Seek professional help from an accredited practising dietitian (APD) or allergy clinic at a large hospital. You will be assessed with a history of your symptoms, how often they occur, how much of the food you can eat before a reaction, and whether anyone else in your family has allergies. A RAST (radioallergosorbent) blood test, a skin prick test and a food diary may also be used.

THE ELIMINATION DIET

A strict elimination diet currently remains the best way to diagnose which foods or chemical components are triggers of intolerance reactions. The elimination diet developed by the Allergy Clinic at Sydney's Royal Prince Alfred Hospital involves three steps:

1. For 4–6 weeks, you eliminate all problem chemicals, both natural and artificial, from your diet and restrict your food to a short list of bland foods like rice, chicken, beef, lamb, pears, flour, sugar, plain unpreserved bread, plain biscuits, potatoes and pasta. It is a monotonous diet, requiring almost all food to be cooked at home. It is also deficient in essential nutrients and should only be followed for a short time under supervision. If the symptoms disappear at this stage, a food intolerance is most likely.

ADDITIVES MOST LIKELY TO CAUSE ADVERSE REACTIONS	
ADDITIVE	**CODE NUMBER**
ARTIFICIAL COLOURS	
Tartrazine	102
Sunset yellow FCF	110
Azorubine	122
Amaranth	123
Ponceau 4R	124
Erythrosine	127
Allura red AC	129
Indigotine	132
Brilliant blue FCF	133
Green S	142
Fast green FCF	143
Brilliant black BN	151
Brown HT	155
NATURAL COLOURS	
Annatto extracts	160b
FLAVOUR ENHANCERS	
L-Glutamic acid	620
Monosodium L-glutamate	621
Monopotassium L-glutamate	622
Calcium glutamate	623
Monoammonium L-glutamate	624
Magnesium glutamate	625
PRESERVATIVES	
Benzoates	
Benzoic acid	210
Sodium benzoate	211
Potassium benzoate	212
Calcium benzoate	213
Sulphites	
Sulphur dioxide	220
Sodium sulphite	221
Sodium bisulphite	222
Sodium metabisulphite	223
Potassium metabisulphite	224
Potassium sulphite	225
Potassium bisulphite	228
Propionates	
Propionic acid	280
Sodium propionate	281
Calcium propionate	282
Potassium propionate	283
Nitrites	
Potassium nitrite	249
Sodium nitrite	250
Sodium nitrate	251
Potassium nitrate	252
ANTIOXIDANTS	
Propyl gallate	310
Octyl gallate	311
Dodecyl gallate	312
Butylated hydroxyanisole	320
Butylated hydroxytoluene	321

2. If the symptoms clear up, you will be asked to take a number of challenges one by one. This may be small doses of purified suspect chemicals like salicylate, benzoate, MSG, colours or sulphite, or whole foods rich in salicylates or glutamates.
3. Finally, the clinic devises a more normal and varied diet for you, allowing food that did not trigger a reaction. Over time, even the offending foods may be eaten occasionally or in small quantities, depending on how much you can tolerate.

ALLERGENS ON LABELS

Food labels carry compulsory warnings for allergy sufferers and declare the presence of the eight common allergy triggers: gluten (from wheat, rye, barley, oats and spelt), crustaceans (prawns, crab, lobster), fish, cow's milk, nuts, sesame seeds, peanuts and soy.

CULPRIT CHEMICALS

There are many problem chemicals in food, both natural and added, that can upset sensitive people. Adverse reactions to food additives do occur, but additives are just one group of all the chemicals known to trigger reactions. Sufferers generally react to both additives as well as natural chemicals. For example, if someone is sensitive to MSG, they will also react to natural glutamates in mushrooms. For the body, there is no distinction between 'natural' and 'artificial'—both substances appear chemically the same and both have to be avoided or minimised by allergy sufferers.

AMINES

Amines are compounds derived from the breakdown of protein or from fermentation. Large quantities are found in cheese, chocolate, yeast extracts, beer and wine and they are also found in tomatoes, bananas, avocados and broad beans.

SALICYLATES

A large group of aspirin-like compounds, salicylates are found in citrus and most other fruit, many vegetables, herbs, spices, honey, tea, coffee, beer and wine. They are also present in mint flavours and eucalyptus oils, so they turn up in perfume, aromatherapy oils, toiletries and toothpaste as well.

MSG AND GLUTAMATES

Glutamates are found naturally and are responsible for the flavour of foods. High concentrations occur in soy sauce, cheeses (parmesan, blue vein and camembert), tomatoes, yeast extracts and mushrooms. As flavour enhancer 621, MSG is added to sauces, stock, gravies, Asian soups, snack foods and instant noodles. MSG generally causes no harm but it can trigger wheezing or skin reactions in glutamate-sensitive people.

COLOURS

Artificial colours like tartrazine, Sunset yellow FCF, erythrosine, amaranth and Brilliant blue FCF are linked to food sensitivity. Tartrazine, in particular, has been extensively investigated for its ability to induce hives and asthma in aspirin-sensitive asthmatics. Use of erythrosine is now limited to maraschino cherries. Many people blame sugar for their kids' behaviour problems, but it may well be the colours that sugar keeps company with in things like lollies, chocolates, ice-creams, soft drinks, cordials and snack foods.

SULPHUR PRESERVATIVES

Metabisulphites 223 and 224 and their related compounds of sulphur dioxide 220 and sulphites 221, 222, 225 and 228 are used in wineries to destroy undesirable bacteria in wine storage vats—sulphur has been used to preserve wine since Greek times. They prevent the darkening of dried fruit and juices and are used to preserve soft drinks, pickled onions and sausages. In sensitive asthma patients they can trigger wheezing and throat tightening, frequently within 1–2 minutes of consumption.

BENZOATES

These occur in cranberries, bilberries and other fruit, vegetables, pepper, herbs, spices, peppermint and honey. Sodium benzoate 211 and potassium benzoate 212 are used as preservatives in soft drinks, cordials and fruit drinks. Both must be avoided by sensitive people.

Alpha-linolenic Acid (ALA)

An omega-3 fatty acid from plants and a precursor to the two longer-chain omega-3 fatty acids, eicosapentaenoic acid (EPA) and docosahexaenoic acid (DHA), needed for the brain and eyes. The richest sources are linseeds and chia seeds, with smaller amounts in canola oil, walnuts, soy beans and green vegetables.

See also Omega-3 and Omega-6 Essential Fatty Acids.

Aloe Vera

Aloe vera juices, gels, ointments, lotions and creams are based on an extract or concentrate of the juice of the *Aloe vera* plant, long used as a traditional medicine and as an external treatment for burns and wounds. Many people take aloe vera juice or gel to treat Crohn's disease, inflammatory bowel disease or arthritis, or simply as a general tonic. Benefits have been reported after taking 50–100 millilitres a day, but there have been few clinical trials and aloe's active ingredients remain undefined. The bitter sap between the outer skin and inner pulp is a strong laxative, hence its reputation as a bowel regulator.

SHOPPER'S GUIDE

Some products contain only minute amounts of aloe, or they have been filtered with activated carbon, which removes many of the active components along with the bitter sap, so it is essential to buy a reputable brand of gel or juice that lists a reasonable percentage of aloe present.

Alzheimer's Disease and Diet

Alzheimer's disease, the most common type of dementia, is caused by physical changes in the brain that usually lead to loss of memory, poor speech, impaired motor skills and other problems that interfere with daily living. Research into the causes and prevention of Alzheimer's disease and mental decline is ongoing. Researchers have investigated whether things such as minimising cell damage by free radicals, reducing inflammation, or maintaining blood glucose levels (even in the absence of diabetes), can stop the build-up of sticky amyloid plaques in the brain and maintain cognitive health.

In the meantime, it's useful to look at the diets of those who have aged well and are mentally alert in their eighties. Certain patterns of eating and certain foods seem to have a protective effect and are worth adopting, especially if there's Alzheimer's in the family.

BRAINPOWER BASICS

Don't forget these brainpower basics that can help slow cognitive ageing.

- ✔ Regular physical exercise to get the blood flowing to the brain and supply fresh oxygen
- ✔ Eating a healthy diet that maximises the intake of vitamins, minerals, phytonutrients and essential fatty acids
- ✔ Keeping your brain active by doing crosswords, puzzles and other difficult mental activities like learning a new language or dancing, where your brain has to think in body spatial mode.

KEY FOODS UNDER STUDY

OMEGA-3 FATS

A few studies have reported a correlation between a high intake of oily fish and dementia, which seems due to one omega-3 fatty acid, docosahexaenoic acid (DHA).

TURMERIC

Turmeric, or its active chemical curcumin, gives Indian curry dishes their distinctive yellow hue and flavour, and may prevent Alzheimer's disease. Recent studies suggest that turmeric may enhance the body's ability to destroy amyloid plaques that build up in the brains of Alzheimer's patients. People in India who eat a traditional diet are four times less likely to have Alzheimer's disease than people in the US.

SUPERFOODS

Eating nutrient-dense superfoods that are packed with antioxidants may help. In particular, blueberries, blackberries and other dark-coloured berries are excellent sources of antioxidants called anthocyanins, the same chemical that gives blueberries their rich colour. They have been shown to increase brain cell communication and may also play a role in reducing harmful inflammation, which can lead to better cognitive function.

CAFFEINE

In laboratory studies, high doses of caffeine reversed the effects of Alzheimer's disease. Mice that were genetically altered to exhibit Alzheimer's symptoms were given the equivalent of 500 milligrams of caffeine. At the end of the study, their cognition had improved to match that of healthy peers. In addition, amyloid plaques had been reduced by half. Taken before symptoms occurred, caffeine seemed to protect the brains of those prone to developing Alzheimer's disease.

See also Anti-ageing Diets.

Amines

Amines are nitrogen-containing compounds, formed from the breakdown of protein or from fermentation. High concentrations are found in matured cheese, chocolate, yeast extract and red wine and lower levels are found in tomatoes, bananas, avocados and broad beans. Amines have the biological potential to constrict arteries and increase blood pressure and are one of the main food triggers for migraines in food-sensitive people.

See also Allergies.

Amino Acids

Proteins are made up of chains of amino acids. Only some 20 amino acids occur in food, but the number of combinations in which they are arranged is infinite. Eight of these amino acids are essential, which means they cannot be made by the body and must be provided by food. These are isoleucine, leucine, lysine, methionine, phenylalanine, threonine, tryptophan and valine. A ninth, histidine, is essential for infants.

The remaining amino acids are inter-convertible and can be made from the essential eight, or from each other. This is because when food proteins are digested, our bodies split them into their individual amino acids, and then reassemble them into the types of human protein we require.

See also **Protein.**

Anaemia (Iron Deficiency) and Diet

If you're tired all the time, it's worth paying a visit to your doctor for a blood test to check whether you have iron deficiency anaemia. Lack of energy, poor stamina, pale skin, an inability to concentrate, frequent headaches, greater susceptibility to infections and feeling the cold are other telltale signs. Iron deficiency is the most common nutrition problem in the world, affecting around 35 per cent of people in developing countries and 8 per cent in affluent countries. Other causes of anaemia include inherited disorders such as thalassaemia and sickle cell disease, chronic diseases like rheumatoid arthritis and some drugs and medications.

Iron deficiency is the most common nutrition problem in the world, affecting around 35 per cent of people in developing countries and 8 per cent in affluent countries.

Women are far more likely to have iron deficiency anaemia than men. Firstly, women's needs for iron are almost double that of men's due to monthly blood loss through menstruation and the demands pregnancy makes on the body—additional stores of iron are needed to provide for the developing baby and increase the woman's own blood supply as blood volume increases during pregnancy. Secondly, many women and teenage girls just do not get enough iron in their diet to meet their needs. This can be for a variety of reasons but very common factors include skipping meals, dieting and just not eating enough red meat or adopting a vegetarian diet without understanding how to meet their iron needs. You can also be at risk if for some reason your body can't absorb iron efficiently, such as those who suffer from coeliac or Crohn's disease.

Q

Why can't I simply swallow a pill?

A

Iron pills are needed during pregnancy when iron requirements are too high to come from food alone, but high doses of iron can cause constipation and nausea. The body's iron is in delicate balance as too little leads to problems, as does too much. Iron overload, or the slow accumulation of iron, can be lethal in someone who has a predisposition to storing excess iron. Known as haemochromatosis, this condition affects one in every 300 Australians and New Zealanders.

PUMP IRON

Our bodies need to pump iron. Not the weights, but the essential mineral we can get from our diet. Iron is an essential part of haemoglobin, the red colouring of blood (along with vitamin B_{12} and folate), which helps carry oxygen to every part of the body. If your iron or haemoglobin count is low, you will feel chronically tired. The best way to increase your iron stores is to obtain iron from food as nature intended.

- ✔ Red meat is the best source of iron and is absorbed well by the body. Generally, the redder the richer, so enjoy that steak or lean lamb chop. Even if you only eat meat occasionally, small amounts (such as a few strips of beef in a vegetable stir-fry) can improve your iron absorption from the vegetables in your meal.

- ✔ The iron in cereal grains, vegetables, legumes, nuts and eggs is not absorbed as well as that in meat. Of these foods, grains make the greatest iron contribution to your diet. In fact, around 30 per cent comes from fortified breakfast cereals and bread.
- ✔ Adding a glass of fruit juice or some tomato or capsicum (all rich in vitamin C) to a meal increases the amount of iron delivered by grains or lentils, as vitamin C aids absorption. Most vegetarian meals, with their emphasis on vegetables and fruit, would automatically contain a lot of vitamin C.
- ✔ Don't forget drinks also play a part. Orange juice doubles iron intakes, relative to water, while milk decreases it by 50 per cent and tea by 75 per cent.

See also **Iron.**

Anaphylaxis

See also **Allergy; Nuts and Seeds.**

This is one of the most severe forms of allergy (usually from peanuts) where the mouth, lips or throat may swell, causing breathing difficulties and, potentially, a fatal collapse.

Anthocyanins

Anthocyanins are an important group of plant chemicals that act as antioxidants and also have a mild antibacterial effect. You'll find them in blue, red and purple coloured fruits (plums and red grapes) and berries (cranberries, raspberries, blueberries and blackberries), as well as eggplant and cocoa.

Anti-ageing Diets

MY TAKE

If you want to age well, I believe it's a case of making every mouthful count. Maintaining a healthy weight by eating lightly (even under-eating) and consuming nutrient-rich foods both help slow the clock. Your anti-ageing goal is to pack as many vitamins, minerals, antioxidants, essential fats and protein as possible into as few kilojoules as possible.

Anti-ageing diets that promise to hold back the clock, slow the ageing process and keep skin youthful have one thing in common—they are invariably based on nutrient-dense, quality foods such as oily fish, leafy green vegetables, orange vegetables, green tea, berries, juices, nuts (especially almonds), seeds such as flax and chia, and herbs and 'memory' spices like turmeric and rosemary. Supplements are also often suggested, such as fish oil, antioxidant vitamins, zinc, spirulina, wheatgrass juice and gingko.

You'll recognise that many of the so-called superfoods are on this list, and for good reason. These foods are rich in important nutrients and maximise your intake of vitamins, minerals and phytochemicals. This is critical, because our body's ability to absorb nutrients diminishes as we grow older, or we simply need more of them to cope with the changes.

Some anti-ageing diets also put you on half-rations. Restricting food intake (cutting your total intake permanently by 20–25 per cent) can extend your life span by 40 per cent (well, it does in animal experiments). While there are no completed studies in people, it seems that restricting your kilojoule intake works by triggering a survival mechanism in the body and reducing blood fats, blood glucose, blood pressure, heart rate and weight. What's more, it cuts the rate at which free radicals are generated.

MY FAVOURITE 'KITCHEN OF YOUTH' FOODS

SALMON, TUNA AND SARDINES

Omega-3 fats from oily fish are the ultimate anti-ageing nutrient. They are an integral part of the structure of your brain and nerve tissues, so work to help keep you mentally sharp. They're good for your eyesight too—the lens of the eye is particularly sensitive to any nutrient deficiency. They also lower blood pressure and triglycerides (a blood fat like cholesterol) and reduce blood clotting. In other words, they prevent stroke, keep your heart merrily ticking away and keep your arteries clear. They also dampen down the swelling and inflammation in conditions like arthritis and inflammatory bowel disease. I can't stress their importance enough. In addition, oily fish is loaded with quality protein, zinc and vitamin D and B_{12}, which are all in high demand as we age. Aim for at least two meals (or preferably more) containing fish each week, both canned and fresh.

BLUEBERRIES

These give you anthocyanins, blue and red plant pigments that can gobble up damaging free radicals that would otherwise wreck DNA genetic material, age the eyes and set the scene for cancer. A 200-gram punnet has a tiny 395 kilojoules and virtually no fat. Eating low-kilojoule blueberries lets you live on 'light rations' yet still enjoy lovely desserts and plenty of vitamins and minerals.

GREEN TEA

This is the favourite drink on the Japanese island of Okinawa, which boasts the highest incidence of centenarians (people living to 100) in the world. Although exact figures are disputed, if you want to live longer and in good health, drinking three to four cups of tea a day is a good idea. More than a dozen studies show tea can reduce the risk of heart problems, may prevent several cancers and can maintain strong bones in older people. Tea's antioxidants, a group called flavonoids, appear to be responsible for the benefits.

SPINACH AND SILVERBEET

These vegetables are rich in two antioxidants called lutein and zeaxanthin, which help protect our vision from age-related eye disorders such as macular degeneration. Regular consumption of spinach (two to three times a week) also seems to enhance memory power. Lutein is now included in most supplements for eye care. And the bonus is that both are rich in beta-carotene, which is converted into vitamin A in the body, and needed for your body's immune system.

TURMERIC

This stands out as the ultimate spice for brain health thanks to its biologically active constituent curcumin, which imparts the golden colour in curries. Turmeric has been shown to do everything from help slow the onset of Alzheimer's disease and dementia, to serving as an anti-inflammatory against arthritis. It's worth adding to your spice rack.

Turmeric grows as a rhizome (an underground stem) and is related to ginger, another anti-ageing food. Make sure your curry powders and pastes are a nice yellow colour. Turmeric is used widely as a food colouring with additive code number 100. Over a lifetime, small quantities may be the fountain of youth.

ROSEMARY, THYME AND OREGANO

Fresh herbs may be helpful in holding back the clock. Rosemary, thyme and oregano are the best researched, but there are no doubt many others that work too. Use herbs lavishly in salads and in your cooking.

LEMONS, LIMES AND OTHER CITRUS FRUIT

These are all rich in potassium, a mineral which counteracts the damage done by salt to the kidneys and heart, and which helps keep blood pressure low as you age. And their acidity and flavour help you cut down on salt. All citrus fruits are packed with vitamin C,

FREE RADICALS

Free radicals are electronically charged, unstable molecules that can easily react with and damage other molecules. They cause damage in much the same way that air turns a cut apple brown. They are also called oxidants because they operate through the process of oxidation. Free radicals are formed both internally and externally. In the body, they are formed as a by-product of metabolism whenever oxygen is involved. Externally, they are left behind by smog, cigarette smoke, pollution, ozone, solvents, pesticides and the sun's ionising radiation. The current nutritional thinking is that when the 'bad guys' (free radicals) outnumber the 'good guys' (the antioxidants), they damage proteins, fatty acids and DNA. If you have more antioxidants to mop up the bad guys, then your body cells stay in good condition.

folate, fibre and phytonutrients known as limonene that can fight off cancer. Use the zest as well as the juice.

YOGHURT

This has been associated with long life span ever since renowned Russian scientist Dr Metchnikoff (1845–1919) claimed it was responsible for the longevity of the Bulgarians in the early 1900s. Metchnikoff believed the 'friendly' live *Lactobacillus* bacteria in yoghurt (known as probiotics today) exerted a key influence on your intestine. Certainly yoghurt's partial pre-digestion makes it more easily digested and absorbed than milk. This means your body takes in more of its protein, B vitamins (particularly riboflavin, needed for healthy skin and eyes) and calcium, which helps prevent osteoporosis.

HERBAL REMEDIES

Gingko biloba, ginseng and garlic have all been suggested to add more years to your life.

HOLDING BACK THE CLOCK

I'm a nutritionist so I have a particular interest in foods that can hold back the clock. But as good as a healthy diet is, I must admit that when it comes to anti-ageing, a healthy lifestyle is more important than eating this or that particular food. Regardless of what you are eating for good health, these six long-life factors are a must.

WALK OR SWIM EACH DAY

Use it or lose it is an important mantra for anyone trying to maintain their brainpower in later life. Just like a muscle, the brain needs exercise in the physical sense, which directs extra blood flow to the brain, and this helps preserve normal brain function. It may also stimulate older nerve cells to form connections that improve the brain's efficiency. Regular exercise outdoors keeps your body and mind young. It helps you unwind and appreciate the world of nature around us. Exercise also helps maintain muscle mass that we lose as we age.

DON'T SMOKE

Smoking adds early lines to your face and 'sucks up' those all-important antioxidants.

Green tea is the favourite drink on the Japanese island of Okinawa, which boasts the highest incidence of centenarians (people living to 100) in the world.

BE MODEST WITH ALCOHOL

It's really a case of less is best. Limit yourself to two standard drinks a day and have a couple of days without alcohol each week. I know many folk who swear off all alcohol for three or four weeks each year to give their liver a rest and do a mini-detox. It's not a bad idea. After the excesses of Christmas, January is a popular time, or you can follow 'Dry July' or 'Feb Fast' for a month if you need support.

AVOID MID-LIFE WEIGHT GAIN

Eating salads and vegetables, saying no to sweets and fast food (most of the time), playing regular sport or walking all help to stop your weight creeping up. People who are obese in middle age have twice the risk of developing dementia as those who maintain an ideal weight.

KEEP UP YOUR NETWORK OF FRIENDS AND SOCIAL CONTACTS

Studies show people with good social networks live longer and stay healthier. Have fun. Enjoy a laugh (it boosts the immune system). Don't take yourself too seriously. Volunteer in your local community or at a charity.

KEEP YOUR BRAIN ACTIVE

Mental stimulation slows memory loss, and it encourages the brain to rewire cells later in life and even create new ones. But make it challenging. If you can keep working and enjoy it, do it. If you are retired, find other challenges. Crosswords, Sudoku, video games, trivia contests, scrabble, art classes or learning an instrument can help baby boomers defend the brain against loss.

Anti-caking Agents

Anti-caking agents help foods such as salt or flavour sachets flow freely when poured, and stop particles clumping together. Examples are sodium aluminosilicate (554) and magnesium carbonate (504).

Antioxidants

A daily diet high in antioxidants is good insurance for your wellbeing. It is a way you can help protect yourself against the two main killer diseases of Western countries—cancer and heart disease—as well as holding back the ageing process and protecting your eyes from cataracts and macular degeneration.

The best way to get them is simply by eating lots of vegetables and fruit. Studies consistently show that people with high intakes of fruit and vegetables, which are packed with antioxidants and other phytochemicals, have lower levels of cancer and heart disease.

DEFINITION

Antioxidants are molecules that act as the body's defence network against damage to cells and genetic material. Like vitamins, there are numerous different antioxidants, each of which act in different ways or on different parts of the body. They help to keep us healthy by neutralising substances called free radicals, which would otherwise damage cells. In this way, they can:

- ✔ Slow down the ageing process
- ✔ Stop LDL cholesterol from being oxidised
- ✔ Preserve eyesight
- ✔ Inhibit the early stage of cancer development
- ✔ Reverse the process of cancer growth and development.

Thousands of antioxidants exist and are produced either in the body or obtained from the food we eat. The best sources are vegetables, fruit, wine and tea, with the three best-known antioxidants (often called the ACE antioxidants) being vitamin C, vitamin E and beta-carotene.

THE ACE ANTIOXIDANTS

VITAMIN C

Its main job as an antioxidant is to regenerate vitamin E, but it also inhibits the formation of carcinogenic nitrosamines in the stomach. It has consistently been shown to reduce cancers of the digestive tract (oesophagus, stomach and pancreas).

VITAMIN E

It prevents LDL cholesterol from oxidation. It is the major antioxidant in all cell membranes, where it maintains the stability of the fatty acids in the phospholipid layer.

BETA-CAROTENE

The precursor to vitamin A in the body, beta-carotene is the best known and most abundant of the carotenoids, a large group of compounds responsible for the yellow and orange colours in fresh produce. Beta-carotene inactivates free radicals, improves immune capacity and inhibits the early stages of tumour development.

OTHER IMPORTANT ANTIOXIDANTS

Copper and manganese (often key components of enzymes) are also important antioxidants, as are the enzymes superoxide dismutase, catalase and glutathione peroxidase, as well as flavonoids, carotenoids and a myriad of natural plant compounds (phytochemicals).

SELENIUM

Selenium works in combination with vitamins C and E. It enhances immune response and affects DNA repair, which can prevent cancer initiation and growth. It is a key component of the antioxidant enzyme glutathione peroxidase, which 'neutralises' peroxidases before they can attack cell membranes.

ZINC

Zinc is part of the enzyme superoxide dismutase, which prevents free radicals from forming peroxides.

BOOST YOUR ANTIOXIDANT INTAKE IN FIVE WAYS

- Eat plenty of fruit. Eat it as a snack, to finish off meals, in smoothies, with yoghurt or ice-cream or with meat and poultry. All fruit will give you antioxidants, but the richest sources are citrus fruit, berries, kiwifruit and rockmelon.
- Give yourself large helpings of vegetables and salads. Go for vegetable soups, cook two or three vegetables with dinner, have salad with your sandwiches or eat raw vegetables with dips and cheese.
- Eat by the rainbow. With vegetables and fruit, the more colourful, the more antioxidants you're getting. Choose red onion over white, dark-green lettuces over pale iceberg, blue-red berries over pale pears or apples etc. Variety is essential as yellow, orange, green, red, brown and blue-purple fruits and vegetables give us different sorts of antioxidants.
- Use herbs and spices liberally. Many everyday kitchen herbs are rich in antioxidants and

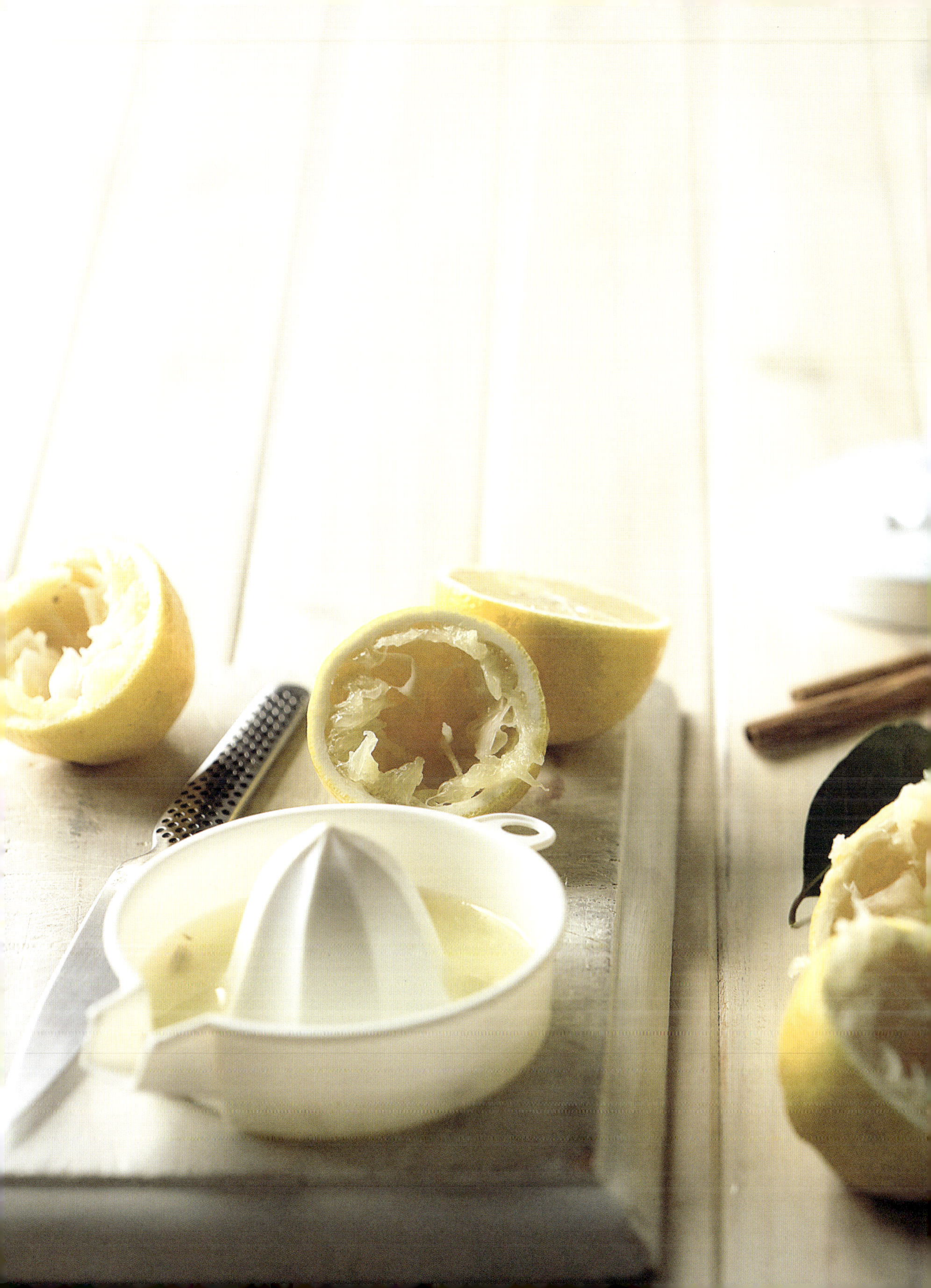

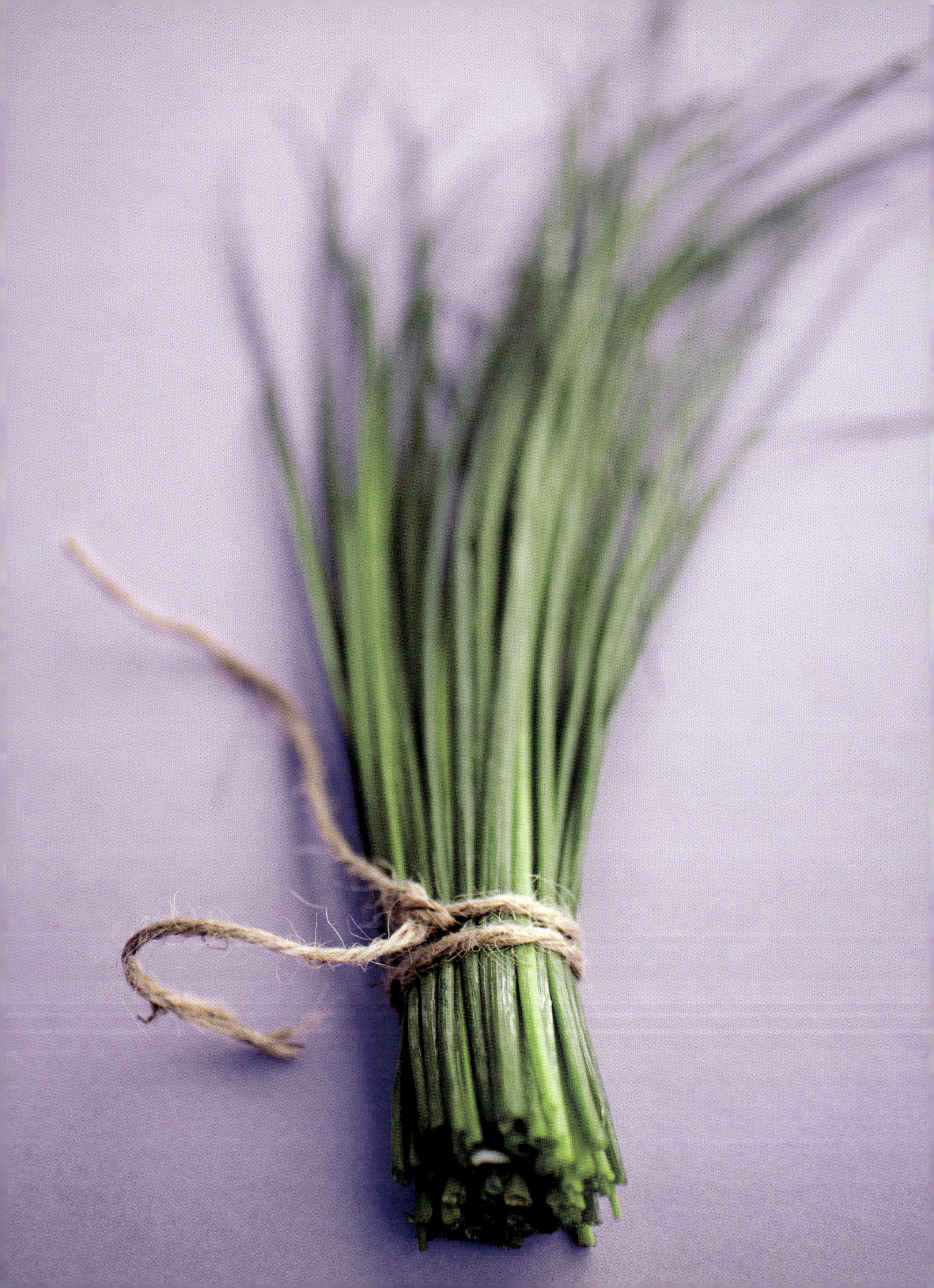

can double or triple your intake. The most widely researched are rosemary, turmeric, ginger, oregano, aniseed, cumin, caraway seeds, cloves, nutmeg and cinnamon.

- Choose tea over coffee, red wine over white. Red wine has nine to 10 times the grape antioxidants of white wine.

ANTIOXIDANT SUPPLEMENTS

It is not enough to simply swallow an antioxidant pill. Food is a complex mix of hundreds of phytochemicals. A supplement will give you only the main antioxidants that have been identified and well researched, and those that can be extracted from food or synthesised. For example, you'll get the ACE antioxidants plus zinc or selenium and then maybe some green tea extract, grape extract or lycopene. By eating fruits, vegetables and wholegrains, you get hundreds of different phytochemicals.

See also **Phytochemicals.**

Appetite and Hunger

Learn the difference between hunger and appetite (or non-hungry eating). Hunger is the body's response to low blood glucose when you haven't eaten for a long time; appetite is when you feel hungry because you've just spotted some food (or even an ad for food), or you think it's near mealtime. Both can feel the same, but only one should be responded to.

THE HUNGER-FULLNESS SCALE

Your stomach is the size of a clenched fist that expands as you eat. If you eat slowly and chew well, your stomach will tell you when it's full. Have a listen. Use my simple scale to tune in to your hunger and fullness levels. Rate how you are feeling on a scale of zero to 10, and mark it on the graph every hour. Keep a record over 4–5 days, and you will soon see your own natural pattern of hunger over the day. Remember, it's normal and natural to feel hungry several times a day—the trick is to match eating your meals and snacks with those times when you're most hungry!

Wait until your hunger is down between zero and 3 before you eat. Stop eating when you reach 5. If you overshoot your fullness and reach between 6 and 10, you'll gain weight.

THE HUNGER-FULLNESS SCALE	
10	I'm ready to burst!
9	I'm absolutely full.
8	I feel like an overstuffed cushion.
7	I'm uncomfortably full.
6	Aaaah, I shouldn't have eaten that last mouthful.
5	I enjoyed that, I feel quite satisfied.
4	What's to eat? I'm peckish.
3	I'm running on empty.
2	Hey there! I'm starving!
1	I'm soooo ravenous.
0	If you don't feed me soon, I'll be too weak to chew!

Apples *See* **Fruit.**

Arthritis and Diet

There is no specific diet that can prevent or treat arthritis (apart from gout, a disease characterised by painful inflammation of the joints), despite the fact that new 'anti-arthritis' diets regularly appear in the news. There are, however, four dietary and lifestyle changes you can make to lessen joint pain and early-morning stiffness.

BE A HEALTHY WEIGHT

Being overweight increases the load on weight-bearing joints such as knees and ankles and decreases mobility. So if you're carrying excess weight, it's time to watch your diet, making portion sizes modest, keeping total fat down and increasing your intake of low-kilojoule vegetables and salads.

GET MORE OMEGA-3 FATS

Studies show that a high intake of omega-3 fats from fish can have a 'calming' effect on arthritis, particularly rheumatoid arthritis, reducing inflammation and aching joints. The simplest and healthiest way to boost your omega-3 intake is to eat oily fish at least three times a week. Regular fish oil intake of 5000 milligrams a day (via liquid oil or capsules) is a good idea.

MOVE IT OR LOSE IT!

Research shows that, after medication, exercise can bring the greatest relief to those who suffer arthritis. It helps to avoid stiffness, strengthen muscles and burn off excess fat. Walking, swimming, yoga, Pilates, tai chi, stationary cycling and dancing are excellent.

EATER BEWARE

View with scepticism any 'new' diet that promises to cure arthritis by eating (or avoiding) certain foods. While they generally cause no harm, any improvement you notice is often due to the fact that you have shed a few kilos and lessened the load on inflamed and sore joints! Remember that food restriction of any kind (including fasting and eating vegetarian) is known to improve arthritis symptoms in the short term by reducing the immune response. And some forms of arthritis can go into remission—if this occurs at the same time as you try a supposed 'cure', then naturally you feel the cure has 'worked'.

ARTHRITIS SUPPLEMENTS AND FOOD MYTHS

Doctors are understandably cautious about recommending supplements, as many desperate people have been ripped off by 'miracle cures' of dubious benefit, according to the Arthritis Foundation. Here are some of the most common food myths.

CIDER VINEGAR

Over the years, numerous claims have been made for cider vinegar, but none of them have stood up to scientific scrutiny. Cider vinegar will not magically 'dissolve' deposits of crystals from around the joints and may actually irritate the lining of the stomach and bowel if consumed in large quantities.

NIGHTSHADE VEGETABLES

Potatoes, eggplants, capsicum and tomatoes belong to the nightshade (*Solanum*) family and have been under a cloud for years. Many sufferers say they cause their arthritis to flare up but there is no proof of this. These claims probably arose because of their association with deadly nightshade, a quite different plant.

Bear in mind that individuals have varying reactions to foods, which may sometimes be due to an underlying food intolerance. Some people will always notice a reaction when they eat a culprit food (e.g. tomatoes or red wine). Others only have trouble if they eat them in large amounts and then there are others who can consume them freely. If you feel that certain foods may be triggering problems, talk to an accredited practising dietitian (APD) or your doctor—they may suggest an elimination diet to test for food sensitivities.

ACID FOODS

Arthritis is not caused by eating foods like oranges, lemons or tomatoes. Even though they taste acidic, their acidity is small compared with the acid levels in our stomachs already. If you find, however, that they upset you, talk to an APD or your doctor.

GLUCOSAMINE

This occurs naturally as a building block that your body needs to regenerate cartilage and lubricate your joints. Commercially, glucosamine sulphate is extracted from the shells of prawns and other shellfish and is now becoming popular as part of arthritis treatments. Many people with arthritis swear by it even though the research jury is still out on this one. If you want to give it a go, check with your doctor as it can interact with some medication, affect blood glucose in those with diabetes and cause reactions in anyone allergic to shellfish.

GINGER

Alternative practitioners have long believed that ginger has anti-inflammatory properties that may help relieve the pain associated with both rheumatoid and osteoarthritis, and now there's research emerging to confirm this. Try it as a refreshing tea and use plenty in your cooking.

Asian Diet

A typical Asian diet is difficult to define as Asia represents an enormous area that is made up of many different diets and cuisines. But in general, it has been inspired by the cuisines of South and East Asia, from countries including China, Japan, Korea, India, Thailand, Vietnam, Cambodia, Indonesia, Malaysia and the Philippines.

NUTRITIONAL VALUE

Despite the diversity, the standout of all traditional Asian diets is the way it makes it so easy to eat your vegetables. Plant food in general—from Asian greens and sea vegetables to legumes like soy—is always the star of the kitchen. Meat, fish, eggs and other animal foods are more of an addition for flavour rather than a staple ingredient. Rice and other grains, noodles, congee and flatbreads are also a feature, and most Asian fare makes divine use of fresh fragrant herbs and spices like chilli, ginger and turmeric.

When comparing the Asian and Mediterranean diets—two notable models for healthy eating—you can see common features. For example, both diets are low in saturated fat and high in vegetables, legumes and grains. The Asian diet is characteristically low in both saturated and total fat. Both also feature regular physical activity, and a strong social element accompanies the sharing of food with family and friends, which may contribute to the high adult life expectancy and low chronic disease rates found in many parts of Asia.

Dairy products such as milk and cheese are generally absent. The major exception to this is India, where moderate amounts of dairy foods are consumed often as yogurt, lassi and yoghurt-based drinks, and soft cheeses.

VEGETARIANS' DELIGHT

If you're seeking a vegetarian way of eating, you can't go past Asian cuisine where many vegetarian traditions prevail (notably in India). Creative cooks have come up with healthy vegetarian dishes that are full of flavour thanks to the liberal use of spices such as chilli, ginger, turmeric, cloves, fresh coriander and mint.

The drawback to the Asian diet is the heavy use of salty sauces such as soy sauce, fish sauce and oyster sauce. It also relies on refined grains, including white rice and noodles. Brown rice is more nutritious so ask for it instead where you can. If it's not an option don't stress, you will still get plenty of fibre and vitamins from the many vegetables and herbs in most dishes.

Aspartame

Aspartame is a sweetener (trade names 'Equal' and 'NutraSweet') consisting of two amino acids joined together. It is 200 times sweeter than sugar but provides no kilojoules. Its sweetness deteriorates after heating, so it is only suitable for cold applications such as in drinks and yoghurt (not cooking). Websites abound alleging aspartame is a 'brain toxin' and is the cause of such things as multiple sclerosis, lupus, chronic fatigue syndrome, brain tumours and diabetes. Virtually all of the information is anecdotal—mainly stories from anonymous sources—and is scientifically questionable.

After saccharin and cyclamate, aspartame is one of the oldest sweeteners and has been extensively studied. When it was first approved in 1981, the US Food and Drug Administration did an exhaustive study into its safety, testing it on humans and animals in amounts many times higher than an individual could consume in an average diet. Australia approved it one year later. Because of the allegations about its safety, aspartame has been re-examined in recent years and the same conclusions have been drawn.

In Australia, three surveys into consumption of sweeteners, especially among high consumers and people with diabetes, have been carried out and not one has ever sounded a warning about aspartame. At present, levels of intake are well below the acceptable daily intake. An adult would have to consume 20 cans of diet soft drink a day to exceed the maximum intake, so there's no evidence to link aspartame to multiple sclerosis, lupus or Alzheimer's disease. With the exception of a few very mild side effects, aspartame appears to be quite safe and isn't among common allergens like milk or fish.

See also
Sweeteners.

Asthma and Diet

No-one knows why asthma is on the increase. It tends to run in families and, in some cases, it is related to a family history of conditions such as hay fever, eczema and allergies. If asthma runs in your family and you want to reduce the chance of your child developing it, breastfeed your baby for at least 6 months, or talk to your doctor or early childhood nurse about using a special hydrolysed formula if breastfeeding isn't possible.

Most people with asthma don't need a special diet. A healthy eating plan based around a variety of foods, including fresh fruit, vegetables, fish, meat, eggs, wholegrains and nuts is essential for everyone with asthma to lead active lives. A nutrient-rich diet can also boost the immune system and help ward off colds and flu—both common triggers of asthma.

It certainly won't hurt to eat plenty of citrus fruits and juices, berries, pineapple, tomatoes and other vitamin C–rich produce. This is one of the key antioxidant vitamins found in the fluid surrounding the lungs, and low intakes of vitamin C have been linked with respiratory problems. Several studies are underway to test its usefulness in asthma, but to date there are no recommendations for how much to consume.

Food is not usually a trigger for an asthma attack; neither are food additives. Many parents cut out dairy foods, believing they create mucus or worsen wheezing. However, there is little scientific backing for this link with three recent intervention trials showing no effect. Unless diagnosed by a skin prick test or radioallergosorbent test, there is no reason to restrict or eliminate dairy from the diet, which will cut out the major source of calcium and is needed for strong bones.

The more likely culprits that trigger asthma attacks are dust mites, pollens, mould and animal fur, colds, changes in the weather and cigarette smoke.

ASTHMA TRIGGERS

SULPHITES

In a small number of sufferers, sulphites can trigger shortness of breath, wheezing and coughing. In Australia and New Zealand, seven sulphite additives (codes 220–225 and 228) are permitted, but the main one used is sodium metabisulphite 223. For kids, keep an eye on fruit juices, cordial, soft drink, dried apricots and apples, pickles and sausages, which can all contain metabisulphite.

FOOD CHEMICALS

A small percentage of people with asthma (less than 10 per cent) are affected by certain chemicals in food, both natural and added. MSG is widely believed to make asthma worse, despite the fact that it has been cleared as a culprit in all studies. Other chemicals are amines (in gravies and deli meats) and salicylates (in juices, fruits, mint). Remember that your response to the food chemical depends on how much of it you eat. You can probably get away with small amounts, but a large amount is likely to produce symptoms.

BEE PRODUCTS

Royal jelly and propolis can trigger an asthma attack and now carry warnings for asthma sufferers.

B

Bananas *See* Fruit.

Barbecuing

Remember, cooking on the barbecue is creation not cremation.

Like many families, we love barbecuing. It's one of the easiest and healthiest meals you can enjoy—just a little lean meat, chicken or fish served with lots of seasonal vegetables such as grilled tomatoes, mushrooms, onions, zucchini, eggplant slices or corn on the cob and, of course, a variety of salads.

However, this high-heat cooking method needs to be controlled so you minimise how much you char (burn) the food. It's not just the meat you need to be careful with; poultry and char-grilled vegetables can burn easily too. When fat drips on hot coals, or any other source of heat, potentially dangerous compounds—heterocyclic amines (HCAs) and polycyclic aromatic hydrocarbons (PAHs) are deposited on the food from the rising smoke and flames. It may taste delicious, but it can set the scene for colorectal cancer later in life.

The good news is that today's barbecues have more than one heat and let you control the temperature as precisely as you can in the kitchen. 'It's about flavour not flames,' chef and author Peter Howard reminded me. 'Remember, cooking on the barbecue is creation not cremation. Turn down the heat and enjoy the juicy, rich flavour of the meat.' To minimise the risk, follow my simple tips for healthy and enjoyable barbecuing.

CHOOSE THE RIGHT INGREDIENTS

- ✔ Choose thinner steaks (no more than 1–2 cm thick), kebabs, lean lamb cutlets and chops, lean mince for burgers and skinless chicken breasts or thigh fillets.
- ✔ Limit processed meats (HCAs and PAHs are formed mostly from fat). If sausages are a family favourite, buy premium quality ones (100 per cent meat) fresh from the butcher or deli—they'll have fewer preservatives and other additives.
- ✔ Add vegetables such as corn cobs, onions, tomatoes and flat mushrooms.

PREPARATION TIPS

- ✔ Trim away any visible fat from steaks, chops and chicken pieces.
- ✔ Marinate the meat and chicken for about 30 minutes before you start cooking with a marinade containing olive oil and lemon juice with herbs like rosemary, thyme and oregano—this tenderises and enhances the flavour of the meat and can reduce the formation of HCAs and PCAs.
- ✔ Precook thick cuts of meat in the microwave or oven and just finish them on the barbecue grill—you'll get all the flavour without the flare.

ZESTY BARBECUED LAMB BACKSTRAPS

This recipe, which has become a family favourite, originally appeared in *The Low GI Diet Cookbook* where it's served with a lentil salad tossed in a tangy lemon yoghurt dressing. I also like these backstraps simply with a big garden salad with lots of ripe red tomatoes and a crusty, grainy roll.

1 tablespoon olive oil
1 clove garlic, crushed
a few sprigs of fresh oregano
zest of 1 lemon
300 g lamb fillet or back strap

Combine the olive oil, garlic, oregano and lemon zest in a bowl. Add the lamb fillets or backstrap and marinate for at least 30 minutes.

Preheat the barbecue to medium–high and barbecue until just cooked. Remove and set aside, covered with foil, to rest for a few minutes. Slice the lamb across the grain about 1.5 cm thick and serve.

COOKING TIPS

- ✔ Keep your barbecue grill and hotplate clean.
- ✔ Cook over a medium heat and avoid open fires or coals where fat can drip on the flames, flare up and burn or char the food.
- ✔ Don't over-cook food; preheat the barbecue before you start cooking and keep your eye on the grill and your mind on the job.
- ✔ Cook red meat like steaks or chops medium, medium-rare or rare—not well done. Burgers and sausages need to be cooked all the way through, so keep the heat down so they don't char on the outside with the longer cooking time.

DID YOU KNOW?
Pan-frying and grilling at high temperatures in the kitchen produce HCAs too.

SERVING TIPS

- ✔ Provide plenty of salads and vegetables.
- ✔ Trim away any charred bits if there was a flare-up (they do happen).

Barley

See Grains and Cereals.

Beans

Beans are the seeds of plants from the *Leguminosae* family. We can eat them immature (pods and all) as snow peas and beans or mature (now called legumes or pulses) as dried peas, beans, lentils and chickpeas. In their mature form they are good sources of vitamins, minerals, fibre, carbohydrate and protein.

See also Legumes.

Beer

Beer is made by fermenting malted grains, usually barley, with brewer's yeast, to produce a brown fermented drink that usually forms a 'head' of foam when it is poured. Hops are added to impart that special bitter quality and flavour.

Historically, beer has been regarded as healthy. This is due in part to the B vitamins that remained present in unfiltered home brews, and in part to the fact that beer was often a safer drink than local water supplies! The water used to make beer was boiled early in the brewing process, destroying any harmful bacteria. The alcohol produced during fermentation, and the addition of bitter hops, helped to preserve the beer, making it the only safe liquid to drink until modern water treatment plants became common.

BEER	% ALCOHOL	GRAMS OF CARBS PER 100 ML	KILOJOULES PER 100 ML
Regular full-strength beer	4.6	2.5–3.6	150–180
Low-carb beer	4.6	Less than 1	120
Light beer	2.7	3.1	119

NUTRITIONAL VALUE

Beer is mostly water and alcohol, with around 3 per cent sugars and dextrin (a type of carbohydrate that's halfway between starch and sugar). Today's modern beers score low in nutrition, despite the fact that their raw materials—malted barley and hops—are quite nutritious. Thiamin or vitamin B_1, for example, is present in yeast and the original grains, but is destroyed during the manufacturing process, or concentrated in the yeast and lost from the beer when it is clarified and the sediment removed. A few of the other B vitamins such as niacin are present, but the levels are low, certainly much less than in breakfast cereal or bread.

There have been calls to fortify beer with thiamin in the past, to counteract the alcohol-related B_1 deficiency known as Wernike-Korsakoff syndrome that occurs in heavy drinkers, but these have never gained government approval.

Varying amounts of minerals such as magnesium, fluoride, selenium and iron are present. Dark beers in particular can carry substantial amounts of iron, but there is little else of nutritional significance.

THE BEER BELLY

At around 5 per cent alcohol, beer appears to have a relatively low alcohol content compared with wine (11–13 per cent) and spirits (40 per cent). There's no fat, no starch and a low-ish 3 per cent of sugars—so where does the beer belly come from?

It is often simply the sheer volume of beer consumed that contributes a significant number of kilojoules. Three schooners (pints) of standard beer pile on 2100 kilojoules, which is equivalent to eight slices of bread.

In the past, the alcohol produced during fermentation, and the addition of bitter hops, helped to preserve the beer, making it the only safe liquid to drink until modern water treatment plants became common.

Unlike wine, beer is often consumed on its own, or with snack foods that are fatty, salty and easy to wash down.

BEER AND COLON CANCER

Colon (bowel) cancer, a killer disease in all affluent countries, is little-known in developing countries. High intakes of junk food are prime suspects, but there is also good research suggesting that a diet low in fibre and vegetables combined with high beer consumption is a contributing factor.

MY TAKE

I recommend going for the light beer—you cut back on alcohol (which is good news for your liver and blood pressure, and reduces the risk of cancer) and save on kilojoules.

LOW-CARB BEER

Low-carb beers such as Pure Blonde and Hahn Super Dry are often sold as a dieter's alternative to full-strength beer. Marketing of these is frequently aimed at women who have traditionally not been big beer drinkers.

You don't have to drink low-carb for weight loss. Low-alcohol beer is just as effective because the two are similar in kilojoules at around 450 kilojoules per 300 ml bottle, or 120 kilojoules per 100 millilitres. Remove either the carbohydrate or the alcohol from beer, and you end up consuming fewer kilojoules (20–33 per cent fewer, depending on the brand).

- ✖ Low-carb beers have around one-third the carbs of regular beer. So if you swap your 375 millilitre bottle of regular beer for a low-carb one, you drop from 10 grams to only 3 grams of carbohydrate. Not a huge saving.
- ✖ Most low-carb beers have the same alcohol content as full-strength regular beers. They're not low in alcohol, which is probably why they appeal as they have a better flavour. So what you save on the carbs, you gain with the alcohol.

See also **Alcohol.**

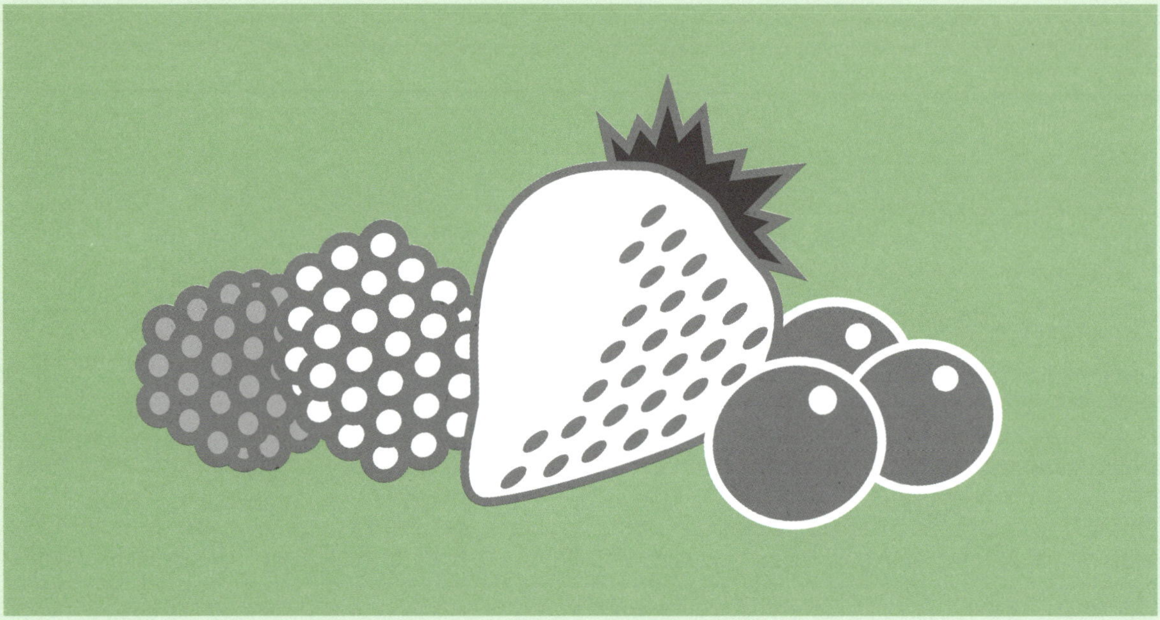

Berries

Berries are among the nutrition powerhouses of the fruit world. They make a guiltless indulgence for anyone watching their weight or fat intake. Served with a squeeze of orange juice and a scoop of low-fat vanilla yoghurt or ice-cream, they make a deliciously light dessert that's also low in kilojoules and fat. For everyday eating, opt for fresh or frozen berries over juices, which are concentrated sources of kilojoules.

NUTRITIONAL VALUE

Nutritionally, berries are in a class of their own. As a group, they are all good-to-excellent sources of vitamin C and they also supply lesser amounts of many essential minerals like potassium, calcium, iron, magnesium and phosphorus. They add a lot of dietary fibre (both insoluble and soluble), which adds to their superfood status.

The purple and red pigments (anthocyanins) function as antioxidants, minimising the effects of ageing, boosting memory and brainpower, and preserving eyesight. Eaten fresh, they're a top supplier of two key B vitamins including folate, which helps prevent birth defects in babies, and niacin, which releases energy from food. They also offer beta-carotene (which gets converted into vitamin A once in the body) and vitamin E. And they won't make you pile on the pounds—half a cup of fresh blueberries gives you 8 grams of carbohydrate, 1.5 grams of dietary fibre and 165 kilojoules.

DID YOU KNOW?

True berries are fleshy fruits produced from a single ovary and their seeds are usually embedded in the flesh. Botanically speaking, this means that bananas, capsicum, eggplant, feijoa, figs, grapes, kiwifruit, persimmon and tomatoes are all examples of berry fruits.

POPULAR BERRIES

BLUEBERRIES

Blue is good for you. As one of today's superfoods, blueberries are bursting with nutrition and flavour, packed with antioxidants and very low in kilojoules. Researchers at the USDA Human Nutrition Centre rank blueberries as number one for antioxidant activity when compared with other fresh fruits and vegetables.

> Berries are among the nutrition powerhouses of the fruit world.

Most blueberries you buy in the supermarket or fresh produce store will be cultivated high-bush blueberries (*Vaccinium corymbosum L*). In the US, it's also possible to buy frozen wild blueberries (*V. angustifolium*). They are about a third of the size of cultivated ones, have a more intense blueberry flavour and retain their shape well in cooking. Interestingly, studies of wild blueberries show they are higher still in antioxidants. If you want to try them, look out for Creative Gourmet's frozen mixed berries, which contain a mix of regular blueberries, wild blueberries, raspberries and cranberries.

CRANBERRIES

The tart, bright-red cranberry is a cousin of the blueberry but you won't find them fresh in punnets very often as some 95 per cent of each year's crop is processed—frozen for sweetened juices, drinks and sauces, dried or used in supplements. Cranberry juice and supplements have been extensively studied as an aid to help prevent recurrent urinary tract infections (UTIs) and incontinence. UTIs are usually caused by *E. coli*, a bacteria commonly found in the intestines. It seems that cranberries contain plant chemicals called proanthocyanidins, which stop bacteria from sticking to the bladder wall and multiplying. Fewer bugs mean less likelihood they can multiply and take hold. You'll need to drink around 300 millilitres (that's a bit over a cup) of cranberry juice a day to lessen the frequency of infection.

STRAWBERRIES

The world's most popular berry, strawberries are packed with vitamin C, potassium, fibre and folate and have a low GI, so enjoy them by the bowlful as a delicious fresh snack or dessert. They boast a number of phytochemicals, naturally occurring plant compounds that are being researched for their medicinal benefits. Because the average serve has very little impact on blood glucose levels, people with diabetes can eat them freely. Remember they are fragile, so store them in the fridge and wash and hull just before using.

EASY WAYS TO ENJOY BERRIES

- ✔ Eat a handful as a fruity snack or to finish a meal.
- ✔ Sprinkle over yoghurt or ice-cream.
- ✔ Fresh berries add a tangy colourful punch over breakfast cereals.
- ✔ Add fresh or frozen berries to a blender with low-fat milk, yoghurt and a small banana (if you want it really thick) and make a smoothie.
- ✔ Make a quick mixed berry *clafouti*—a custard dessert where fruit (traditionally cherries) is mixed with a batter—using your favourite berries, egg, flour and a little sugar.

See also **Bran; Oats.**

Beta-glucans

A natural gum of oats and barley prescribed for its ability to lower blood cholesterol.

Beverages

One of my favourite sayings is 'don't drink in the kilojoules'. If you're wondering why it's hard to shift that extra layer of fat, check out what and how much you're drinking. According to US researcher Professor Barry Popkin, the beverage industry has been successful in marketing the idea of always drinking: drink when you are active, drink when you are resting and relaxing, and drink when you go to a party. With functional beverages now hitting the marketplace you can also drink for extra energy, drink for better skin, drink for more vitamins, and drink for extra antioxidants. And all these drinks come with a bonus—extra kilojoules.

Popkin says that today, many Americans drink more than twice as many 'caloric' beverages as they did 40 years ago. Instead of drinking mostly water, tea, coffee, whole milk and a limited amount of beer and hard alcohol as they did then, for around 420–840 kilojoules a day, the average American today downs around 1680 kilojoules each day from beverages. Over two-thirds of this increase is coming from soft drinks and fruit juices. The story is much the same in Australia and New Zealand where it is estimated that the beverages we are drinking contribute around one-fifth of our daily intake of kilojoules (that's about 1700 kilojoules for someone with an 8700 kilojoules intake).

MY TAKE
Think before you drink. Remember, some beverages have as many kilojoules as a meal.

Research is now linking what we drink to the obesity epidemic as well as weight gain, abdominal obesity, diabetes and heart disease. It seems that drinks are less filling than solid food and don't register with our brain's appetite control centre. So it's easy to swallow large amounts of juice or soft drink (these two drinks combined supply over half of all the sugar we consume).

Here are my guidelines for what's good to drink and what's not so good.

THE BEST DRINKS

WATER

It has no kilojoules, no extra sugar and no sodium. An inexpensive water filter jug removes the taints and off-flavours without taking out the fluoride, which is good for your teeth—it really does make water taste nice. Chill your water or serve it with a slice of lime or lemon. Carry a refillable water bottle when you are out and about.

WEAK GREEN OR BLACK TEA

Tea is a major source of flavonoids—natural compounds that can keep your heart healthy and may even slow the ageing process. It also contains theanine, an amino acid unique to tea that keeps you alert yet relaxed. Tea does contain caffeine, but only at around half the level found in coffee, so it's a healthier choice. Enjoy two or three cups a day with milk or lemon.

HERB AND FLORAL TEAS

These infusions add zero kilojoules unless you sweeten them. Some have medicinal properties; for example, chamomile induces sleepiness, or peppermint and ginger act as natural stimulants.

FRUIT JUICE

Limit juice consumption to one small glass (about 200 millilitres) of unsweetened juice a day—it's healthy but it's fruit in a concentrated form without the fibre. I recommend you buy 100 per cent fruit juice and dilute it 50/50 with water or ice-blocks. This way it's still refreshing but lower in kilojoule density. Check the label—don't buy 'fruit juice drinks' or 'fruit drinks', which contain a lot of added sugar and only a small percentage of real fruit juice. Always check that you are buying pure fruit juice.

Juice bars have made juice trendy. You can get vitamin-packed orange and carrot juice with a shot of wheatgrass, apple, celery and ginger, or a pineapple smoothie in minutes. But the servings are supersized. A standard foam cup of juice packs in 1040 kilojoules. Order the smallest size or share with a friend. And remember to eat two serves of whole fruit each day as well.

Growing bodies
Low-fat milks suit families with kids over the age of two. Children need four serves of dairy foods a day, which can come from milk as well as yoghurt and cheese.

LOW-FAT MILKS

Most of these milks are enriched with extra calcium so you get half the fat and 30 per cent more calcium per glass. They're good value. You don't need to go to skim (very low-fat or no-fat) versions unless you're being super-strict on fat intake, or love drinking milk but are on a weight-loss diet.

LOW-FAT, CALCIUM-ENRICHED SOY, ALMOND, OAT AND RICE DRINKS

Make sure the drinks are fortified with calcium (most are) otherwise you'll short-change yourself on calcium.

FRUITY FRAPPES AND SMOOTHIES

Smoothies made with low-fat milk, yoghurt or ice-cream (or soy alternatives), fruit and perhaps some wheatgerm or chia, provide an excellent source of bone-building calcium. They'll also provide long-lasting energy, as they are usually low GI. But they're supersized, so regard them as a complete meal, not just a snack or thirst quencher.

HOW MUCH OVER THE DAY	
Water	4–6 glasses
Milk	1 glass
Teas	2–3 cups
Unsweetened juice, diluted	1 small glass (optional)
Other	1 glass/cup (optional)
Wine	1 glass (optional)

OCCASIONAL DRINKS

SPORTS DRINKS

Sports drinks are useful if you're an endurance athlete exercising hard for more than an hour at a time. The rest of us weekend warriors will do fine on plain water. However, if you need to replenish lost sweat quickly, sports drinks do a good job with their formulation of lower sugar content (at 5–6 per cent, which is half that of soft drinks) plus added sodium and potassium.

SPORTS WATERS

At only 1–2 per cent sugar, sports waters are like drinking water with a splash of sugar and flavouring. Forget the claims about added B vitamins often what's added is just enough to make an enticing claim on the label, rather than a difference to your life.

VITAMIN WATERS

Lightly sweetened but full of fanciful claims promising 'clarity', 'focus' and 'recharge', these are vitamin-enriched, flavoured drinks with 5–7 per cent sugar, the same as most sports drinks. While their labels list healthy-sounding things like vitamins, guarana, taurine, cranberries or pomegranate, they're full of caffeine, colours, flavours and preservatives.

Regard them as a cross between a sports drink and an energy drink. They've got the sugar level of a sports drink, but the vitamins and caffeine of an energy drink!

ICED TEA

Lightly sweetened (4–5 per cent) and low on carbonation, commercial iced teas are great thirst quenchers. Make your own using cold, brewed black tea, a little sugar, lemon slices and mint leaves. Iced tea is not as rich in polyphenols (antioxidants) as hot tea.

DRINKS THAT ARE NOT SO GOOD

SOFT DRINKS

Once reserved for parties and special occasions, fizzy, sugary drinks are now everyday staples in supersizes. The small 200 millilitre Coke 'waist' bottle of the 1950s has been superseded by 375 millilitre cans, large 600 millilitre Coke 'buddies' or even 900 millilitre fast-food cartons to go. Yet soft drinks give us no nutrients apart from water and load us up with kilojoules—a 375 millilitre can of regular soft drink will hit you with 41 grams of sugar (10 teaspoons) and 655 kilojoules.

Over the past 20 years, soft drinks have gradually replaced milk as the main drink of teenagers. Apart from the fact that they lack calcium, they are not bone-friendly for another reason—it seems the phosphoric acid interferes with calcium absorption. The phosphoric acid makes them overly acidic which, together with their high sugar level, is a harmful combination for teeth.

Diet or zero-sugar versions that are sweetened with aspartame, acesulphame K or sucralose are handy if you want to cut back on your sugar intake, but they too can erode enamel and dentine. And you don't want to be on a high intake of sweeteners of any sort—despite their safety record to date. Stick to one or two diet drinks a day.

ENERGY DRINKS

These sound as if they're doing you good, crammed with healthful-sounding ingredients like B vitamins, taurine, amino acids and guarana. But the truth is they're really just a fizzy drink with added caffeine plus guarana (actually a plant that contains caffeine). The combination of caffeine with alcohol (i.e. a Vodka Red Bull) is not a good one—one picks you up while the other settles you down! Steer clear of these.

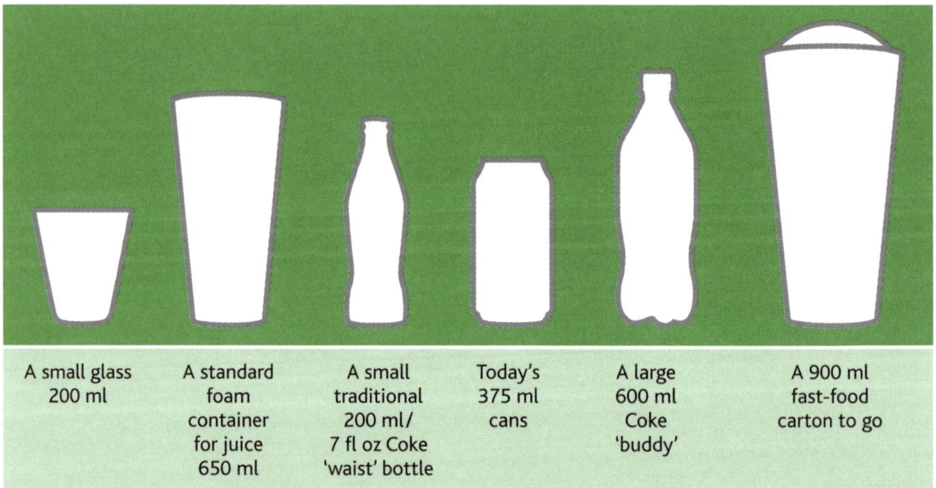
A small glass 200 ml
A standard foam container for juice 650 ml
A small traditional 200 ml/ 7 fl oz Coke 'waist' bottle
Today's 375 ml cans
A large 600 ml Coke 'buddy'
A 900 ml fast-food carton to go

TAKEAWAY COFFEE

These can be a real trap. Gourmet coffee chains such as Starbucks, Jamaica Blue and Gloria Jeans offer the tempting combination of supersize sofas, supersize serves and killer kilojoule syrups. A jumbo latte with caramel syrup plus whipped cream packs in a hefty 1000 kilojoules and 10 grams of fat, not forgetting the 31 grams (around 6 teaspoons) of sugar. It's rather like drinking the equivalent of a regular-size Mars Bar.

Coffee in moderation is fine—there are even early reports that it may reduce your chances of Parkinson's disease. But too much caffeine can leave you sleepless, jittery and with an upset stomach. If you are a regular milky coffee drinker, it's a good idea to opt for a 'skinny' latte, flat white or cappuccino. A full-cream version of these has 2 grams of fat and 190 kilojoules. Limit yourself to no more than two real coffees (this means a cappuccino or short black made from espresso) or four instant coffees each day.

HOT CHOCOLATE

If you choose a hot chocolate with whipped cream (the one that comes in the tall glass) you get a whopping 41 grams of sugar and 24 grams of fat. This is not a mere beverage—this is equivalent to a mini-meal!

MY TAKE

Adults should drink water or a small glass of juice (or wine, if preferred) with meals. Serve kids milk with their meal (full-fat up to the age of two, and then reduced-fat or light after that). The best fluids for in-between meals are water, milk, tea or herbal infusions.

Bloating

Bloating is a tricky one as there are numerous causes for a distended and uncomfortable abdomen—some serious, others not. For most people, it tends to be a consequence of wind. Other causes include constipation or a sluggish bowel, a full bladder, fluid retention or pregnancy. In the week before a period starts, bloating is one of several uncomfortable symptoms many women experience.

If you have chronic bloating accompanied by other worrying symptoms, make an appointment with a gastroenterologist to check for underlying problems such as irritable bowel syndrome, coeliac disease, Crohn's disease, lactose intolerance or fructose malabsorption.

SUSPECT FOODS

Self-help for bloating and flatulence starts by taking a good look at your diet. First of all, cut back on gas-producing triggers.

- ✖ Cruciferous vegetables like cabbage, broccoli and cauliflower along with onions and garlic
- ✖ Legumes including beans, chickpeas and lentils
- ✖ Very starchy foods like bread, pasta, rice, corn (including popcorn), pastries and cakes
- ✖ Fatty foods including fried foods and rich creamy sauces and desserts
- ✖ Highly spiced foods like curries
- ✖ Fizzy (carbonated) drinks including sparkling mineral water, beer and Diet Coke

WHAT YOU CAN DO

- ✔ Eat regular meals.
- ✔ Chew your food slowly—watch you're not swallowing air when chewing.
- ✔ Drink plenty of fluids.
- ✔ Exercise every day.
- ✔ Avoid constipation by eating plenty of fibre-rich foods.
- ✔ Avoid sorbitol, a sweetener found in large quantities in sugar-free gum, mints, diet cordials and pear or apple juice.

See also **Coeliac Disease; Fibre; Flatulence; Fructose Malabsorption; Irritable Bowel Syndrome; Lactose Intolerance.**

Blood Pressure and Diet

High blood pressure (or hypertension) is a dangerous condition. It predisposes you to a stroke, heart attack or kidney damage, which is why your doctor will take action if they notice that you have high blood pressure at a routine check-up.

Blood pressure is a measure of the heart's force when pumping blood through the arteries. It is at its highest when the heart contracts (the systolic measurement, around 120 millilitres of mercury in a healthy adult) and its lowest when the heart relaxes (the diastolic measurement—around 80 millilitres). This is expressed as a normal blood pressure of 120/80.

More than three million Australians over the age of 25 have high blood pressure. It's a silent condition that can go undetected for years until it suddenly causes a stroke or heart attack. It used to be accepted that our blood pressure rose automatically as we aged. Today, researchers believe that it need not happen if we lead a healthy lifestyle.

The tendency to develop high blood pressure is largely genetic. If your parents had high blood pressure, or suffered an early heart attack or stroke, you are a likely candidate for high blood pressure yourself. But it's believed that a tendency will not appear unless one or more of the following five factors trigger the mechanisms that cause high blood pressure:

- Excess weight—forcing the heart to pump harder
- Alcohol intake—responsible for about one in 10 blood pressure cases
- High salt intake
- Stress
- Sedentary lifestyle.

SALT AND YOUR BLOOD PRESSURE

The role of salt in high blood pressure has been suspected since the beginning of the last century. Populations who consume little or no salt do not suffer high blood pressure, and heart attacks and strokes are rare. Moreover, the blood pressure in such populations does not rise with age as ours does. New Guinea Highlanders, Yanomamö Indians (in the Amazon rainforest on the border between Brazil and Venezuela) and Solomon Islanders survive with little salt, yet live in excellent health because of the kidney's ability to conserve rather than excrete sodium. Their diets, like those of our early ancestors, supply a mere 200 milligrams of sodium per day.

By contrast, people in the Northern Akita province of Japan traditionally have one of the saltiest diets in the world, consuming over 9000 milligrams per day in the form of miso soup, pickled vegetables and salted fish. Approximately 40 per cent of adults in this region have high blood pressure, and stroke is the most common cause of death. Health authorities have been working hard since the 1990s to decrease salt intake in the region.

THE SALT-FREE RICE DIET

During the 1940s, a salt-free, rice-based diet called the Kempner diet became famous as a way of lowering high blood pressure. The diet, a spartan regime of only unsalted boiled rice plus fruit and juices, was successful in about 70 per cent of cases.

Not all cases of high blood pressure improve when salt is eliminated (for reasons nutritionists do not fully understand). However, when it works, avoiding salt is a valuable aid in the treatment of high blood pressure in conjunction with drugs such as ACE inhibitors and angiotensin antagonists. In some cases of mild hypertension, reducing salt intake can lead to medication being reduced or withdrawn.

THE DASH DIET

A dietary approach is gaining momentum and, unlike those bestseller diet books, it's one that has solid research to back it up. Called the DASH diet—Dietary Approaches to Stop Hypertension—it is rich in vegetables, fruit, low-fat dairy foods, nuts and wholegrains and has very little saturated fat. The diet also includes fish (for omega-3s, which lower blood pressure) and poultry. What you cut out are sweets, drinks containing sugar, bad fats and junk food.

The earliest report of success on the DASH diet was published in the prestigious *New England Journal of Medicine* way back in 1997. Since then, a number of follow-up studies have confirmed the results, showing that this diet has successfully lowered blood pressure in people with hypertension.

WHY IT WORKS

Nutritionists believe there are three good reasons behind the success of the DASH Diet.

- ✔ It gives you lots of minerals such as potassium, calcium and magnesium, which all seem to protect against salt's damaging effect.
- ✔ It is high in fibre.
- ✔ It helps you shed weight, which in turn decreases blood pressure.

The diet includes daily servings of grains, plenty of raw and cooked vegetables and fruit, low-fat or fat-free dairy foods, lean meat, chicken, fish and some fats as well as nuts and seeds four to five times a week.

A DAY ON THE DASH DIET

- **BREAKFAST**—A bowl of natural muesli with low-fat milk topped with low-fat Greek yoghurt and half a cup of blueberries; small glass of juice.
- **LUNCH**—Chicken, tabbouli and salad wrap made with a wholemeal mountain bread wrap filled with ⅔ cup cooked, sliced chicken breast, ½ cup shredded lettuce, ½ cup tabbouli, tomato slices and a thick spread of avocado. Alternatively serve as a salad with two crunchy rye crispbreads like Ry-King, which are salt free; glass of low-fat milk.
- **DINNER**—Zesty, slow-roasted salmon (marinated in lime zest and juice, olive oil, ginger and garlic) served on a bed of wilted spinach with ½ cup buckwheat noodles and a large mixed green salad (at least 3 cups of salad with plenty of colourful capsicums); bowl of fresh fruit salad with low-fat yoghurt; water.
- **SNACKS**—You can have up to three snacks a day depending how hungry or active you are.
  Snack 1: Fresh fruit, or a tub of fruit salad, or a small handful of dried fruit.
  Snack 2: Glass of milk, or a tub of low-fat yoghurt, or a skinny cappuccino or café latte.
  Snack 3: Small handful of unsalted nuts or trail mix.

HELPFUL MINERALS

Potassium is a complementary mineral to sodium and plays a major role in normalising blood pressure. You should aim for as high an intake of potassium as possible.

Calcium has been shown to lower blood pressure in both animals and humans. A high calcium intake from sources such as dairy foods can protect against salt sensitivity in some adults. US research reports that as long as the calcium intake is high, people can eat a higher sodium diet with little ill-effect on blood pressure.

Magnesium works with calcium, sodium and potassium in a number of bodily functions including building bones, controlling muscle contractions and regulating the heartbeat. Magnesium occurs in many healthy foods, such as wholegrains, green vegetables, milk, meat, nuts, bananas and fruit.

See also Salt.

CALCULATE YOUR BMI

Your BMI = your weight (in kilograms) divided by your height (in metres) squared. For example, someone who weighs 70 kg and is 1.75 m tall: 70 ÷ (1.75 x 1.75} and you have a BMI of 22.8. There are many BMI calculators on the internet that will do the maths for you.

BMI	CLASSIFICATION
Less than 18.5	Underweight, risk of health problems are increased.
18.5–25	Healthy weight range.
25–29.9	Overweight or pre-obese, risk of health problems are increased.
30 and over	Obese, risk of health problems are greatly increased.

BMI and Body Fat

The Body Mass Index, or BMI, is the most commonly used way to assess your weight. It is a formula that determines whether your weight falls into the healthy weight range—a range of weight for your height that is consistent with the lowest rate of death. To calculate it, you will need to know your weight in kilograms and your height in metres. You divide your weight by your height squared.

LIMITATIONS

The BMI has limitations that you should keep in mind when assessing your own weight. It was designed to apply to adults (both women and men) aged 18 and over and is therefore not suitable for children. It also does not take into account muscle mass, just overall weight, so it over-estimates someone like a body builder, rating them as overweight when they simply have a high ratio of muscle to fat.

MY TAKE

Remember that there is no single weight perfect for your height, but there is a weight range where your chances of good health are highest—this is the healthy weight range (BMI of 18.5 to 25).

Bone Food *See* Calcium; Osteoporosis.

Brain Food *See* Alzheimer's Disease and Diet; Anti-ageing Diets; Food and Mood.

Bran and Bran Cereals

I find bran a handy ingredient to quickly boost the fibre content of any diet. A tablespoon over cereal or yoghurt or thrown into a smoothie is the simplest way to increase your fibre intake quickly. It's not equivalent to the nutrition gained from wholegrains, but it doesn't require much change to your usual eating habits or food preferences. It's also easy to sneak into muffins, a Bolognese sauce or a hearty casserole.

NUTRITIONAL VALUE

The term 'bran' refers to the outer protective layers of any cereal grain. The bran is there to protect the seed, so all brans are concentrated sources of fibre and high in minerals, particularly phosphorus, silica, magnesium and potassium as well as lesser amounts of iron, zinc and calcium. However, most of these minerals are not biologically available to the human body because of another bran component called phytic acid (phytates), which binds to the minerals and prevents them being absorbed from the digestive tract. This is a problem if you eat straight bran, but yeast leavening in wholemeal breads and the heat applied during the manufacturing of breakfast cereal release much of the bound minerals.

NUMBER CRUNCH

A heaped tablespoon of wheat bran (weighing 7 grams) gives you 1 gram of protein, a trace of fat, 2 grams of starch, a trace of sugars, 3 grams of fibre and 60 kilojoules.

WHEAT BRAN

At over 40 per cent fibre, unprocessed wheat bran has one of the highest fibre contents of all foods, around six times as much as wholemeal bread and twice that of bran cereals. Being rich in insoluble fibre, it is effective in relieving constipation, keeps the digestive system healthy and may help protect against diverticulitis and cancer of the bowel. This laxative action is due to bran's ability to absorb water in the bowel, which increases the size and softness of the faeces. But the particle size of bran is critical—if it is too finely ground, much of this water-holding ability is lost.

Unprocessed wheat bran has been a popular addition to breakfast meals since fibre first attracted scientific interest in the 1970s. It is also processed into breakfast cereals like All-Bran or Bran Flakes (which are much easier to take in) and incorporated into fibre-increased breads, biscuits and muesli bars.

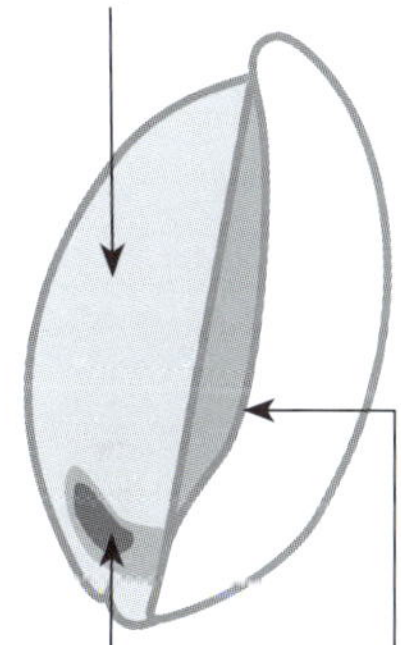

A Wheat Kernel

OAT AND BARLEY BRAN

These are very similar. Both contain around 17 per cent fibre, mostly soluble fibre known as beta-glucan, which helps lower blood cholesterol levels and keep your heart healthy. Both of these brans are much more palatable than wheat bran, but their laxative effect is not as strong.

RICE BRAN

With 26 per cent fibre, rice bran lies in between and has a mix of both sorts of fibre. It's also high in oil with a golden colour and pleasant nutty taste. It's useful for gluten-free diets, as are psyllium husks. In sharp contrast to the other brans, it contains gamma-oryzanol, a natural antioxidant, as well as other phytosterols that can lower the 'bad' LDL cholesterol. It also has fat-soluble forms of vitamin E known as tocotrienols, adding a nutritional bonus.

DAILY INTAKE

Oat and barley bran have been proven to lower cholesterol, but the amounts you need to eat are large—around 1 cup (100 grams) every day. While this is impossible to consume in a single meal, you can spread it over the day by having a couple of tablespoons at breakfast, whirling some into a milkshake and baking the rest into oat-bran muffins. But don't forget that you still need to modify the fats in your diet to lower your cholesterol level.

For unprocessed wheat bran, two heaped tablespoons (30 grams) is usually sufficient to ensure bowel regularity and prevent constipation. Just remember to increase your intake gradually and make sure you drink plenty of water.

Adding a lot of wheat bran to your diet can cause a loss of valuable minerals through the bowel. In a balanced diet, such a loss is unlikely to lead to mineral deficiencies but could pose problems with nutritionally inadequate diets. Large amounts of bran (more than 1 cup a day) can also cause flatulence (wind), stomach cramp and diarrhoea. It is not recommended for elderly people, pregnant and breastfeeding women, and growing children, whose requirements for minerals are high.

Another danger in eating too much bran is the pesticide residue that remains after grain crops are sprayed to prevent insects. Because bran is derived from the outer layers of the wheat grain, it has been found to be higher in pesticide residue than flour. It is better to get most of your fibre from bran cereals, which are processed and have the harmful chemical residues removed.

Bread

Wholemeal, rye, multigrain, high-fibre, gluten-free, sourdough, soy and linseed—there are lots of interesting breads to choose from these days.

NUTRITIONAL VALUE

Whatever its colour, bread is a nutritious food that is low in fat and contributes filling carbohydrate and protein. With the high extraction rate for milling white flour in Australia (just under 80 per cent), it's a good source of three B vitamins—thiamin, niacin and folate—which we need for energy release. Wholemeal and grainy breads are superior for their fibre, minerals and vitamins, but even a slice of white bread spread with peanut butter or jam makes a healthier snack than cracker biscuits or salty packet snacks like potato crisps.

The basic ingredients of all breads are flour (which can be white, wholemeal, rye or a mixture), water, yeast and a little salt. Other ingredients include skim-milk powder, gluten (wheat protein), a little fat (often listed as vegetable oil on the label), cracked (kibbled) grains, seeds, sugar, malt and mould-inhibitor, generally calcium propionate. Despite the many different types or shapes of bread, all bread is similar in nutritional terms and can be classified into four main categories according to the base flour it's made from—white, wholemeal, rye or multigrain. Cheese rolls or olive breads have more fat, while fruit loaves have slightly more sugar.

NUMBER CRUNCH

A sandwich slice of wholemeal bread (30 grams) gives you 3 grams of protein, 1 gram of fat, 11 grams of starch, a trace of sugars, 2 grams of fibre and 260 kilojoules.

CHOOSING THE RIGHT ONE FOR YOU

Ideally, your everyday bread should be a wholegrain type, either a smooth wholemeal or a chewier multigrain or heavy rye. Save the crusty white bread for the weekend or eating out. Remember, not all your bread needs to be wholegrain. Nutritionists recommend that you eat at least half your grain foods as wholegrains. As a general rule, look for the word 'wholegrain' on the label or more than 7 per cent fibre.

WHOLEMEAL

If you prefer a soft, smooth bread, this is a good choice over white bread as it contains more fibre, B vitamins for energy release, minerals and antioxidants. You may see these breads labelled as wholegrain, wheatmeal or whole wheat—they all mean the same thing. Bread made with 100 per cent wholemeal flour contains all the components of the wheat grain but it's been milled to a fine texture.

MULTIGRAIN OR MIXED GRAIN

There are two different types of multigrain bread. The heavier breads are darker in colour and more dense in texture. These are usually based on wholemeal flour, with added whole or cracked (kibbled) wheat or rye grains, which stand out in the slice and add a chewy texture. These are nutritious choices. The lighter multigrain loaves are based on white flour with only a sprinkle of softened cracked grains. These appeal to kids and are a good compromise between the softness of white bread and the wholesomeness of grains. They're a good stepping stone to heavier breads for adults too. For both types, the actual pieces of grain slow down the rate of carbohydrate absorption, making these breads low GI. Check the percentage of wholegrains on the label. Ideally go for one with over 50 per cent wholegrains or compare brands and buy the one with the highest.

SOY AND LINSEED

These breads are made by adding soy grits or soy flour and linseeds (flaxseeds) to a white or wholemeal bread dough. Originally promoted to menopausal women (based on the theory the soy contains beneficial phytoestrogens), these are excellent breads which are high in fibre and a source of the plant omega-3 alpha-linolenic acid (ALA) and folate, which is important for pregnant women or women wishing to conceive. Thanks to the seeds, these tend to be higher in fat (8 or 9 per cent compared with 2–3 per cent for non-seed breads) and have a moist texture, which keeps well.

RYE

This grain is closely related to wheat and is traditionally consumed in northern European countries such as Denmark, Sweden, Germany, Poland and Russia. It produces a heavier, darker bread compared with wheat, so is often mixed with white wheaten flour to produce a light rye bread (usually 30 per cent rye, 70 per cent wheat). Dark rye breads such as black bread, pumpernickel or *schinkenbrot* are generally 100 per cent rye. It's also popular in the form of rye crispbread. Rye has a low GI, is high in soluble fibre and contains more antioxidants than wheat. It is a good choice health-wise, and it adds variety to your breads. Note: it contains gluten so it NOT suitable for gluten free diets.

FIBRE-INCREASED WHITE

These breads have boosted fibre content, without affecting the colour, taste or texture. The sources of fibre are usually soy hulls or white lupin hulls or Hi-Maize, a unique flour high in resistant starch that acts like fibre in the body. White fibre-increased breads are not as nutritious as the wholemeal variety because they don't contain all the parts of the original wheat grain, therefore lacking the B vitamins, minerals and phytonutrients from the bran and germ. It matches the fibre content of a wholemeal, but that's all. This puts it above regular white bread and is a good compromise for children who refuse to eat wholemeal bread.

DID YOU KNOW?

The thickness of bread slices has become bigger over the past five years. Today we don't tuck into the thin slice we ate as kids (about 30 g). These days, a slice of bread is often thick enough to qualify as toast (at around 50 g). This applies particularly to fruit loaf, which comes in trendy, thick café-style slices (60 g).

WHITE

Traditional white bread is made from white flour and has two vitamins added to it (thiamin and folate), as well as iodine from iodised salt. These days, however, white bread comes with all sorts of additions— you can purchase white breads that are also high in invisible fibre, low GI, or boosted with omega-3, iron or other vitamins and minerals. These breads appear to have it all—soft, smooth, square sliced bread with no 'bits' yet offering those important extras! Remember, though, that you're not getting the benefits of a true wholemeal with all the grain. You may get some fibre and a handful of added vitamins, iron or calcium but none of the other grain antioxidants that keep us healthy. Often the quantity you get from the bread is only a fraction of what you'd find in a food that's a rich source.

FLAT BREAD, LAVASH AND MOUNTAIN BREAD

Go for the wholemeal, rye or barley-based versions of these where possible.

PRODUCT	AVAILABLE CARBOHYDRATE (g)
1 thin slice, white bread	15
1 toast slice, white bread	25
1 medium (200 g) potato	20
1 cup cooked white rice	30
1 cup cooked spaghetti	30
1 small (100 g) can baked beans	12
50 g pack corn chips	32

BREAD AND WEIGHT LOSS

Bread is a food that's rich in starchy carbohydrates (45 per cent). For this reason, it's often eliminated by people trying to lose excess weight—especially those on a high-protein/low-carb diet plan. But bread is no higher in carbs than other common starchy foods, and it contains less than many popular junk foods. The benefits of cutting out bread are often because you simultaneously cut out the butter or margarine and toppings that go with it.

It's not wise to eliminate all carbohydrates. Our bodies need a minimum amount to fuel the brain (which relies entirely on glucose for energy), and to balance out the protein and fat. Choose a minimum of three serves of healthy carbohydrates a day such as a wholegrain, soy and linseed or rye bread, rye crispbread, brown rice or a high-fibre cereal. These have plenty of fibre to fill you up, are low in fat and low GI—all good things that help you achieve and maintain a healthy weight.

Breakfast

The word breakfast literally means to 'break the fast' from the eight to 12 hours since your last meal. Your brain and muscles are crying out for starter fuel to spring them into action and face the day ahead. But these days, around one in five Australians regularly miss breakfast on some days of the week. Young adults aged between 19 and 24 were the worst offenders, with approximately 40 per cent eating breakfast fewer than 5 days a week, and a further 15 per cent rarely or never eating breakfast.

SHOPPER'S GUIDE
A good cereal will have:

- ✔ **High fibre**—check the list of ingredients for wheat bran, whole wheat, whole barley, oats and brown rice. Oats and corn are always wholegrain but wheat, rice and barley are often refined. Look for at least 10 per cent fibre; bran cereals (i.e. All-Bran, Sultana Bran) have 15–30 per cent, while Corn Flakes and Rice Bubbles are down at a low 2 per cent.
- ✔ **Low sugar**—look for one with less than 15 per cent sugars or less than 25 per cent sugars when a cereal includes dried fruit (e.g. Sultana Bran, muesli). You can't tell from the nutrition information panel how much of the sugar is from the fruit and how much has been added, so I allow more for the natural sugars from sultanas and raisins. Compare brands and buy the one with the lowest.
- ✔ **Less sodium (salt)**—go for 600 mg or less per serving. A low-salt cereal should have less than 120 mg per serving. Compare brands and buy the one with the lowest.

YOU NEED THE BOOST

Eating breakfast has been identified as one of seven healthy habits that promote long life and good health. But there are more immediate and practical reasons not to skip breakfast.

MEMORY AND CONCENTRATION

People who eat a balanced breakfast can concentrate better and are more efficient at their work than those who skip breakfast. Children especially benefit during morning lessons at school.

METABOLISM

Research shows that breakfast speeds up the metabolism, which helps to burn food faster. A group of French researchers asked volunteers to eat identical meals at 9 am, 5 pm and 1 am and measured how well their bodies metabolised the kilojoules from the meal. They found that the morning meal was disposed of far more efficiently than the afternoon meal, while the evening meal was burnt up the least efficiently. This gradual decline in the metabolic rate throughout the day is controlled in some way by our body's natural clock or circadian rhythm. It explains why many shift workers tend to gain weight when on night shift, despite the fact that their daily food intake is no different from that of day workers.

BREAKFASTS TO SUIT YOUR LIFESTYLE

No time to eat in the mornings? Try these quick and easy ideas for breakfast (if you exercise regularly or have a physical job, you may need to scale up the portions).

AT HOME

- ✔ Have a liquid meal. Pour one cup of milk in a blender or food processor with fruit, 3–4 tablespoons of yoghurt or a scoop of ice-cream and a pinch of nutmeg. Whirl for 30 seconds until smooth and frothy. For a high-fibre shake, add 1–2 tablespoons of bran cereal or wheatgerm. Drink and run.
- ✔ Pour a bowl of muesli or bran cereal with low-fat milk and sliced banana. Look for wholegrain cereal that is a good source of fibre, and preferably one with less than 15 per cent sugars.
- ✔ Grab a muffin or toast topped with grilled cheese, a poached egg or a small can of baked beans.

IN THE CAR, ON THE TRAIN OR BUS

- ✔ Bolt out the door with a sandwich you've made the night before and a carton of flavoured milk.
- ✔ Pack a breakfast or muesli bar and drinking yoghurt in your bag.

EAT OUT BEFORE WORK

- ✔ Try thick fruit loaf toasted and topped with ricotta or cottage cheese together with a skim cappuccino or latte.
- ✔ Order grilled cheese and tomato on grainy toast with an English breakfast tea.
- ✔ Snack on a snack pack of fruit and tub of yoghurt.

GLUTEN-FREE OR WHEAT-FREE OPTIONS

Avoiding wheat, oats and barley at breakfast is not easy! Look for cereals based on rice or corn (maize) but always check ingredients to be sure. Fresh fruit salad with a bowl of puffed rice or flaked corn cereal topped with a tablespoon of rice bran or psyllium is also a good option. Add cow's milk or soy milk for extra goodness. Or if you have a few extra moments, cook up some eggs with grilled tomato on gluten-free toast.

BREAKFAST CEREALS: READ THE LABEL

Forget the marketing claims on the front of the pack and read the ingredients label. Ingredients have to be listed in descending order by weight—the ingredient with the highest proportion is listed first. Things to look for include:

- ✔ How high up the list the sources of added sugars (such as sugar, honey, malt, glucose or dextrose, fructose) and salt are
- ✔ Whether any of the sugars come from fruit like sultanas or apricots
- ✔ If words like 'whole' or 'wholegrain' are in the first two ingredients listed; this means

Q

How can I tell if muesli and breakfast bars are high in sugar?

A

It is difficult to give firm guidelines on the acceptable amount of sugar. Reading the label does not help as it does not distinguish between natural sugars from fruit and from added sugar. Diabetes Australia encourages its members to first check out fat, fibre and glycemic index (GI) and then look through the ingredients list to work out where the sugars come from. If the sugars are derived from nutritious ingredients such as fruit, these foods are generally healthier than those where sugar is added; for example, sucrose, glucose, dextrose or corn syrup.

these cereals contain more fibre and more of the natural components of the grain, including vitamins, minerals and phytochemicals

✔ Add up the percentages of the key ingredients, which must be stated if they make a claim e.g. 'with blackcurrant'.

If you want to check out your family's favourite cereals, all major breakfast cereal manufacturers post this information on their websites. It's very easy to find and much easier to read than peering at the small print on the pack. I suggest you focus on comparing information in the 'Per 100 g' column as serve sizes vary considerably.

MY TAKE

Watch the serving size—a standard serve of cereal used to be 30 g, which is 1 cup of bubbles or flakes or 2 breakfast biscuits. But some manufacturers have decided a serve is now 45 g in an effort to claim the 'highest fibre content' or the 'most vitamins'. Muesli is particularly heavy and can range from 45 g to 60 g.

Just Right

	Per 100 g
Energy (kJ)	1490
Fat, total (g)	1.6
- saturated (g)	0.4
Carbohydrate (g)	71.8
- sugars (g)	28.7
Fibre (g)	7.9
Sodium (mg)	30

INGREDIENTS: WHOLEGRAIN CEREALS (63%) (WHOLE WHEAT, ROLLED OATS), SULTANAS (17%), SUGAR, TRITICALE (6%), DRIED APRICOT PIECES (3.5%) (DRIED APRICOT [PRESERVATIVE (220)], WHEAT FLOUR, FRUCTOSE, STABILISERS [1422, 466], PALM OIL, HUMECTANT [GLYCEROL], DEXTROSE, WHEAT FIBRE, FOOD ACID [CITRIC ACID], NATURAL FLAVOUR, COLOUR [160E]), BARLEY MALT EXTRACT, SALT, HONEY (0.1%), MINERAL (IRON), VITAMINS (NIACIN, RIBOFLAVIN, FOLATE, THIAMIN).

Sultana Bran

	Per 100 g
Energy (kJ)	1410
Protein (g)	9.5
Fat, total (g)	1.7
- saturated (g)	0.4
Carbohydrate (g)	62.9
- sugars (g)	22.7
Fibre (g)	14.9
Sodium (mg)	270

INGREDIENTS: WHOLE WHEAT (38%), SULTANAS (25%), WHEAT BRAN (26%), SUGAR, BARLEY MALT EXTRACT, SALT, HUMECTANT (GLYCEROL), MINERALS (IRON, ZINC OXIDE), VITAMINS (NIACIN, RIBOFLAVIN, VITAMIN B6, THIAMIN, FOLATE).

Weet-Bix

	Per 100 g
Energy (kJ)	1490
Protein (g)	12.4
Fat, total (g)	1.4
- saturated (g)	0.3
Carbohydrate (g)	67
- sugars (g)	3.3
Fibre (g)	11
Sodium (mg)	290

INGREDIENTS: WHOLEGRAIN WHEAT (97%), RAW SUGAR, SALT, BARLEY MALT EXTRACT, MINERALS (ZINC GLUCONATE, IRON), VITAMINS (NIACIN, THIAMIN, RIBOFLAVIN, FOLATE).

Breastfeeding *See* Pregnancy and Breastfeeding.

Buckwheat *See* Grains and Cereals.

Butter *See* Spreads.

C

Caffeine

Caffeine is a natural stimulant found in varying amounts in coffee, guarana, tea, cocoa and chocolate. It is also added to cola soft drinks, energy drinks and many anti-sleep tablets. Chemically, caffeine is a methylxanthine compound that acts on the central nervous system, speeding up the heartbeat and rate of breathing, dilating blood vessels (except in the brain) and relaxing smooth muscles. It boosts alertness and concentration and overcomes the perception of fatigue—all key reasons for its enduring popularity in our fast-paced world.

Caffeine postpones exhaustion and enhances physical performance effectively, and is commonly used by athletes. Up until 2004, its use was wide enough for the International Olympic Committee to routinely test for caffeine on the basis that excessive intake is considered an artificial enhancement. Caffeine also triggers the release of fatty acids into the bloodstream, which provides an alternative fuel to glycogen and partially explains its ability to quieten hunger.

Caffeine is absorbed into the bloodstream within an hour of consumption and metabolised within 3–7 hours. It is not stored by the body, but passes out via the urine. The coffee you have at an afternoon break is unlikely to keep you awake at night, but drinking one just before bed probably will.

YOUR DAILY FIX

On a daily basis, most people can handle 300 milligrams of caffeine without experiencing any significant health problems (this is equivalent to four cups of instant coffee or three shots of espresso—a standard latte, short black or cappuccino has one shot). However, some people are very sensitive to caffeine and find that just one cup is enough to keep them awake at night, or even set them on edge.

During pregnancy, it's probably wise to limit caffeine to the equivalent of one or two cups of instant coffee (about 150 milligrams) a day. Reports of caffeine causing miscarriages or low birth weight in babies have not been supported with moderate consumption levels, but may occur if the intake of caffeine is high.

These days, it's not just coffee and tea you need to watch. Caffeine turns up in some surprising places including energy drinks like Red Bull or V, and chocolate bars or corn chips with guarana (the chief ingredient being caffeine, despite being marketed as 'natural caffeine' and supposedly 'safe').

DON'T OVERDO IT

Those who drink coffee all day may well be suffering caffeine overload, but a tolerance to caffeine can build-up over time and many people are able to ingest large amounts without noticing problems. But others will complain of things like insomnia, an upset

KICKING THE HABIT IN FOUR EASY STEPS

Most caffeine junkies don't realise they are physically dependent on caffeine until they try to go without. If you go cold turkey for a day or two, you may find yourself with a headache that is sometimes accompanied by nausea. You may feel a little nervous or shaky and you may be tired, yawning and unable to concentrate. Symptoms are the worst on the first two days. They usually subside 4–7 days after stopping, but are often bad enough to prompt heavy caffeine users to return to drinking their favourite caffeine-containing brew. The best way to reduce your caffeine intake is to cut back gradually and allow your body to adapt without going into withdrawal.

Step 1: Start on a weekend or on holiday when you won't be under pressure.

Step 2: Begin by replacing one or two cups a day with tea, herbal tea, coffee substitute (made from roasted barley, chicory or dandelion root), or decaffeinated coffee. In particular, replace the coffee you'd normally have in the late afternoon or evening that could interfere with your sleep. Alternatively, switch to tea instead of coffee as this will approximately halve your caffeine intake.

Step 3: Drink more water.

Step 4: Keep cutting back each day until you drink no more than four cups of instant coffee or one cappuccino (espresso) a day.

stomach, heartburn and a rapid heartbeat (tachycardia), and you can be sure it's because they've been drinking too much caffeine. Nervousness, irritability and anxiety ('coffee jitters') are other telltale side effects of excess caffeine.

Some people never notice any side effects—that is, until they have to go without. For some, going camping or fasting for a blood test is all they need to get hit by caffeine withdrawal. You get the massive headache that doesn't go away and incredible tiredness, and while this might only last for a couple of days, it's bad enough to send you screaming for a coffee fix (which works quickly and effectively). Other people get warning signs from caffeine habituation, which is what the experts call that addictive quality of caffeine—they don't go so far as to use the word 'addiction'.

For me, two coffees in a row is enough caffeine to get my heart seriously beating, and make my stomach unhappy. I just don't go there anymore.

PRODUCT	CAFFEINE CONTENT (mg)*
COFFEE	
1 shot (30 ml) espresso	60
Long black, 2 shots (60 ml)	120
Turkish, 2 shots (60 ml)	80–120
1 cup percolated/plunger/ drip	60–120
1 cup instant coffee	60–80
1 cup decaffeinated	2–5
1 cup cappuccino, latte, flat white made with 1 shot (30 ml) espresso and topped with hot steamed or frothed milk	60
TEA (no milk)	
1 cup tea from leaf or teabag	10–50
1 cup green/Jasmine/ Chinese tea	30–50
1 cup peppermint/ chamomile herbal infusion	0
1 cup rooibos	0
DRINKS	
250 ml can energy drink	80
375 ml can cola soft drink, diet and sweetened	35–45
375 ml can cola soft drink, decaffeinated	0
300 ml carton coffee-flavoured milk	40
1 cup cocoa	5–20
CHOCOLATE	
30 g dark chocolate	20–30
30 g milk chocolate	2–10
OVER-THE-COUNTER STIMULANTS	
No Doze	100

*Keep in mind that figures like these give average values only. The caffeine content in coffee, for example, varies depending on the type of beans, how it was made and how strong it is. In tea, the type of tea leaves and how long it was brewed for are contributing factors.

HEART PROBLEMS

Anyone with a pre-existing heart condition should be very cautious about consuming too much caffeine. In 1999, a 25-year-old woman died from caffeine induced cardiac arrhythmia after consuming a 'natural energy' guarana health drink containing a high concentration of caffeine.

BIRTH DEFECTS

Researchers are divided on the dangers of consuming caffeine during pregnancy; the studies are not conclusive and most reports clear caffeine of posing any major health risk when taken in moderation. However, if consumed in excess, health risks certainly rise. One of the difficulties with caffeine studies is that it's hard to isolate caffeine from other problem-causing habits. Studies repeatedly find that many heavy coffee drinkers are also heavy smokers, drink more than a moderate amount of alcohol and have high levels of stress.

DID YOU KNOW?

Alex Watson, a fencer from Australia who competed in the 1988 Summer Olympics in Seoul, was banned due to an elevated level of caffeine in his system.

BRITTLE BONES

High intakes of caffeine promote the loss of calcium by 'dragging' calcium out of the body via the urine. If you continually overdo caffeine, your bones will eventually suffer, which may predispose you to osteoporosis in later life. The results of several studies reveal, however, that this applies when calcium intake is already low; coffee posed no increased threat to women who consumed at least one glass of milk a day.

ULCERS

Caffeine increases the amount of acid produced by the stomach, which can irritate the stomach lining or worsen any existing ulcers. Cutting back is a good idea here.

Calcium

Calcium is one of the most vital nutrients. We all know it plays a key role in building strong bones and preventing osteoporosis (brittle bones), but it performs a lot of other important functions in the body as well. Of the body's calcium, 99 per cent is stored in the bones and teeth. The remaining 1 per cent is distributed in body fluids and soft tissue and plays an essential role in blood clotting, muscle functioning, conduction of nerve impulses and fluid balance. Calcium also helps to regulate blood pressure.

The calcium level of the blood is kept constant by a delicate balancing act between the bones and blood. When calcium levels in the blood drop too low and not enough is taken from food, it is drawn out of the bones. A little bone loss each day can result in osteoporosis by the age of 60.

Our bones need 150 milligrams of calcium a day to keep up the renewal process. But because the absorption of calcium is often inefficient and hindered by many food components, we must take in at least 500 milligrams of calcium. If calcium is not available from food, the storehouse in our bones will gradually be depleted. More than 60 per cent of women consume less than the recommended dietary intake of calcium. They frequently cut out calcium-rich dairy foods in order to cut kilojoules, avoid cholesterol and saturated fats, or because of a dairy intolerance.

DAILY REQUIREMENTS

It's not only growing children who need calcium; here's what to aim for at various stages of life.

Women aged 19–50	1000 mg
Women over 50 (past menopause)	1300 mg
Pregnant women (last trimester)	1100 mg
Breastfeeding women	1000 mg
Men aged 19–70	1000 mg
Men over 70	1300 mg
Girls aged 12–18	1000–1300 mg
Boys aged 12–18	1000–1300 mg
Children aged 9–11	1000 mg
Children aged 4–8	700 mg

THE HEALTH BENEFITS

Calcium's role in the prevention of osteoporosis—the disease of thinning bones—and ensuring bone strength is undisputed. But this miracle mineral is proving to be valuable in a host of other health benefits as well.

OSTEOPOROSIS PREVENTION

The best protection against osteoporosis is to build strong healthy bones in the teen and early adult years, when peak bone mass is reached (the bones become less capable of storing calcium as you get older). Weight-bearing exercise such as walking, jogging, dancing and lifting things is also very important. Just as muscles become stronger when used, bones develop strength when muscles pull on the skeleton.

ALLEVIATING PMS

New research suggests premenstrual syndrome, or PMS, may be due to a disturbance in the body's calcium regulation. When a group of women were given a calcium supplement every day over a period of 3 months, they noticed significant improvements in their PMS symptoms such as irritability, depression and anxiety, particularly by their third cycle. What is not clear is if PMS is a sign of poor calcium status or if it interferes with calcium metabolism, so more research is needed to determine this. In the meantime, if you suffer the monthly blues it makes good sense to evaluate how much calcium you're getting and consider boosting your intake with either a better diet or a calcium supplement.

KIDNEY FUNCTION

Too much calcium in the diet was often blamed for the formation of kidney stones. Those unfortunate enough to suffer a kidney stone were often advised to adopt a low-calcium diet in the hope they would avoid another. Recently, evidence to the contrary has been mounting, and shows that diets high in calcium can actually protect us from kidney stones.

Oxalate, a compound found in foods like wholegrains, legumes, fruit and vegetables, plays a major part in the formation of kidney stones. Dietary calcium is able to attach to oxalate in the intestine and prevent it from being absorbed, hence reducing the chance of it reaching the kidney to cause mischief.

BLOOD PRESSURE BENEFITS

When researchers compare the diets of different populations, those containing the most calcium are linked to lower blood pressure. This remains true even when age, weight and alcohol intake—all factors that may affect blood pressure—are considered. The benefits of calcium appear to relate to how much you have in your diet; around 600–700 milligrams of calcium each day (just over half the recommended intake of 1000 milligrams) seems to give the most benefit to blood pressure.

Choosing dairy foods as your source of calcium also appears to have added benefits. The famous Dietary Approaches to Stop Hypertension (DASH) trial showed that by adding low-fat dairy foods to a diet high in fruit and vegetables, blood pressure could be reduced to the levels only previously achieved with medication.

COMBATING CANCER

The case for calcium as a protective nutrient against colon (bowel) cancer is growing. Research shows that a diet high in calcium is associated with not only a reduced colon cancer risk, but also improvement in the blood markers doctors use to gauge any future cancer development. Calcium is believed to reduce the risk of colon cancer by either binding to or neutralising potential cancer-causing compounds found in the bowel contents.

BEST FOOD SOURCES

Your best sources of calcium are milk, cheese and yoghurt. Without these three dairy foods in your diet, it is impossible to meet even the lowest requirement of 700 milligrams. Lactose, the natural sugar in milk, enhances the absorption of calcium, making milk not only one of the richest, but also one of the most readily available sources of calcium for your body.

Soy milk fortified with calcium (for example, So-Good, Vita Soy and CalciPlus) is a good substitute for milk for those unable to consume dairy products, as are other non-dairy alternatives like oat milk, rice milk and almond milk—providing they are fortified with calcium.

Smaller amounts of calcium are found in foods like sesame seeds, sardines and salmon (if you eat the small, softened bones), nuts, prawns, dark-green vegetables and figs. However, their calcium is not as well absorbed as that from milk due to the presence of oxalates (found in vegetables) and phytates (in bran and wholegrain cereals and breads). They can top up your intake but are not to be relied on as your sole calcium source.

MY TAKE

Remember, cream and butter might be dairy foods, but they are not good sources of calcium. I aim for three serves of calcium rich foods a day. This translates into having a glass of milk plus a carton of yoghurt and a wedge of cheese. Dark-green veggies, nuts and seeds top up my intake.

Tofu can be another reasonable source of calcium, depending on how it was processed. If set with calcium chloride or calcium sulphate, it has around 120 milligrams of calcium per 100 gram block. If not (as with soft and silken tofu), the calcium content is negligible.

ABSORBING CALCIUM—WHAT TO WATCH FOR

SALT

A diet high in salt can accelerate bone loss. Every 2000 milligrams of sodium removed by the kidneys in the urine (based on the average salt intake) takes with it 60 milligrams of calcium. Over 10 years, the job of eliminating this salt load from the body would remove 150–200 grams of bone calcium, an amount equal to 15 per cent of the skeleton.

More than 60 per cent of women consume less than the recommended dietary intake of calcium.

CAFFEINE

At high levels, this acts as a diuretic and flushes more calcium through the kidneys. It is wise to cut down your caffeine intake.

FIZZY OR CARBONATED DRINKS

These are associated with softer bones in teenagers. A Harvard University study reported that physically active teenage girls who drank soft drinks were five times more likely to have a fracture than active girls who didn't drink soft drinks.

ANTACIDS

Aluminium interferes with calcium absorption, so be wary of antacids containing this element.

VITAMIN D

Formed via a reaction of sunlight on the skin, this vitamin is essential for the absorption of calcium. Around 15–20 minutes of sun a couple of times a week is thought to be enough for us to generate our vitamin D. You'd think we get plenty in a country like Australia, but there's increasing recognition that significant numbers of the population do not get enough vitamin D. Elderly people in nursing homes who never venture outdoors and religious women who traditionally cover themselves from head to toe will need a food source of vitamin D. Vitamin D is found in cod-liver oil, oily fish, eggs, table margarine, butter and cheese. Alternatively, a calcium supplement containing vitamin D can be used.

MAGNESIUM AND POTASSIUM

These minerals can help preserve bone calcium. Potassium is believed to act in place of calcium to neutralise acids in the body. Magnesium helps transport potassium into bones, so it is able to carry out this task and contribute to the mineral content of the skeleton. Diets high in fruits and vegetables are rich in both of these minerals.

CALCIUM SUPPLEMENTS

Nutritionists agree it is best to obtain your calcium from food, where it is cheapest, safest and best absorbed. But supplements are useful if you do not eat calcium-rich dairy foods or are at risk of osteoporosis. Then you'll need to take two or three tablets, ideally spread over the day, in addition to calcium-fortified soy drinks or juices.

For the rest of us, calcium supplements can be used to top up our daily calcium needs, bridging the gap between what we get from food and what's recommended.

READ THE LABEL

Labels often list the quantity of the calcium compound such as calcium carbonate (the most common form of calcium), calcium gluconate, calcium orotate, calcium citrate or calcium amino acid chelate—and that's not the same as pure calcium, which is what our bodies need. A tablet with 1500 milligrams of calcium carbonate, for example, provides only 600 milligrams of the good stuff. Supplements containing calcium carbonate are absorbed better with food or immediately after eating, while those containing calcium citrate, calcium lactate or calcium gluconate are well absorbed and can be taken any time, with or without food.

Check how much elemental or pure calcium you are actually getting from each tablet. Make sure it's 200 milligrams or more, otherwise you're wasting your money. Also, make sure your supplement contains vitamin D, which plays a key role in calcium absorption. Without it, the calcium won't make it into your bones. So look for a combined supplement, with 5 milligrams of cholecalciferol (the chemical name for vitamin D) or vitamin D_3 (which it's sometimes referred to as), which is equivalent to 400 IU or 10 milligrams. Ideally, your supplement should also contain magnesium and potassium as both these minerals help build and preserve healthy bones.

Remember:

- ✔ It's recommended to take calcium supplements just before bed, as calcium uptake by bone peaks during the night.
- ✔ Effervescent tablets contain sodium bicarbonate and should not be taken by people on low-salt diets.
- ✔ If you also take iron supplements, take them at a different time from your calcium, as they can interfere with each other.

WHO NEEDS EXTRA?

You need to take a supplement if you think you're likely to get osteoporosis. This includes:

- ✔ Anyone with a family history of osteoporosis or bone fractures at an early age
- ✔ Those with a low body weight in their late teens and early twenties including models, ballet dancers, elite athletes and anorexia sufferers
- ✔ Women who have gone through menopause or are currently on hormone replacement therapy
- ✔ Anyone taking medications to halt osteoporosis.

DID YOU KNOW?

Contrary to popular belief, white spots on fingernails are not caused by a deficiency in calcium, or any other nutrient. White flecking is thought to occur where there's damage to the nail bed, and is a likely explanation for people who have jobs where their fingers are bumped and bruised.

Calories

In nutrition, the calorie (or the kilocalorie) is a unit used to measure the chemical energy in food and the mechanical energy expended by the body. In the metric system it has been replaced by the kilojoule.

See also Energy Measures.

Cancer and Diet

In Australia, cancer claims more than 40,000 lives each year and is the second leading cause of death after heart disease in both Australia and New Zealand. Statistics show that over the last 40 years it has been slowly on the increase.

The geographical distribution of types of cancer tumours and the changing patterns of cancer in migrants both point to nutrition as being a key factor in cancer development. Colon (bowel) cancer is a killer disease in all affluent countries including the US, Australia,

New Zealand and northern European nations, yet it is little-known in developing countries. High intakes of junk food are prime suspects, but there is also good research suggesting that a diet low in fibre and vegetables combined with high beer consumption is a contributing factor.

Cancer of the breast follows the same worldwide trend. A high-kilojoule, affluent diet from childhood onwards appears to alter the endocrine system, causing girls to menstruate earlier. Studies of women with breast cancer show that they tend to menstruate earlier than average. And women who are overweight are at greater than normal risk of breast cancer. Scientists now believe that large fat stores may produce an abnormal balance of hormones, which favours the growth of breast cancers.

Even within the same country, differences in cancer rates are apparent. In the US, religious groups such as Seventh Day Adventists and Mormons have much lower cancer rates—attributed in part to their high intake of vegetables and fruit and lower smoking levels. Australian researchers have compared the diets of native-born Australians with southern European migrants. People coming from Greece, Italy and Yugoslavia have low rates of cancer of the pancreas, bowel and rectum. Their high intake of fibre and antioxidants from vegetables, beans, bread and pasta and their low consumption of animal fats are two anti-cancer factors in their favour. They also drink little beer. By contrast, cancers of the pancreas, bowel and rectum are common in Australians. The researchers found that the longer the migrants lived in Australia, the more their cancer rates increased, approaching those of Anglo-Australians. After an average residence of 16 years (and the adoption of much of the diet and lifestyle of Australians), southern European migrants were suffering a similar level of cancer to Australians.

MAJOR CAUSES OF CANCER DEATHS

- Women—lung, breast, bowel.
- Men—lung, prostate, bowel.

The reverse pattern has occurred when natives of Japan, which has one of the world's highest rates of stomach cancer, migrate to the US, where this type of cancer is uncommon. In studies of successive generations of Japanese, the incidence of stomach cancer dropped from very high to very low, even though there was no intermarriage with Americans. Thus, the grandchildren of the original migrants end up with the same stomach cancer rate as Americans. Unfortunately, they also develop the higher American rates of bowel and breast cancer.

FOOD

There are at least four basic mechanisms by which food can influence the development of cancer. The most obvious occurs when a carcinogen (a cancer-causing substance) is present in food. One such example is aflatoxin, a poisonous compound produced on mouldy peanuts and grains such as maize. It is known to cause liver cancer in animals and has been correlated with human liver cancer in Africa.

Certain food components can activate the body's metabolism to produce substances that 'switch on' cancer development. Excess saturated fat stimulates the production of bile, which is needed to emulsify and digest it. The extra bile alters the bacteria that live in the bowel, causing them to produce carcinogens or promote the action of other cancer-causing substances.

Some food components can impede or enhance the delivery of carcinogens to their target organs. One of fibre's actions is to speed the transit of food through the digestive tract and this lessens the contact time with any carcinogen that's ingested and the inner lining of the bowel. And finally, food factors may alter the susceptibility of our body's cells to cancer.

WHAT YOU CAN DO

AVOID BECOMING OVERWEIGHT

Obesity raises the chances of hormone-dependent cancers of the breast, cervix, endometrium and prostate. So, limit consumption of energy-dense foods and be physically active every day.

CHOOSE THE GOOD FATS

Cut back on saturated and industrial trans fats. There is good evidence from both animal and human studies that excess consumption increases the risk of several cancers.

EAT MORE FRUIT AND VEGETABLES

Full of many antioxidants, studies show that people who eat lots of fruit and vegetables have a lower risk of cancer of the stomach, oesophagus and possibly others. Vegetables of the cruciferous or mustard family (broccoli, cabbage, cauliflower, turnip and horseradish) are especially helpful against bowel cancer. They contain sulphur compounds known as indoles and isothiocyanates, which can induce anti-cancer enzymes and block carcinogens.

CANCER AND FOOD ADDITIVES

Some additives have been banned because they caused cancer in animals (often only at very high doses). Others are thought to be protective through their actions as antioxidants or by reducing mycotoxins in food. Nature produces its own natural toxins or carcinogens in far greater numbers. For example, beetroot, lettuce, spinach and radish contain nitrates; potatoes contain alkaloids. The bottom line is both processed and fresh foods can contribute.

EAT MORE FIBRE

Fibre plays a key role in the prevention of cancer of the bowel and breast. Wheat bran in particular has been shown to be effective against bowel cancer, through its laxative effect and the production of fatty acids such as butyrate.

CUT BACK ON SMOKED AND CURED FOODS

Minimise salt-cured and smoked foods such as hot dogs, salamis, corned beef, sausages, bacon and ham. Such foods contain nitrates and nitrite compounds, which can form nitrosamines in the stomach. These are among the most potent agents of stomach cancer in animals. However, nitrites are also made naturally in the body by bacteria that inhabit the bowel, so it may be impossible to protect ourselves completely from exposure to them. The good news is that vitamin C inhibits their formation, protecting against stomach cancer.

DRINK ALCOHOL IN MODERATION

Alcohol, particularly if combined with smoking, is associated with cancers of the mouth, throat, oesophagus and rectum (especially for beer consumers). It is more harmful for women than men.

QUIT SMOKING

Approximately one in five deaths from cancer is due to smoking. Smoking causes a long list of cancers—lung (it's responsible for around 90 per cent of lung cancers), throat, mouth, nose, ovary, bowel, bladder, liver, pancreas, kidney, oesophagus, tongue, cervix, bone marrow and stomach. It is also important to avoid passive smoking by not breathing in other people's cigarette smoke.

MINIMISE BROWNED AND CHARRED FOODS

Cooking meat, chicken, fish and vegetables at high temperatures (over 150°C) can create potent end products called polynuclear aromatic hydrocarbons and heterocyclic amines. So, when grilling, barbecuing or toasting, do not produce over-done meat or burnt toast—this will cut the risk of colorectal cancer.

Candida and a Yeast-free Diet *See* Yeast.

Carbohydrates

After water, carbohydrate is the most widely consumed nutrient in the world. One of the three main macronutrients (protein and fat are the other two), carbohydrates come mainly from plants (cereal grains, fruits, vegetables and legumes). Milk and foods made from milk also contain carbohydrates in the form of milk sugar or lactose and yes, that includes breast milk.

Some plant foods contain large amounts of carbohydrates (rice, corn and potatoes), while others such as beans, broccoli and carrots have much smaller amounts. Foods rich in carbohydrates include:

- Cereal grains like barley, oats, quinoa, rice, rye, sweet corn (maize) and wheat—this includes foods made from these ingredients such as bread, breakfast cereals, pasta and noodles
- Starchy vegetables like potatoes, sweet potato, taro, yams and green peas
- Legumes (or pulses) like all dried or canned beans (kidney, black and cannellini), chickpeas, lentils and split peas
- Fruit (fresh, frozen, dried or juiced) including everyday favourites like apples and pears; stone fruits like apricots, nectarines, peaches and plums; citrus fruits like oranges and grapefruit; grapes; kiwi fruit; and tropical fruits like bananas and mangoes
- Dairy foods (from cows, sheep and goats) like milk, ice-cream and yoghurt.

Carbohydrates are classified into two major groups: starch and sugars. During digestion, starch and sugars are broken down into their simpler components, which are absorbed into the bloodstream to become glucose. Not all carbohydrates are digested and absorbed at the same rate. Slow-release (low-GI) carbohydrates from foods like pasta, kidney beans, All-Bran, traditional rolled oats, apples, pears, bananas, grapefruit, milk, yoghurt and grainy breads produce smaller fluctuations in your blood glucose and insulin levels. I talk more about this in the section on blood glucose (page 60).

STARCH

Starchy carbohydrate is the major carbohydrate component of cereal grains (and foods made from them, like bread and breakfast cereals), root vegetables, legumes and baked goods such as cakes and biscuits. Corn flour (wheat starch), arrowroot and tapioca are purified starches valued for their ability to thicken sauces. In uncooked foods like flour or raw grains, carbohydrates occur in tiny granules, which are insoluble in water. Before we can digest them, the foods must be cooked or processed, which causes the granules to absorb water and swell, releasing their contents and permitting access for digestive enzymes.

SUGARS

Glucose—glucose is the form of carbohydrate that circulates in the bloodstream (called blood glucose or blood sugar) and is the primary fuel for our brain. It is found in sweet fruits such as berries, grapes and bananas and some vegetables like corn and sweet potato.

STARCH	% CARBOHYDRATE
Flour, white	73
Rice Bubbles, Corn Flakes	71–76
Cracker biscuits, crispbread	55–70
Flour, wholemeal	52
Scone, plain	51
Biscuits, plain sweet	49
Bread, white	45
Bread, wholemeal	38
Crumpet	38
Fruit loaf	36
Rice, white, cooked	28
Pasta, cooked	25
Cake, plain	22–34
Sweet corn	17
Potato, boiled	13
Sweet potato, boiled	13
Baked beans, kidney beans	11
Rolled oats, cooked	9
Banana	3–7
Pumpkin, boiled	3

SUGARS (includes added sugar, honey and naturally occurring sugars)	% CARBOHYDRATE
Sugar	100
Honey	82
Sultanas	76
Golden syrup	75
Boiled sweets	74
Jam	67
Dates, dried	66
Chocolate, milk	56
Apricot, dried	41
Chocolate biscuit	41
Fruitcake	40
Nutri-Grain cereal	35
Liqueur	28–32
Ice-cream	22
Biscuits, plain sweet	22
Banana	16
Grapes, white	15
Apple	12

Glucose sports drinks are easily absorbed by endurance athletes in need of quick fuel. Being only half as sweet as sucrose, they are often given to patients without producing nausea. However, there is no other advantage in using glucose over sucrose as a sweetener.

Fructose—also known as fruit sugar, fructose is found in ripe fruits, some vegetables and honey. It is 70 per cent sweeter than sucrose.

Sucrose—sucrose is a double sugar of one molecule each of glucose and fructose. It is familiar as white table sugar and is the main component of brown sugar, golden syrup, molasses and maple syrup, and also occurs in many fruits.

Lactose—also known as milk sugar, lactose is found in milk from humans, cows, goats, sheep, buffalo and other mammals.

Maltose—also known as malt sugar, maltose is produced when starch is broken down, or in the malting of barley or wheat grains.

NUTRITIONAL VALUE

Carbohydrates have one major function in the body: to provide energy to feed our brains and fuel our muscles. Although protein and fat can also be used to generate

Q

If I want to lose weight, should I eliminate all carbohydrates after 5 pm?

A

As yet there is no scientific evidence to support the 'carb curfew' theory. Cutting out carbs like potato, pasta or rice with dinner is simply a way of cutting down on kilojoules. That's all. So out of a total dinner intake of say 1200 kj for grilled steak, potato and a salad, you can knock off over 50 per cent if you cut out the potato. That's why you lose weight! But there's no point in eating an unbalanced meal—it only sets you up to snack the night away because you're still hungry. A steak or fish fillet with non-starchy vegetables is not a balanced meal. Add a small carbohydrate portion and you'll feel a lot more satisfied.

> **DID YOU KNOW?**
>
> No single food except breast milk can supply all the nutrients needed for health and growth. Most foods are a combination of several nutrients. Bread is often labelled a carbohydrate, yet the average loaf of bread contains about 45 per cent carbohydrate, 9 per cent protein, 2 per cent fat, 3 per cent fibre, 1 per cent vitamins and minerals and 40 per cent water.

energy, carbohydrates are preferred. In fact, the brain, nervous system and red blood cells must have a constant supply of carbohydrates (as glucose) to keep working. Carbohydrates (glucose) are also the primary fuel source for a growing foetus. And where would we be without carbohydrate foods to fill those hollow legs of active, growing children?

Carbohydrate foods also bring many essential nutrients into your daily diet including fibre and B vitamins (from grains), vitamin C and antioxidants (from fruit and vegetables). Unlike protein and vitamins, there are no precise recommendations for how much you should eat. In fact, intake varies enormously around the world, with the different levels still compatible with good health.

Compare the high-carb traditional Japanese rice- and noodle-based diet (where around 70 per cent of their kilojoules comes from carbs) with the almost carb-free fish and seal meat diets eaten by the Inuit living in Iceland—less than 10 per cent of their kilojoules comes from carbohydrates. These days, it's generally agreed that for most of us, a healthy intake can be anything ranging from 40 to 60 per cent of our total energy each day. How much carbohydrate you eat is ultimately up to what works for you. For most of us eating a Western diet, this is typically about 200 grams a day for women and 300 grams a day for men.

> **Q**
> **Are bread and potatoes fattening?**
> **A**
> No single food on its own can make you fat. Often what is eaten with the bread or potato—butter, peanut butter, sour cream or cheese—adds more kilojoules than the humble slice or spud itself. Carbohydrate-rich foods have often been blamed for weight problems, but the evidence points to sedentary lifestyles, eating out more frequently and too much of everything!

It's recommended to spread portions of carb-rich foods evenly over the day; 50–60 grams of carbohydrate at any one sitting is a good average for most of us. On your dinner plate, that's the equivalent of 1¼ cups of cooked pasta.

BLOOD GLUCOSE

Carbohydrate foods are the biggest determinants of your blood glucose (sugar) levels. If your blood glucose drops too low, you can feel dizzy, shaky and unable to concentrate. So carbs are critical for your mood and brainpower, as anyone who's been on the Atkins virtually zero-carb diet will testify.

The emphasis nowadays is more on carbohydrate quality. Choose the healthy and less-refined low-GI carbs that trickle glucose into the bloodstream, stabilise blood glucose and insulin levels, help keep you feeling fuller for longer and help you maintain a healthy weight.

The glycemic index (GI) is simply a dietary tool that's used to rate the glycemic character or quality of the carbohydrate in individual carb-rich foods like bread, breakfast cereal, rice, pasta and apples. Understanding the GI is fundamental to a healthy diet for people with diabetes or for those looking for healthy weight loss or peak sports performance.

LOW-CARB EATING

If you do want to cut back on carbs (and it's a very popular weight-loss strategy), my recommendation would be not to go lower than 120 grams of carbohydrate a day. Here's what this might look like.

FOOD GROUP	SERVES	EXAMPLES	CARBOHYDRATE (g)
Vegetables	5	1 starchy (1 medium potato or ½ cup peas) 4 leafy or non-starchy (broccoli, beans, lettuces, salad vegetables)	20 15
Fruit	2	1 pear ½ cup blueberries	20 10
Whole grains	3	1 small bowl muesli 1 slice grain bread ½ cup brown rice, cooked	15 15 15
Milk	1	1 glass, 250 ml	10
TOTAL	11		120

Sweets and sugary foods are extras—they are not necessary for good health but in small quantities they add flavour and enjoyment to other foods.

FIVE TIPS FOR HEALTHY CARB CHOICES

- Cut out the 'junk' (high-GI) carbs like soft drinks, lollies, chips, cakes and biscuits.
- Don't give up all bread; buy a solid grain bread or dense wholemeal or rye loaf and eat one or two slices a day to keep you full and stop you picking between meals.
- Swap your breakfast cereal for one made from oats (muesli or porridge) or whole wheat (wheat flake biscuits, wheat flakes) or bran (All-Bran, bran flakes)—the fibre will also keep your bowels in good order.
- At dinner the best choices are pasta or starchy vegetables like peas, lentils, chickpeas, sweet potato, carrots or corn—many types of potato and rice are fast digesting (high-GI) so keep portions modest, one medium potato or ½ cup of rice will balance out your meal nicely.
- Eat two pieces of whole fruit (or fruit salad) a day, and don't drink fruit juice that has had its fibre removed and is easy to over-consume.

See also Glycemic Index.

Carob

Carob powder comes from the dried, ground pods of the carob tree, an evergreen native to the Middle East. With its chocolate-like flavour, it is an obvious substitute for cocoa powder and is quite nutritious. It is lower in fat than cocoa powder and contains no caffeine or theobromine, the stimulants of cocoa. And it is far less bitter. Carob bars or blocks, however, are another matter. Even though they may be made with vegetable oil and honey or raw sugar, they end up having just as much fat and kilojoules as chocolate.

Carotenoids

This is a group of 500–600 naturally occurring compounds that give fruit and vegetables their yellow-orange colour and act as antioxidants. The best studied are beta-carotene, lycopene, lutein, zeaxanthin and beta-cryptoxanthin.

Carrageenan

A red seaweed (also known as Irish moss), carrageenan is most commonly found off the coast of Ireland. It may be eaten as a vegetable; however, it is best known for the gum extracted from it, which is used as a food thickener—additive code 407.

Carrots *See* Vegetables.

Cellulose

See also Fibre.

Cellulose is a component of insoluble dietary fibre that forms the structure of plants. Unlike grazing animals, humans can't digest it.

Cereals *See* Grains and Cereals.

Cheese

Cheese has to be the most convenient protein food around. I find it's a really handy stand-by in the fridge, whether I want a creamy ricotta on a grainy cracker for a quick snack, a grab-and-go tasty cheddar and salad sandwich for lunch, melted mozzarella over tomatoes on toast for a light meal on a cold day or a Greek salad with crumbled feta with my dinner. With more than 400 varieties to choose from, there's a cheese for every eating occasion. Add to that enormous variety cheese's absolute convenience factor, and it's easy to see why cheese consumption has been increasing steadily in Australia over the past 40 years. The average Australian currently consumes almost 250 grams of cheese each week.

NUTRITIONAL VALUE

Like me, you may find it useful to think of cheese as simply being a form of concentrated milk—a 40 gram wedge of cheddar (about two slices) has nearly the same food value as a small (250 millilitres) glass of milk, except for the extra salt. It has been made for thousands of years and is in fact one of the most effective ways of preserving milk. When milk sours either naturally or because acid ingredients are added, it forms the curds that are the basis for cheese.

Apart from carbohydrates (the lactose is lost in the watery whey that's left behind during the manufacturing process), cheese provides us with all the goodness of milk. All cheeses are good sources of protein, for example, but the actual amount varies depending on the variety. Some, such as cheddar cheese at 26 per cent protein, are up there with lean meat, while cottage cheese, at 16 per cent, is closer to eggs. Gram for gram, reduced-fat cheese will have more protein than the regular version. The protein (mostly casein) is of excellent value, supplying all the amino acids essential for our health.

Cheese is also one of our best sources of bone-building calcium in a form our bodies absorbs well. It's also an important source of riboflavin (a B vitamin we need for healthy skin and eyes), vitamin B_{12} (important for vegetarians) and, in full-fat cheeses, vitamins A and D. Here's how the numbers stack up: eating a 40 gram wedge of cheddar cheese a day can supply 23 per cent of your protein needs, 29 per cent of your calcium, 26 per cent of your vitamin D, and around 20 per cent of your vitamin B_{12}, riboflavin and vitamin A.

Cheese is also a tooth-friendly food. It appears that eating cheese reduces mouth acidity and helps maintain a pH level that is safe for teeth while its calcium and phosphorus help to toughen teeth by protecting the enamel from demineralisation and weakening the tooth surface.

MY TAKE
Keep trips to the specialty cheese counter for special occasions—most people will only need a small portion of a beautiful quality cheese to finish a meal served with crackers and fresh fruit or muscatels.

FAT, SALT AND PROCESSING

Sadly, with these valuable nutrients come very large amounts of fat (mostly saturated). Low-fat types like cottage cheese and ricotta have long been a mainstay of dieters and heart patients, but anything else from the cheese counter (apart from the reduced-fat types) can quickly blow your fat budget for the day. So, when a cheese platter is produced, remember that moderation really matters. It is all too easy to overdo it when it is so more-ish.

Salt can also be a worry with cheese, especially from high-salt options like parmesan, pecorino, stilton, gorgonzola and feta. Salt is essential to cheese manufacture and is difficult, if not impossible, to reduce significantly. It not only determines the flavour and texture of cheese but controls the ripening by suppressing the growth of undesirable micro-organisms. Mozzarella, Swiss, cottage and ricotta have relatively low salt contents (less than 1 per cent), but the flurry of salt-reduced cheddars that appeared on the market in the 1980s have now dwindled.

Much of the cheese sold in supermarkets is processed cheese. With its bland flavour and rubbery texture, it's a winner with most kids, and parents can be comforted by the knowledge that it compares well with natural cheddar for calcium and protein. Its significantly higher salt level is what worries nutritionists. Processed cheese is made by heating a blend of cheddars and emulsifiers until thickened, and is then pumped through filling machines to be packed into blocks or formed into slices, cheese sticks or shapes.

NUMBER CRUNCH

A wedge of cheddar cheese weighing 40 grams gives you 9 grams of protein, 12 grams of fat (of which 8 grams is saturated fat), 240 milligrams of sodium and 588 kilojoules.

Compare some of these popular cheeses (right) with milk and yoghurt for fat, protein and sodium.

CHEESE	FAT (g)	PROTEIN (g)	SODIUM (mg)
¼ cup reduced-fat cottage cheese	1	5	75
¼ cup cottage cheese	2	5	170
¼ cup ricotta	4	3	60
40 g reduced-fat cheddar	6	14	230
40 g goat's cheese	8	8	120
200 g tub plain yoghurt	8	11	145
2 tablespoons grated mozzarella	9	11	170
40 g cheddar	10	13	240
40 g edam	11	11	285
40 g processed cheddar cheese slices	11	8	695
2 processed cheddar cheese sticks	12	6	640
2 tablespoons grated parmesan	11	14	425
1 cup full-cream milk (250 ml)	11	8	118
40 g blue-vein	12	10	540
40 g camembert	12	8	240
40 g gouda	12	10	325
40 g Swiss	13	11	127
40 g regular cheddar	14	11	244

HOW MUCH IS A SERVE?

When nutritionists say a serving of cheese, they mean about 40 grams, which is equivalent to drinking a 250 millilitre cup of milk or eating a 200 gram tub of yoghurt in terms of the protein, fat and calcium; see the table on page 63:

- ✔ A wedge of cheddar cheese
- ✔ 2 slices of cheddar cheese
- ✔ 2 slices of processed cheese
- ✔ 2 cheese sticks
- ✔ 7 small cheese cubes
- ✔ 2 tablespoons grated mozzarella
- ✔ 2 tablespoons grated parmesan
- ✔ 5 cubes feta cheese
- ✔ ¼ cup ricotta or cottage cheese.

See also Allergies, Intolerances and Diet; Lactose Intolerance; Pasteurisation; Pregnancy and Breastfeeding.

Cheese consumption has been increasing steadily in Australia over the past 40 years. The average Australian currently consumes almost 250 g each week.

Chia *See* Grains and Cereals.

Chicken *See* Poultry.

Chilli

Around 25 per cent of the world's population gets a daily dose of chilli. It is eaten in many ways, ranging from harissa paste in Morocco and tomato-lime salsas in Mexico to fiery jungle curries in Thailand and bottled chilli sauce, a condiment which can give oomph to a stir-fry or noodle soup.

DID YOU KNOW?

Chillies are one of a number of oral irritants in our diet. Pepper, ginger, mustard and horseradish fall into the same category, but chilli is the strongest and most widely consumed.

NUTRITIONAL VALUE

Chillies pack a mighty punch in terms of nutrition. They have a strong concentration of vitamin C—around two or three times greater than citrus fruit—and are high in fibre and minerals such as potassium and some B vitamins. But the quantity consumed is usually fairly small, and the overall nutritional contribution in a meal ends up being minor (although for chilli aficionados, it may be significant). Red chillies are at a more mature stage of ripeness than green chillies, and offer plenty of beta-carotene, a prominent antioxidant and precursor to vitamin A. Dried chillies have less vitamin C than fresh or bottled, but are still rich in beta-carotene, other related carotenoids and minerals.

Chillies are known to raise the metabolic rate, one of the reasons why a curry often warms you up. This has been promoted as an advantage to dieters, as a body with a super-speed engine burns fuel faster. In any case, chilli and chilli sauces can certainly give pep to an otherwise bland diet meal.

Many chilli lovers swear they stimulate the secretion of saliva and gastric juices and act as a digestive aid. If used in large enough quantities, they also appear to have antibacterial qualities,

BEAT THE CHILLI BURN

If the going is too hot, eat a yoghurt–cucumber mix or drink milk like the Indian yoghurt drink *lassi*. These will coat the mouth with a layer of fat and dilute the chilli. Capsaicin is fat-soluble, so drinking water or sucking on ice doesn't help, as it doesn't dissolve the irritant.

which are valued in hot climates where refrigeration is often absent. And all of this for almost no kilojoules! Ointments and lotions with capsaicin have also had success as an external remedy for nerve pain and itching. Capsaicin blocks substance P, which is part of the body's pain and inflammation chemistry.

Chocolate

Chocolate is the world's favourite flavour of ice-cream, cake, sweet sauces and milk shakes—those who say they don't like it are few and far between! Each new study on the alleged benefits of chocolate's antioxidants is greeted with glee (and headlines), and gives chocoholics and health-conscious consumers the green light to indulge.

ANTIOXIDANT BENEFITS

Cocoa and dark chocolate have been found to be abundant in flavonols or polyphenols, which is the general term for this whole class of related antioxidants, including those found in tea and red wine. These cocoa flavonols are platelet inhibitors, which research now shows have a mild anti-coagulation and anti-inflammatory effect. They can also keep arteries elastic, lower blood pressure, prevent cholesterol from being oxidised and even help prevent cancer. But it's still early days in the research department and not all chocolate is created equal. This research applies to dark chocolate, where the level of cocoa solids is high, over 70 per cent. Milk chocolate has much less, and the milk may actually interfere with the absorption of the antioxidants into the body. White chocolate contains none at all. Some manufacturers have modified their dark chocolate with slightly lower cocoa solids to create a less-bitter taste, but retain the high level of important flavonoids.

MAKING CHOCOLATE

Chocolate is made by roasting and husking cocoa beans, which are then crushed into small pieces called nibs. Rollers grind the nibs to a fine paste, which melts the cocoa butter—the natural fat of cocoa beans—producing a thick, dark aromatic liquid known as cocoa liquor or paste. To make cocoa powder (drinking chocolate), some of the cocoa butter is extracted, leaving hard, dark cakes of cocoa that are ground to become cocoa powder. To make solid chocolate, the cocoa liquor is combined with extra cocoa butter, sugar and sometimes flavouring such as vanilla, and emulsifier (usually lecithin), then blended and smoothed in a process called conching.

NOT A GUILTLESS SWEET

Antioxidants aside, chocolate remains a rich, high-fat and high-sugar concentrated food that packs a lot of kilojoules into a small piece. This is great for hikers on long treks in need of a small, energy-dense snack, but for most of us, consumption should be limited. The average 50 gram bar of chocolate supplies 1100 kilojoules, which is twice as much as you get from 50 grams of steak (410 kilojoules) or even 50 grams of fried potato chips at 500 kilojoules. That 50 gram bar slaps on 15 grams of fat plus 25 grams of sugar. The good news is that, even though the fat is mainly saturated, much of the saturated fat is in the form of stearic acid, which has little effect on blood cholesterol. So even if you are following a heart-healthy diet, you can still happily eat a piece—in moderation of course.

But however much you'd love to hear it, chocolate does not qualify as a superfood alongside vegetables, fruit and wholegrains. It's a treat food to be had in very small doses. And small means small—about 20 grams (three small squares) a day is the limit to maintain a healthy diet.

WHAT CHOCOLATE IS THAT?

LIGHT CHOCOLATE

There are four ways chocolate manufacturers can 'lighten' a bar of chocolate, and some give a nicer result than others. It could be aerated or whipped while it's still warm so tiny bubbles of air are trapped inside to produce a less dense bar with fewer kilojoules. It could be filled with a light centre like Turkish delight, nougat or mousse. The sugar or fat may be replaced with polydextrose or another bulking agent, and isomalt or sucralose that add fewer kilojoules (this is how Cadbury Lite does it), or it may be packed in a smaller size so you eat less weight.

All these ways allow you to get that lovely chocolate taste and save on fat and sugar. But ask yourself whether the trade-down is worth it—I have to admit, I'd rather eat a little of the real thing than lots of a light substitute. By focusing on the food and savouring it slowly, you will feel satisfied.

DARK CHOCOLATE

Dark chocolate contains cocoa liquor, sugar, cocoa butter, flavouring and emulsifier. Although it tastes semi-sweet, it actually contains more sugar than milk chocolate, as extra is needed to mask the bitterness of the cocoa bean. It's been largely used for cooking and baking until the recent interest in antioxidants, which has seen many health-conscious people start eating it. It is labelled with its percentage of cocoa solids ranging from 40 to 80 per cent. The higher the percentage, the greater the concentration of cocoa and more bitter the taste.

The average 50 g bar of chocolate supplies 1100 kJ, which is twice as much as you get from 50 g of steak (410 kJ) or even 50 g of fried potato chips at 500 kJ. That 50 g bar slaps on 15 g of fat plus 25 g sugar.

MILK CHOCOLATE

This is primarily an eating chocolate and tastes milder than dark chocolate due to the addition of around 25 per cent milk solids (or milk powder).

WHITE CHOCOLATE

White chocolate does not contain cocoa liquor and is not regarded as 'true' chocolate by many people. Those who suffer migraine headaches as a result of eating chocolate can often eat white chocolate without any problems, as the active component stays with the cocoa liquor. The fat and kilojoules content is similar to that in milk chocolate.

CARBOHYDRATE-MODIFIED CHOCOLATE (OR DIABETIC CHOCOLATE)

This is made with sorbitol or mannitol (sugar-related compounds) instead of sugar. Unfortunately it still has the same number of kilojoules as ordinary chocolate, so is of no real benefit to the majority of diabetics who need to lose weight. Its taste is very much inferior to the real thing.

Cholesterol and Diet

Cholesterol is not fat—it's a waxy substance made by all animals. It's a necessary part of the structure of cell membranes and is used to synthesise our sex hormones, adrenal hormones, vitamin D and bile acids. About three-quarters of the body's cholesterol is produced by the body; only one-quarter comes from cholesterol in food.

Cholesterol from food does not automatically become cholesterol in your blood. Eating large amounts of cholesterol (say from eggs) does not raise the blood cholesterol level of healthy people. When there is an abundance of food cholesterol, the body makes less from its own resources or gets rid of more. Conversely, eliminating cholesterol-rich foods such as egg yolk, liver, kidney and shellfish produces a fall of only 10 per cent in blood cholesterol levels, which is too small to be effective.

Blood cholesterol is raised by too much saturated fat and by being overweight. Fat people either convert too much fat into blood cholesterol or do not excrete enough cholesterol. High blood cholesterol is one of the main risk factors for heart disease, along with smoking, high blood pressure, carrying excess weight, family history and a sedentary lifestyle. So it pays to have your doctor check your cholesterol regularly (particularly if you're over 50) and help you look at ways to keep it down.

High cholesterol is usually defined as over 5.5 millimoles per litre (mmol/L). However, if you already have heart problems or have one or more risk factors, your doctor may prefer to keep it lower at 4.5 mmol/L or less. You need to discuss any blood tests with your doctor to work out the best course of action for you.

KNOW YOUR CHOLESTEROL

In the bloodstream, cholesterol is carried as particles called lipoprotein cholesterol. The two critical ones are 'high' or 'low' due to their density and composition. It's the ratio of HDL to LDL that you need to worry about, not just the level of total cholesterol.

HIGH-DENSITY LIPOPROTEIN CHOLESTEROL (HDL)

The 'good' cholesterol, HDL appears to protect against heart disease. It clears cholesterol from the arteries and removes it from the body.

LOW-DENSITY LIPOPROTEIN CHOLESTEROL (LDL)

The 'bad' cholesterol, LDL is correlated with heart disease and contributes to the fatty build-up on artery walls.

HOW TO LOWER YOUR CHOLESTEROL

Here are my top tips in order of priority—the most important steps are at the top.

Maintain a healthy weight—often just losing some excess weight will automatically bring your cholesterol and blood pressure down.

CHOLESTEROL CONTROVERSY

EGGS

Egg yolks were once limited to two a week on a cholesterol-lowering diet, along with other foods like liver, kidney, brains, prawns and calamari (squid). However, recent research has found that the number of eggs eaten doesn't significantly raise cholesterol—the real culprits are saturated and trans fats, as well as being overweight. Now you can happily eat six eggs a week as long as you don't drown them in butter or rich sauces. Pan cook them in a little olive oil or simply poach or soft boil. Enjoy!

GRAPE SEED OIL

Not all fats are equal. Nut and seed oils give us healthy fats that actually help keep cholesterol in check. Grape seed oil is rich in polyunsaturates (around 60 per cent), while macadamia and olive oil are rich in mono-unsaturated fats. The National Heart Foundation ranks these three oils equally in terms of their cholesterol-lowering ability. Some nutritionists believe diets higher in mono-unsaturated fats, like *The Mediterranean Diet*, are a better way to go. Keeping all three in your pantry will offer you variety in your cooking as well as doing your heart and blood vessels a favour.

A DAY ON A DIET TO LOWER BLOOD CHOLESTEROL

- BREAKFAST— Bowl of muesli, oat cereal or porridge with low-fat milk topped with a sliced banana or grated apple; tea, herbal tea or fruit juice.
- LUNCH—Large salad with tuna or salmon or lean meat or barbecued chicken with an oil-vinegar dressing and sprinkled with nut-seed mix; 1–2 slices grain bread or crispbread or rice salad or a sandwich made with any of the above; fresh pear or apple; mineral water.
- DINNER—Vegetable or bean soup; char-grilled salmon cutlet or ocean trout fillet or vegetarian dish made with beans or nutmeat; baked potatoes in their jacket; broccoli, carrots and beans with sterol spread; low-fat dessert like yoghurt with fruit, stewed fruit and custard, reduced-fat ice cream or baked apple; glass of red wine (if you wish).
- SNACKS—Handful of mixed nuts, nut and fruit bar, low-fat yoghurt or toasted, thick fruit loaf with sterol spread.

Steer clear of saturated and trans fats—these are the 'bad' fats that raise cholesterol. You'll find them in fried fast foods, salty snack foods, commercial pies, pastries and biscuits, chips, fries, doughnuts, fatty meat and deli meats like salami, bacon and sausages.

Eat small quantities of 'good' fats, which are mono-unsaturated and polyunsaturated—these are found in oils, soft spreads/margarines, nuts, seeds and avocado. Allow 1–2 tablespoons of oil for cooking and salads plus 1 tablespoon of spread/ margarine a day.

Eat three serves of sterol-enriched foods each day—such as Logicol or Pro-activ spreads.

Eat a handful of unsalted nuts (30–50 grams) a day.

Eat plenty of soluble forms of fibre such as pectins, gums, beta-glucans and saponins—these can speed up the removal of cholesterol via the bowel. Soluble fibre is found in oats, oat bran, barley bran, rice bran (not wheat bran), dried beans, lentils, barley, fruit and vegetables.

Eat generous serves of vegetables and fruits for their antioxidants—red wine, tea and dark chocolate also add antioxidants, but you don't need lots of these; one or two serves is OK.

Buy wholegrains whenever you can—shop for grainy bread, muesli, oat cereals, cereals marked wholegrain and brown rice.

Keep active—regular moderate exercise is essential for a healthy heart. It burns up kilojoules and can boost the levels of protective HDL cholesterol in the blood. Avoid sudden or over-exertive exercise that can strain an unfit heart.

EVERY DAY YOU MUST HAVE:

- ✔ 1 tablespoon oil (olive, rice bran, canola, flaxseed, sunflower or maize)
- ✔ 3 teaspoons sterol spread (Logicol, Pro-activ)
- ✔ 2 cups low-fat milk
- ✔ 5 or more serves of vegetables and salads
- ✔ 1–2 pieces fruit.

See also Sterol.

Choline

This is a vitamin-like compound made in your body, which can, at times, also be supplied by your diet. It functions as a component of the neurotransmitter acetylcholine and of lecithin, important in fat and bile metabolism. The Adequate Intake (AI) for choline is 550 milligrams per day for men and 425 milligrams for women (lower values are recommended for children and higher values are required by pregnant or lactating women). A balanced diet contains twice the amount of choline recommended, so supplements are rarely needed. Excellent sources of choline include eggs, wheatgerm and liver. Soy beans, peanuts, cabbage and cauliflower also have some. Excessive choline consumption can result in side effects like a fishy body odour and intestinal upsets.

Chromium See Minerals.

Cinnamon Cassia

I love cinnamon for its aroma and flavour, but now research has revealed that one kind of cinnamon, cinnamon cassia, may help lower blood glucose levels in people with diabetes. In recent years, lab research has suggested that cinnamon cassia, which contains around 5 per cent of coumarin, a polyphenol that is the starter compound for the blood thinner Warfarin ('true' cinnamon doesn't contain coumarin), may make body cells more sensitive to insulin. Small studies in healthy people and people with diabetes have also shown that this type of cinnamon (usually given in supplement form) can reduce the rise of blood glucose after eating. But the jury is still out—some results have been promising while others have found no benefit on either glycated haemoglobin or fasting blood glucose. What's needed are a couple of well-planned, well-controlled, long-term clinical trials.

In the meantime, be generous with the cinnamon in your desserts such as creamy rice, baked custard, apple crumble, apple strudel and stewed pears. Sprinkle it over your breakfast porridge instead of sugar. It may help, and there's no downside.

Cinnamon is probably not the only spice with such good news. Other spices like cloves and nutmeg may well turn out to have similar benefits. We already know that most spices are extremely rich in nutrients such as beta-carotene, certain B vitamins and natural antioxidants, but the tiny amounts used in cooking are not usually significant sources of nutrition. If you use them, be generous in how much you use.

CINNAMON AND CINNAMON CASSIA

According to spice expert Ian (Herbie) Hemphill, 'true' cinnamon (*Cinnamomum zeylanicum*) is a very thin under-layer of bark from a quite young piece of branch, while 'cassia' cinnamon (*C. cassia*) is the complete thickness of the bark from the fully grown tree. There are some significant differences in aroma and use. The aroma of cinnamon is delicate, sweet and subtle, and it's virtually impossible to use too much in your cooking. Cassia, on the other hand, has a highly fragrant cinnamon aroma when it is ground, but you need to use it in moderation; too much spoils the flavour and even a few extra grams in some dishes might be rather unpalatable.

Citrus Fruit

There are many good reasons to eat an orange, grapefruit, mandarin, tangelo, pomelo, lemon or lime every day. As a group, citrus fruit stands head and shoulders above other fruit. I find navel oranges are the ideal eating orange, but you may like to try exotic citrus types such as the Minneola tangelo (a cross between a mandarin and grapefruit), blood oranges and the lemonade lemon.

NUTRITIONAL VALUE

Not only are citrus fruits full of vitamin C but they are valuable for folate (a B vitamin that can prevent birth defects), beta-carotene, a number of phyto-chemicals such as carotenoids and flavonoids, plus the soluble type of fibre which helps to lower cholesterol. One orange is estimated to have nearly twice the recommended intake for vitamin C, 18 per cent of the intake for folic acid and 8 per cent of the fibre. They are also low in fat and kilojoules.

If you want to maximise the fibre, eat whole citrus fruit rather than drink the juice. It takes about three oranges to make one glass of orange juice, but you will miss out on the fibre, which is left behind with the pulp.

Citrus fruits, particularly oranges, offer plenty of the mineral potassium and are low in sodium. They also contain small amounts of calcium, thiamin, niacin, vitamin B_6, phosphorus, magnesium, copper, riboflavin and pantothenic acid.

Citrus fruits contain a large range of bioactive phytochemicals. For example, an orange has more than 170 different phytochemicals and more than 60 flavonoids, many of which have been shown not only to have antioxidant effects but also to contain anti-inflammatory, anti-tumour and blood clot–inhibiting properties.

The best-studied phytochemicals are hesperidin, naringin and limonene, which are responsible for citrus' sharp taste. Of the flavonoids, there are coumarins (shown to have anti-cancer properties in experimental studies), mono-terpenes, tri-terpenes and phenolic acids. Liminoids are the most abundant of the terpenes, a major phytochemical class in citrus, which stimulates a detoxifying enzyme system and inhibits tumour formation.

NUMBER CRUNCH

One orange weighing 200 grams gives us 1 gram of protein, a trace of fat, 13 grams of sugars, no starch, 4 grams of fibre and 285 kilojoules.

BE ZESTY

Don't overlook the rind or zest. Both the rind (zest) and juice contain the flavonoid limonene, an antioxidant that's showing promise as an anti-cancer agent. There's also new research from the US that shows the rind has the potential to lower cholesterol. Regardless of whether or not this ends up being proven, it's another good reason to add grated lemon rind to muffins, grilled fish, steamed green beans and chicken dishes.

EASY WAYS TO ENJOY CITRUS

- ✔ Coat pork or chicken fillets with grated orange rind, orange juice, garlic and Dijon mustard before cooking.
- ✔ Start your day with a freshly squeezed grapefruit juice or a grapefruit simply cut into quarters.
- ✔ Add a slice of lemon or orange to iced water for a subtle refreshing flavour (you'll drink more water too).
- ✔ Lemon and honey in hot water can make a soothing and relaxing tea before bed.
- ✔ Chop citrus segments into salads.
- ✔ Use orange, lemon, lime or grapefruit juice to make a dressing with olive oil, Dijon mustard and black pepper. This is great over chicken or rice salads with added orange segments.

Clear Fluid Diet *See* Diarrhoea.

Cocoa

Cocoa (or cacao) is the dried and fermented oily seed of *Theobroma cacao*, from which cocoa solids and cocoa butter are extracted. They are the basis of chocolate. Cocoa can also refer to dry cocoa powder, which is made by grinding cocoa seeds and removing the cocoa butter, creating bitter cocoa solids.

Cocoa powder contains high levels of flavonoids, specifically flavanols, which may have beneficial cardiovascular effects on health. This mainly applies to raw cocoa and, to a lesser extent, dark chocolate, since flavonoids degrade during chocolate manufacture. Cocoa is relatively low in fat compared with chocolate, and delivers an intense flavour to cakes, desserts and drinks.

Cocoa and chocolate are common Fairtrade commodities. This means they are grown sustainably and farmers and workers in the developing world operate in decent working conditions with guaranteed prices and fair terms of trade.

Co Enzyme Q

This is a substance also known as ubiquinol, which is found in most foods, particularly fish, red meat and oils. It can be synthesised in the body, is needed for oxygen production by cells and is essential for mitochondria, which converts fuel into energy. It works in synergy with vitamin E to keep LDL cholesterol from being oxidised. It is often promoted as a supplement for heart health.

Coeliac Disease and Diet

Coeliac [seel-ee-ack] disease is the result of a permanent intolerance to gluten, and affects around 1 per cent of the population. If left untreated, it damages the delicate inner lining of the bowel, preventing food from being digested and absorbed properly. This can result in malnutrition, iron deficiency and an increased risk of other diseases including lymphoma and osteoporosis. Symptoms most often reported are those relating to an 'irritable bowel'—bloating and tummy pain, diarrhoea, weight loss, vomiting and fatigue. However, some people show no symptoms at all.

Thanks to better screening, coeliac disease is being increasingly diagnosed so these days it is more common than in the past. The same dietary treatment is needed for anyone who suffers from dermatitis herpetiformis (commonly referred to as coeliac skin).

New research in Australia suggests that for around 15 per cent of the general population, gluten may also trigger gut symptoms such as bloating, wind and pain, as well as fatigue in people who do not have coeliac disease. In addition, there is a whole range of people who don't have the condition but want to avoid gluten, believing that it causes digestive upsets, wind, bloating and loose motions. Both groups are primarily responsible for the rise in gluten-free products, representing a huge new market. The downside can be a restrictive gluten-free diet, which is hard to follow, and lacking in good nutrition.

Diagnosing coeliac disease

If you have one or more of the signs or symptoms I have mentioned, see your doctor for a check-up. The only way to diagnose coeliac disease is with a blood test and small intestinal biopsy, and gluten must be present in your diet in order for these tests to be accurate. Starting on a gluten-free diet before the test could easily result in being misdiagnosed. If you do have coeliac disease, following a strict gluten-free diet for life is critical and must be followed very carefully.

FOODS TO AVOID

Gluten is part of a protein found in wheat, rye, barley and triticale (a cereal which is a cross between wheat and rye). When mixed with water, gluten forms an elastic-like substance, which expands when a dough rises.

Gluten is common in many foods including flour, bread, cereals, pasta, cakes, biscuits and porridge—all of which are basic foods in our daily diet and quite difficult to avoid. Even small quantities of flour or starch thickeners in commercial foods can be a problem and must be checked.

Rice and corn (maize) are gluten-free and should be substituted for gluten-containing grains wherever possible.

SHOPPING FOR GLUTEN-FREE FOODS

The presence of gluten in any food ingredient or component of an ingredient (including additives) must now be declared on the label, no matter how small the amount. Foods labelled as 'gluten free' must not contain any detectable gluten (less than 0.003 per cent). Foods labelled as 'low gluten' must not contain more than 0.02 per cent gluten.

It's still wise to double-check labels for ingredients that could be sources of gluten. These include wheatmeal, bran, semolina, malt and cereal filler.

It's also important to check the ingredient list for additives like starch or thickener (additive code numbers ranging from 1400 to 1450). Many manufacturers have moved to thickeners derived from maize or potato. If it doesn't tell you, there should be a warning 'contains gluten' on the label. Some people can also react to the flavour enhancers 620–625 and the enzyme or flour treatment agent 1100.

AVOIDING DEFICIENCY PROBLEMS ON A GLUTEN-FREE DIET

Avoiding most grains can leave you short on fibre and some of the B vitamins. So try to include brown rice, rice bran or psyllium in your diet and make sure you eat plenty of vegetables and fruit. Talk to your doctor about a calcium or iron supplement, particularly if you have had diarrhoea for some time.

See also **Gluten.**

Coffee and Coffee Substitutes

Like many people, I enjoy the odd cappuccino—that aroma and adrenalin hit is just wonderful. Plus with café society booming, sharing a latte or short black is a great way to catch up with friends or colleagues, especially when you're pressed for time. Coffee was first prepared in Arabia and Ethiopia around 1000 AD in the same way it is today—roasted, ground and then brewed. The practice of drinking coffee spread to Europe in the 1500s, and coffee houses (or cafés in France) were established in the late 1600s.

Despite the many different blends available, coffee beans can be divided into two types. Arabica beans have a rich flavour and less caffeine, but are more difficult to grow and are therefore more expensive. They are grown mainly in Indonesia, East Africa and South America. Robusta beans, as the name suggests, come from tougher plants with greater resistance to pests and diseases and are faster-fruiting. However, they produce less flavour and aroma than Arabica beans, and are more bitter. They are grown mainly in Africa.

Most coffees are blends of several beans from different regions and it is the skill of blending that produces characteristics like body, aroma, acidity and colour.

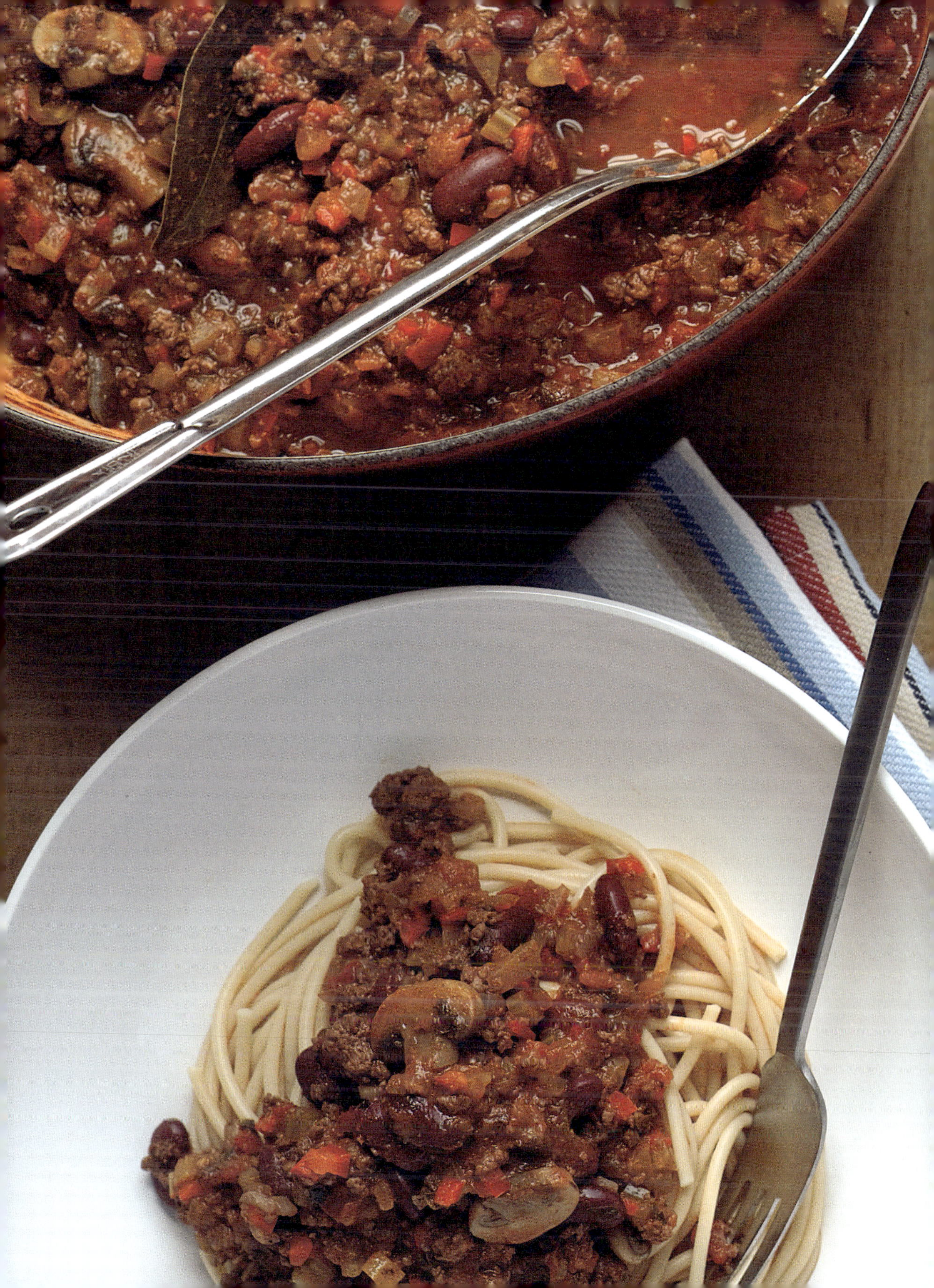

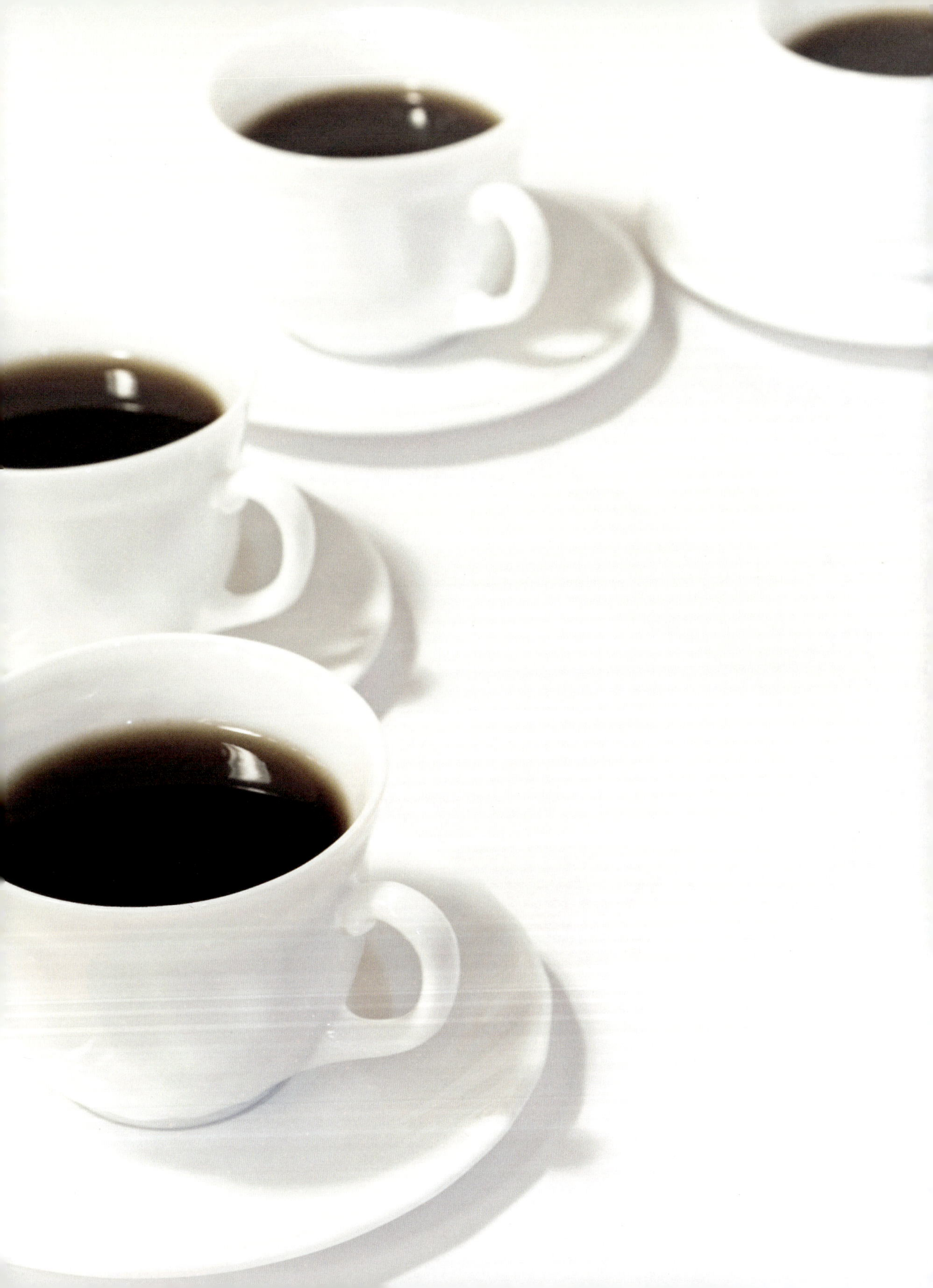

COFFEE AND YOUR HEALTH

While the general consensus is that coffee in moderation does not cause health problems, there are a few issues that crop up. Research from the Netherlands points to unfiltered brews as a problem. Studies revealed that unfiltered European-style coffees such as Turkish, Greek and plunger coffee (French press) are rich in sediment and can send cholesterol levels soaring. Any type of coffee that is prepared without a filter may carry substances called diterpenes, which are found in oil droplets and fragments of beans floating in the coffee. These are the culprits that can raise cholesterol.

The Dutch researchers concluded that drinking 5 cups a day could send cholesterol up by 1 millimole per litre, which is significant when the ideal level is 5.5 millimole per litre or less. Espresso coffee has a similar, though smaller, effect. Drip-filtered coffee made with a paper filter and percolated coffee contains negligible amounts of diterpenes and so poses no problem.

Too much caffeine can also be a problem if you over-indulge. It can leave you feeling sleepless and jittery, and with an upset stomach. Limit yourself to no more than two 'real' coffees (such as a cappuccino or short black made from espresso), or four instant coffees each day.

The good news is research suggests that coffee in moderation may help prevent type 2 diabetes, Parkinson's disease and liver disease (cirrhosis). Researchers are still not entirely sure how, but it seems that the weight-loss properties of coffee may be the key—coffee can reduce glucose concentration, increase insulin sensitivity and slow the absorption of glucose in the intestine. There is less evidence on the health benefits of the antioxidants in coffee compared with those in tea.

WHAT COFFEE IS THAT?

ESPRESSO (SHORT BLACK)

This is a strong brew of a shot (30 millilitres) extracted in 25–30 seconds. A well-made espresso is characterised by a dark, golden *crema*. Always drunk black, it is produced by forcing near-boiling water through ground coffee under pressure and is the basis of all other coffees.

CAFE MACCHIATO

A macchiato is a single shot of espresso with a dash of textured, creamy milk.

CAPPUCCINO

The most popular way to drink coffee in Australia, this is one-third espresso, one-third steamed milk, and one-third frothed milk, often with cinnamon or flaked chocolate sprinkled on top.

CAFFE LATTE

A single shot of espresso with three times the volume of steamed (not frothed) milk.

FLAT WHITE

This is ideal for those who enjoy the strength of the cappuccino but not the foam that goes with it. Served in a cup of around 160–180 millilitres capacity, it is one shot of espresso and steamed milk, with 1–2 centimetres of creamy milk on top.

MOCHA

An espresso with equal portions of chocolate powder and frothed milk, this is sweeter and not as intense in coffee flavour.

LONG BLACK (LUNGO)

A long black is an espresso shot pulled on top of a cup of boiling water.

RISTRETTO

Meaning 'restricted' in Italian, a ristretto is normally only the first 15 millilitres of extraction, and therefore restricted in the amount of coffee extracted to better capture the sweetest, most intense characters of the coffee. The term 'double ristretto' is capturing 30 millilitres of espresso, made up from two 15 millilitre shots.

DECAF

Decaffeinated coffee is made by removing the caffeine from green beans before roasting. One method uses a well-tested solvent, methylene chloride, but then the problem of how to remove all traces of the solvent remains. Another method, which is more expensive, is to use water to dissolve out the caffeine. Whichever way it is done, there is some loss of flavour and aroma. If you drink a milky coffee it's probably still pleasant, but coffee aficionados will not find it to their taste.

COFFEE SUBSTITUTES

Coffee substitutes such as dandelion tea, Caro, Ecco, Cafix and Pero are a useful drink for people who are affected by caffeine's over-stimulating effects. They are made from roasted malted grains like barley, wheat or rye, or from roasted chicory or root vegetables (e.g. dandelion, beetroots or carrot) with molasses or maltodextrin. The roasted ingredients are steeped and the liquor separated and concentrated under vacuum before drying. Some coffee substitutes are high in fibre. If you like your coffee weak with milk, I think you'll find them fine—but not if you love your espresso.

See also **Beverages; Caffeine.**

Colds, Flu and Diet

When the cold and flu season strikes, it often seems as if every second person has a sniffle, cough or runny nose. You won't be surprised to learn that the common cold accounts for more time lost from work and school over winter than any other complaint. Most of us suffer two or three colds a year, so it's worth knowing the best way to treat them.

If you are laid up with a cold, here's my best grandmotherly advice to help you get over it quickly.

REST

Go to bed! There's no point soldiering on. You're better off not going to work or school and spreading the virus around. Stay warm and get as much sleep as you can.

MEDICATE

Consider taking cold and flu tablets or paracetamol (check with your doctor first if you are currently taking other medicines, and don't mix paracetamol and cold and flu tablets without medical advice).

HYDRATE

Drink lots of fluids. Diluted juices, weak teas, clear soups and water are all valuable ways to hydrate when you're sick. There's interesting research proving what our mothers have known for a long time—soup is especially good; the hot liquid seems to liquefy the mucus and relieve stuffiness. It certainly won't hurt and you'll get minerals too.

MY TAKE

At the first sign of a sore throat or sniffle, try my old-fashioned lemon and honey drink—it really helps! Dissolve a spoon of honey in a little hot water and top it up with the juice of a freshly squeezed lemon. Stir, and enjoy!

VITAMIN C

A dose of 500 milligrams can help shorten the duration of a cold, although it can't prevent it entirely. Additionally, 10 milligrams of zinc and 1 gram of echinacea can also help. I prefer the powder to the tablets.

STEAM

Twice a day, do a steam inhalation over a sink or bowl of hot water, or a vaporiser with a few drops of tea tree or eucalyptus oil to clear the nasal passages. A warm saltwater gargle can help to remove phlegm. A teaspoon of 10+ manuka honey (antibacterial) can also help with a sore throat.

INFECTION CONTROL

Take some simple measures to reduce the likelihood of passing your bug on to other family members. Wash your hands regularly, especially before eating, and dispose of used tissues in a plastic bag.

SEEK MEDICAL HELP

If you're not better after four or five days, or if you're short of breath, see your doctor. You may need antibiotics or you could have pneumonia.

Colours

See Food Colours; Hyperactivity and Diet; Additives.

Confectionery

Sweeties, lollies, cough lollies, candy—whatever you call them, confectionery is a huge group ranging from boiled sweets to chocolate, fudge, toffee, soft jellies, jubes, Turkish delight, nougat, coconut ice and liquorice.

Nutritionally, confectionery is a no-no, being largely made from sugar with added colours and flavours. It contains no vitamins, minerals or protein, but is very high in sugar. Along with the heat of manufacture and the low water content, the sugar acts as a preserving agent, which is why they keep so well without any refrigeration. It's often sugar in chewy, sticky form that clings to the teeth or bathes the tooth enamel, which provides a food source for the bacteria that live in our mouth to ferment to acid. It's little wonder that lollies are often banned by dentists!

'Natural' or not, a 50 g serve (about six snakes) still packs in 710 kJ and 39 g of carbohydrates (all sugars).

Apart from chocolate and fudge or caramels, most confectionery has little fat—a quality often featured on packaging as '97 per cent fat-free'. So if you're craving something sweet, but don't want the kilojoules of chocolate, reach for a jube or mint as it will be much lower in kilojoules.

MY TAKE

Sweets have long been used as rewards. How many of us recall receiving a jellybean for being well behaved or putting up with a needle at the doctor's? This reward system really goes into overdrive when it comes to fundraising. But it's something that makes my blood boil, as it's a no-win deal for your family's health. If you are organising a fundraiser try using some of these practical products instead:

- ✔ *Small tube or roll-on bottle of SPF30+ sun cream*
- ✔ *Apple slinky machine*
- ✔ *Filtered, portable water bottles*
- ✔ *Iron-on name labels.*

'NATURAL' CONFECTIONERY

Sales of natural jellies, snakes and fruit jubes made with no artificial colours, flavours or preservatives are booming. Parents feel they're doing something right by buying lollies made red with natural anthocyanins instead of the more suspicious azorubine (additive 122) or Allura Red AC (additive 129). Yellow and orange hues are derived from turmeric or paprika rather than tartrazine (additive 102). Purple tones are extracted from grape or elderberry, not Brilliant Blue FCF (additive 133).

Yet whether it's Allen's (owned by Nestlé) or the Natural Confectionery Company (owned by Cadbury-Schweppes), you'll consume the same kilojoules and sugar per lolly. Natural or not, a 50 gram serve (about six snakes) still packs in 710 kilojoules and 39 grams of carbohydrates (all sugars), although there's less than a gram of fat.

COMPARE

Regular snakes

INGREDIENTS: GLUCOSE SYRUP, SUGAR, GELATINE, THICKENER FROM WHEAT (1420), FOOD ACID (CITRIC ACID), FLAVOURS, COLOURS (102, 110, 122, 123, 133).

Natural Snakes

INGREDIENTS: GLUCOSE SYRUP, SUGAR, GELATINE, WHEAT STARCH, FOOD ACID (CITRIC ACID), NATURAL FLAVOURS INCLUDING ORANGE ESSENTIAL OIL, FRUIT JUICE CONCENTRATE, NATURAL FOOD COLOURS (TURMERIC, ANTHOCYANINS, PAPRIKA OLEORESIN, GRAPE SKIN EXTRACT).

Constipation and Laxatives

Constipation is a common problem—almost one in five people over the age of 30 has constipation at some stage during their life. Straining to pass small, hard stools causes a build-up of muscular pressure in the bowel. Eventually, constant pressure causes weak spots or 'blow-outs' in the wall, which can become inflamed and painful. This is how haemorrhoids and diverticular disease develop.

Many people rely on laxatives in the form of powders, granules, tablets, syrups or suppositories. Apart from the expense, laxatives (whether bulking agents, stool softeners, osmotic agents or stimulants) can become habitual and may even be harmful over a long period of time. I recommend you forget laxatives, and get your system regular with a high-fibre diet. A bowel motion each day is not essential (every second day is fine), but it is important that your stools are soft and easy to pass. Straining to pass a bowel motion should be avoided—aim for a soft consistency rather than regularity! Check the Bristol Stool Chart online for details.

Fibre offers the safest, simplest solution to relieve constipation. It increases the bulk of the stool, giving the faeces the correct soft consistency so they can be eliminated without effort. Bowel motions are passed more easily and more frequently and it also helps you stay healthy in numerous other ways. It is also important for pregnant women to eat plenty of fibre as, due to hormonal changes, the bowel often becomes sluggish and less able to work. This is exacerbated if you take iron supplements.

BEAT CONSTIPATION

- ✔ Drink plenty of water each day. Fibre absorbs a lot of water (around 70 per cent of the weight of bowel motions is water).

- ✔ Substitute high-fibre meals and snacks for any low-fibre choices you now eat. The easiest foods to start with are breakfast cereals, bread and snacks like wholemeal crispbreads and fruit. Next, try to eat a meal with beans or lentils every second day.
- ✔ Forget fruit juice, which lacks the fibre of whole fruit. Instead drink water or weak tea and eat a piece of fresh fruit, preferably with the skin on.
- ✔ Regular exercise helps maintain bowel tone and internal muscles. Walking is all you need to do.
- ✔ Forget strict diets that often supply so little food that they induce constipation. Stick to eating low-fat, high-fibre foods and three balanced meals a day.
- ✔ Allow yourself enough time to relax when you need to pass a motion. Rushing and straining too hard increases the pressure in the blood vessels around your anus, setting the scene for haemorrhoids.
- ✔ Finally, if high-fibre eating and fibre supplements do not relieve your constipation, seek the advice of your doctor, especially during pregnancy when constipation is common, or in children. Do not prescribe laxatives yourself for more than a week—some are irritants and may damage the nerves of the bowel.

Cooking Techniques

The aim of healthy cooking is to retain the most vitamins and minerals, remove the saturated fat from meats and chicken and make recipes taste good without adding salt or sugar. However, no matter how careful you are, all forms of cooking deplete nutrients to some extent—heat inactivates three heat-sensitive vitamins (vitamin C, thiamin or vitamin B_1, and folate), while water leaches out minerals. The trick is to minimise the loss, and some cooking methods are better at this than others.

As a rule of thumb, the quicker the cooking time and the less water used, the more the nutrients will remain in the food. On the other hand, cooking improves the digestibility of fibre and proteins and also increases the availability of lycopene and other fat-soluble vitamins. Mineral levels such as zinc or magnesium are not affected by cooking.

Healthy cooking doesn't require you to become a gourmet chef or invest in expensive cookware. Here I've set out 12 basic cooking methods for preparing foods in healthy ways without adding excessive amounts of fat or salt.

STEAMING

Whether you opt for a double boiler or a foldable metal basket that fits into a pot, steaming ranks at the top of the cooking methods. It minimises loss of vitamins, cooks quickly and needs no fat. It's the ideal way to cook vegetables, much better than boiling, where nutrients are leached out into the cooking water. Steam ovens rate highly too. They inject steam into a cooking chamber and cook food quickly without discoloration or softening, while retaining good flavour.

MICROWAVING

Microwaving cooks the fastest and requires little or no water, and no salt. Forget the rumours about microwaves destroying the goodness in food. Like radio waves, microwaves are a form of electromagnetic energy. Microwave cooking works by vibrating the water molecules within the food so they heat up. It is as safe as cooking on a conventional stovetop.

COOKING WITH WINE

Wine, vermouth, sherry, madeira and port make wonderful marinades or sauces. They impart a mellow flavour and zest, and are evaporated during cooking. Just how much is removed will depend on cooking time—the longer you cook it and the higher the temperature, the greater the evaporation and the less alcohol retained in the final dish. If you add it towards the end of your cooking, the resulting dish will have a much higher alcohol content (in some cases as much as 85 per cent of the alcohol can remain) than if you add the alcohol at the beginning and heat it for an hour or so. If you want a substitute for alcohol, stock with garlic and chopped fresh herbs, soy sauce, or Worcestershire sauce can be used in savoury dishes. In sweet dishes use orange juice with grated orange zest, dark grape juice, apple juice or a light sugar syrup with a dash of bitters and good lime cordial.

It's best to use containers that have been specially designed for microwave heating or stick to glass, ceramic or paper. Don't use plastic containers that are high in polyvinyl chloride (PVC), such as margarine or ice-cream containers. The plastic molecules may pass into the food.

FAST BOILING

Short, rapid boiling is better than long simmering for vegetables. The more water and the longer the cooking time, the more nutrients you lose. Ideally bring the water to the boil first, then add your vegetables and cover the pan (this speeds up the cooking time).

STIR-FRYING

Stir-frying delivers a lot more heat than a conventional pan so your food cooks faster and doesn't stew in its own juices. Go for a non-stick surface so you don't have to use a lot of oil—you can even stir-fry with just a spray of oil or a little stock or water. Remember to dice or slice your ingredients to a uniform size so they cook at the same rate.

SAUTÉING

Frying in oil piles on the fat. In fact, half the kilojoules in a fried chicken breast come from the oil it is cooked in. Additionally, the high frying temperatures are quite destructive of nutrients. But sautéing (cooking quickly in a little oil and tossing frequently) is fine. Use a little oil, or brush or spray the pan first. A good tip is to warm the pan a little before adding the oil; this way it spreads better and you can use less.

POACHING

To poach foods, gently simmer ingredients in a liquid such as water, broth, wine or juice until they're cooked through and tender. The food retains its shape during cooking. For stovetop poaching, choose a covered pan that best fits the size and shape of the food. You want to just cover the food with the poaching liquid.

GRILLING

Grilling on a slotted tray or barbecue plate allows any fat to drip away from food and also creates its own flavour. An electric health grill is a great idea for quick steaks or melts when space is limited. Some grills cook from the top and bottom at the same time, so your meat cooks faster. You can use them for toasted sandwiches too.

BARBECUING

This high-heat method needs to be controlled so you minimise how much you char (burn) the food. When fat drips onto hot coals (or other source of heat), potentially dangerous compounds are then deposited on the food from the rising smoke and flame. If you use the barbecue hotplate, watch the amount of oil you add or you'll end up frying the food in fat, not barbecuing it.

ROASTING

Roasting uses dry heat at a high temperature to cook the food. For poultry and meat, make sure you place a rack inside the roasting pan so that the fat can drip away during cooking.

SLOW COOKERS

When the weather gets cold, it's time to bring out the electric slow cooker or a heavy-based casserole dish that you can leave on low in the oven or over a gentle heat. The direct heat from the pot, lengthy cooking and steam created within the tightly covered container combine to destroy bacteria and make the slow cooker a safe process for cooking foods. Always defrost meat or poultry completely before putting it into a slow cooker.

OVEN BAGS

These work like a mini-slow cooker so you steam your meat in an individually sealed bag in the oven. Best of all, you simply throw the bag out once you've finished.

WRAP AND COOK

I am a fan of wrapping fish fillets or single chicken breasts in baking paper (the French call this method *en papillote*), or even bamboo, banana leaves, fig leaves, grape leaves, corn husks, spinach leaves or cabbage leaves. Include lots of fresh herbs and place in the oven or on the barbeque. Although you don't get any browning with this method, it seals in the flavour and works wonders with lean, fat-free cuts.

Copper *See* Minerals.

Couscous *See* Grains.

Cravings

Do you get a craving for chocolate in the afternoon? Or for something sweet after dinner? No-one knows for sure why we get cravings but they play havoc with the best diet intentions. Cravings may come from a dietary imbalance, but few of us crave healthy foods like carrots or spinach. The fact that most cravings are for junk food tells us that there are other reasons behind cravings.

To help you decide the cause of your particular craving, think of what's going through your head when you crave a chocolate bar at 3 o'clock in the afternoon. Are you feeling lethargic? Bored? Stressed? In need of a reward? All these are indications you are using food to meet an emotional need. Food works well as a comforter, which is why we turn to it so often. But in the long run, it's best to satisfy these feelings with the right thing, rather than food. In our well-fed world, it's unlikely that we have a genuine nutrient shortage.

MY TAKE

The best insurance against cravings is to eat a balanced diet and drink at least eight glasses of water a day. Keep alcohol to a minimum as it can trigger binge eating. Don't avoid sugar, but have it with other healthy food, as in jam on grainy bread or canned fruit with a scoop of ice-cream, rather than lollies, chocolate or sweet biscuits. If you're craving a sugar fix late at night, two diet modifications seem to help—increase the size of your protein serves (more fish, meat, eggs or tofu), and replace high-GI refined carbs (white rice, white bread, potato and biscuits) with low-GI alternatives, and keep to a moderate portion.

PHYSIOLOGICAL CRAVINGS

Cravings can be triggered by a shortage of a particular nutrient in the body, but not in most cases. It's a theory that's been around for a while, but no-one has come up with really good solid proof, apart from a few studies on pregnant women.

The theory is that if you're running low on copper, for instance, your body sends out signals for you to seek out foods rich in copper. Cocoa happens to be quite rich in copper, so one of the reasons behind a chocolate craving is said to be a shortage of copper. Of course, there are many other reasons for a chocolate craving and most of them have nothing to do with getting more nutrition! The same theory is often applied to cravings for Vegemite yeast spread (your body is low on B vitamins), seafood (iodine), milk or cheese (calcium) and nuts (selenium, manganese and other trace minerals).

PREGNANCY

During pregnancy, cravings are notorious and many women report eating a range of foods they normally wouldn't, from pickled cucumbers to miso soup, day after day. At the opposite end, aversions are equally common. Many women are unable to face strong-smelling foods such as coffee, tea, alcohol, meat or even vegetables like cabbage or swede. Several studies have reported biological explanations for pregnancy cravings—adjustments in fluid and electrolyte balance, hormone fluctuations, bigger blood volume and rapid tissue growth, but these don't occur at other times of our lives.

CAVING TO THE CRAVING

If you suddenly experience an urgent feeling for a healthy item like blueberries or a tossed green salad, then go with it. But if it's for a chocolate bar, use the steps here to see if it's genuine or not. Cravings often satisfy an emotional need for a particular texture or mouth feel. Try to work out if the things you crave fit into a specific characteristic and what emotion you're tapping into.

CRAVING	TEXTURE OR 'MOUTH FEEL'	EMOTIONAL TRIGGER
Chocolate	Rich and smooth	A need to indulge
Lollies, sweets	Sugary	A need for better balance
Bread, pastries, doughnuts	Doughy/starchy	A need for comfort
Salty crisps	Crunchy	Feelings of anger, hostility
Ice-cream, thick shake, iced coffee	Creamy	Related to childhood memories

Crohn's Disease and Diet

Crohn's disease, (which includes ulcerative colitis—both known as inflammatory bowel disease or IBD) causes inflammation in the small intestine. It normally occurs in the lower part of the small intestine (the ileum) but can affect any part of the digestive tract. The inflammation causes pain and diarrhoea. Despite a great deal of research, the cause of IBD is unknown, but it is not caused by diet or allergies to certain food components. However, some people find that dietary modifications help them to manage the symptoms.

LOW-FIBRE DIET

When IBD is active, most people find a bland, low-fibre diet helps to ease diarrhoea and reduce abdominal cramping.

LOW-FAT DIET

People with Crohn's disease who experience steatorrhoea (diarrhoea that contains undigested dietary fats) may benefit from a low-fat diet.

LOW-LACTOSE DIET

The milk sugar lactose is broken down by the enzyme lactase, commonly found in the lining of the small intestine. Some people with Crohn's disease may lack this enzyme, so limiting milk and milk products may be helpful. Lactose intolerance can be diagnosed with a simple test—consult with your doctor.

People with IBD also need to drink plenty of fluids to prevent dehydration. There is no need to take vitamin supplements if the overall diet is a healthy and varied one. However, some people find fish oil supplements and probiotics can help.

Anyone with IBD should discuss their diet with their doctor or an accredited practising dietitian.

D

Dairy Foods and Alternatives

Milk, yoghurt and cheese are needed for their readily absorbed calcium, along with their protein, riboflavin, and fat-soluble vitamins A and B_{12}. It is believed they may also help protect against bowel cancer.

The average adult should aim to eat three to four serves of milk, yoghurt or cheese a day, to achieve the recommended intake of 1000 milligrams of calcium. If you cannot tolerate dairy products, look for soy, almond, oat or rice beverages, but make sure they are fortified with calcium so they're equivalent to milk.

ONE SERVE

- 1 cup (250 millilitres) milk
- 1 tub (200 grams) yoghurt
- 1 cup (250 millilitres) custard
- 2 slices (40 grams) cheese
- ½ cup (125 millilitres) evaporated milk.

DID YOU KNOW?

As a group, dairy products (excluding butter) supply around 20 per cent of the protein and vitamin A consumed in Australia, a huge 60 per cent of the calcium, 30 per cent of the riboflavin, 15 per cent of the fat and 10 per cent of the kilojoules.

THE LOW-FAT ALTERNATIVE

Dairy products like butter, cream and full-fat cream cheeses are high in saturated fat. Reduced-fat dairy foods are the healthy choices, and have a role to play in keeping blood pressure down and helping with weight loss. If you have high cholesterol, you are best to go with the low-fat options.

These days, most low-fat milks and yoghurts are a far cry from the days of thin, watery skim-milk products. Dairy technology and the use of gelling agents and emulsifiers give a rich, smooth 'mouth feel' and pleasant texture. The protein, calcium and important B vitamins remain unchanged.

Sadly, cheese is one dairy product that is difficult to produce in a low-fat form, and is one of the foods most often missed on a low-fat diet. Cheddars with 25 per cent less fat are commonly found in supermarkets, but glorious triple brie and blue-vein varieties remain full-fat.

Studies by Professor Michael Zemel (Professor of Nutrition and Medicine at the University of Tennessee) have highlighted the role of calcium in moving fat cells out of the body's adipose stores and facilitating weight loss. Overweight women who consumed three serves of low-fat milk or yoghurt a day, as part of a low-kilojoule diet, lost more weight than women on the same kilojoule intake without the dairy foods. However, it's still early days—other researchers haven't been able to duplicate his findings, so the jury is still out. In the meantime, low-fat milk and yoghurt are valuable foods for any diet plan, being low GI, high in protein, filling and nutrient-dense.

Growing bodies

Children under two need full-fat products as full-fat milk, yoghurt and cheese are a good source of fat-soluble vitamin A.

See also Cheese; Milk; Yoghurt.

DASH Diet *See* Blood Pressure.

Detox Diets

The theory behind detoxing is that we can 'cleanse' and 'purify' our body by removing wastes and eliminating toxins (which are never defined in any real detail). Many claim to 'work like an intestinal broom'. This will supposedly get the bowel working efficiently and rejuvenate the liver, based on the underlying naturopathic concept that your health will improve once your digestive tract is working correctly. By following a strict regime based around water, juices, raw vegetables and teas (and eliminating all caffeine, alcohol, refined carbohydrates, meat and dairy), the toxins will magically be flushed out and glowing health and energy will be your reward. A detox is touted to improve a whole range of common conditions such as indigestion, heartburn, poor immunity, fatigue, headaches, allergies, muscle aches, acne, dry skin and eye puffiness. The claim that sucks most women in is the promise of weight loss, radiant skin and clear eyes.

Despite all the hype, there's no proof that a detox diet really does clean out the body, or that the average person needs to detox at all. That said, given our overconsumption of processed foods and alcohol, a few days of moderate eating can do us all good—but it's not a formal detox. Detox diets are not the solution to permanent weight loss either. They are only quick fixes (often promoted to 'kick-start' your diet), that don't help re-educate your eating patterns. Once people finish detoxing, most go happily back to their former (fattening) way of eating and the weight comes back on.

There's no proof that a detox diet really does clean out the body, or that the average person needs to detox at all.

Many detox diets are simply a healthy but minimalist eating plan, followed for 2–10 days, which for most of us is fine. Others require you to take a number of herbal extracts and supplements such as digestive bitters, goldenseal and elecampane for the stomach, milk thistle and dandelion for the liver, acidophilus for the intestines, mild laxatives such as senna, cascara or rhubarb, fibre sources such as psyllium, slippery elm, resistant starch, aniseed, liquorice, uva ursi, Irish moss or agar for the colon. There are also many detox kits sold through pharmacies (at great expense) that you can embark on for a torturous 14 days.

Detoxing often has a laxative or diuretic effect, which can be harmful, and should not be done by people with diabetes or compromised kidneys, pregnant or breastfeeding women, or those with irritable bowel syndrome or anaemia. Even if you are in good health, do not follow a strict detox for more than 7 days.

There's no doubt detoxing is a popular weight-loss approach. The key appeal is that it's a quick fix—you only have to endure it for a short, finite time. It's also simple, there's no counting kilojoules, and it totally eliminates all the 'baddies' like alcohol, caffeine, sugar, meat and highly processed foods. Detoxing is like a modern-day penance; you can atone for your sins of overindulgence and excess, and feel saintly and virtuous.

LEMONS AND DETOXING

The Lemon Detox attempts to ride on the tail of lemon's long association with weight loss. For 10 days, you don't eat at all, but exist on a sweet lemonade-style drink made with lemon juice, cayenne pepper and a special syrup called the Madal Bal Natural Tree Syrup, an expensive, high-sugar product derived from palm and maple trees. You also get a herbal laxative tea to drink, which further increases weight loss. Even with the sugar from the syrup, your intake is less than 1700 kilojoules a day (the average intake is around 8700 kilojoules), which means it's a semi-fast.

There's no proof a lemon detox semi-fast does what it claims to do. The liver and kidneys are highly efficient organs that have evolved to break down and remove toxins from the bloodstream without the need for a detox. You might feel better because you've cut out 'junk' and boosted your intake of antioxidants, fibre and vitamins, but you can achieve this by eating a healthy, balanced diet.

Dextrose

This is an alternative name for glucose, the simple sugar that is the building block of starch and a constituent of sugar.

See also Glucose.

DHA

Docosahexaenoic acid (DHA) is concentrated in tuna oil, while other fish oils, fish and seafood supply smaller amounts. Breast milk is rich in DHA, and newborn babies utilise it to develop brain, nerve and eye tissue.

Diabetes and Diet

Diabetes is a breakdown in the body's ability to utilise blood glucose (sugar) efficiently. The body fails to produce enough of the hormone insulin or to use the little insulin it does generate. Insulin is needed to transport glucose into the muscles. Left untreated, the glucose builds up in the bloodstream, resulting in high blood-glucose levels that increase the risk of heart disease and may cause serious damage to the kidneys, nerves, skin and eyes. Ideally, blood glucose levels should be kept within normal and safe levels of 4–8 millimoles per litre (mmol/L).

TYPE 1 DIABETES (INSULIN DEPENDENT)

Representing approximately 10 per cent of all cases of diabetes, type 1 usually occurs in childhood or young adulthood, though it can occur at any age. In developed nations, it is one of the most common childhood diseases. It is an auto-immune disease that occurs when the pancreas no longer produces enough insulin to convert glucose into energy. It is not caused by obesity or lifestyle factors. Treatment involves lifelong, daily insulin injections or insulin pumps, regular blood-glucose testing, a healthy diet and regular exercise.

TYPE 2 DIABETES (NON-INSULIN DEPENDENT OR MATURE-AGE ONSET DIABETES)

This is the most common type of diabetes, accounting for approximately 85–90 per cent of all cases. It develops when the pancreas is not producing effective insulin and is promoted by lifestyle factors such as an unhealthy diet and lack of exercise, contributing to obesity. Treatment for most people (at least initially) mainly involves regular blood-glucose testing, eating a healthy low-GI diet and taking regular exercise. Some people may require tablets or insulin. Type 2 diabetes typically occurs in adults over the age of 50, but it is increasingly occurring at a younger age due to rising rates of obesity, sedentary lifestyles and an ageing population. According to AusDiab, the first national diabetes and lifestyle study that began in 1999, one in four Australians now has diabetes, or is at high risk of developing it in the next 5–10 years.

GESTATIONAL DIABETES

This is a form of diabetes that occurs in pregnancy and in most cases disappears after the baby is born. It occurs in about 16 per cent of pregnancies (the mother does not have diabetes before pregnancy), but the incidence among some high-risk groups can be as high as 30 per cent. These high-risk groups include Aboriginal and Maori women, as well as those from India, China, Asia and the Pacific Islands. Gestational diabetes increases the risk of pregnancy complications and significantly increases the likelihood of the woman developing type 2 diabetes later in life.

INSULIN RESISTANCE

This is a condition where the body becomes insensitive to the hormone insulin. The body produces insulin but the tissues and muscles don't recognise it. The body then responds by making more, building up levels of both insulin and blood glucose in the bloodstream, which is unable to move into the tissues to generate energy. It is linked to a sedentary lifestyle, being overweight, and having high blood fats and high blood pressure. Regular exercise and a low-GI diet that's also low in saturated fat will help make muscles more sensitive to insulin. Insulin resistance is key part of Metabolic Syndrome or Syndrome X.

RISK FACTORS FOR TYPE 2 DIABETES

You are more likely to develop type 2 diabetes if you:

- ✔ Are over 50 and have high blood pressure
- ✔ Are over 50 and overweight
- ✔ Are over 50 and one or more members of the family has diabetes
- ✔ Had gestational diabetes while pregnant
- ✔ Have heart disease or have had a heart attack
- ✔ Have recorded a borderline blood-glucose level
- ✔ Have polycystic ovarian syndrome and are overweight
- ✔ Are over 35 with a Maori, Pacific Island, Aboriginal or Torres Strait Islander background
- ✔ Are over 35 and from the Indian sub-continent or have a Chinese background.

If you fit any of these categories, it's time to modify your lifestyle and to speak to your doctor about an annual test for diabetes or pre-diabetes.

A DIABETES-FRIENDLY DIET

Having diabetes doesn't mean you need to buy special foods. A healthy diet for diabetes is much the same as a healthy diet for all of us—it needs to be a balanced, low-GI diet that is high in fibre and wholegrains, moderate in salt and sugar, and low in saturated fats. It should incorporate a variety of vegetables, fruits, nuts, legumes, lean meats, fish and low-fat dairy foods.

EAT REGULARLY

Have regular meals and snacks. Spread your carbohydrates throughout the day to give a steady supply of glucose to your muscles and organs (or match it to your insulin). Don't skip meals.

BE A HEALTHY WEIGHT

Lose your excess weight, especially if it's around your middle. This can improve your blood glucose and even lessen the number of tablets or injections you need each day. If your weight is fine, aim to maintain a healthy weight as you get older.

CHOOSE FOODS LOW IN SATURATED FAT

People with diabetes are five to six times more at risk of heart disease, often having high blood triglyceride levels (a blood fat), high blood pressure, clotting and circulation problems. So it's essential to cut back on saturated fats in an effort to keep heart disease (one of the major complications of diabetes) at bay.

GO FOR THE HEALTHY FATS

Substitute saturated fats with mono-unsaturated fat from olive and canola oils, avocados and nuts or polyunsaturated fat from sunflower oil or polyunsaturated spreads.

INCREASE OMEGA-3S

Omega-3 oils from fish, seafood and lean meat keep the blood free-flowing and improve insulin resistance. A modified-fat diet, which is low in saturates and high in omega-3 and mono-unsaturated fat, is considered an alternative approach for some diabetics and is easier to stick to than a conventional low-fat diet.

FILL UP ON FIBRE

Aim for plenty of fibre—vegetables, salads, baked beans and lentils, wholemeal bread, bran cereals and oats.

CHOOSE LOW-GI CARBS AND KEEP PORTIONS MODERATE

Try to include some slow-digesting carbohydrates like pasta, beans, bran cereals, grainy breads, pumpernickel, oat bran muffins, yoghurt and certain fruit (apples, cherries, grapefruit, peaches, pears and plums) in your meals and snacks. These low-GI foods demand much less insulin for their absorption and don't produce a high rise in blood-sugar glucose levels.

HEALTHY LIFESTYLE FACTORS

MOVE MORE

Regular daily exercise like walking or swimming is essential. This will help shift abdominal fat and make your muscles more sensitive or receptive to insulin.

> **One in four Australians now has diabetes, or is at high risk of developing it in the next 5–10 years.**

LEARN MORE

Anyone newly diagnosed with diabetes should make an appointment to see a dietitian or sign up for a diabetes education course, usually located at large hospitals.

SUGAR AND DIABETES

Sugar is not the cause of diabetes. Research shows that a moderate amount of common table sugar (sucrose) has only a moderate effect on blood glucose. In fact, the effect of sugar on blood-glucose levels is similar to or even better than many starchy foods like rice, bread and potatoes.

Eating modest amounts of sugar in healthy foods like breakfast cereal, yoghurt, custard and low-fat ice-cream should not upset or spike blood glucose levels. The sugar found in baked beans, tomato sauce and other cooking sauces also has little effect on blood-glucose levels. Your goal is to minimise large amounts of added sugar. Sugar is not a good choice when it is eaten in concentrated forms such as soft drinks and lollies, especially on an empty stomach. In high-fat foods like pastries or desserts, sugar makes fat palatable and easy to overeat.

A moderate amount of sugar in diabetic diets (30–50 grams or 6–10 teaspoons per day) does not lead to poor blood-glucose control or weight gain. Keep in mind, however, that this moderate amount includes all sources of refined sugar you consume such as white, brown, raw, treacle, golden syrup, soft drinks, desserts, cookies, breakfast cereals or a teaspoon of sugar added to a cup of tea or coffee.

See also Glycemic Index; Metabolic Syndrome.

Diarrhoea and Diet

A clear fluid diet is the best form of treatment for gastroenteritis and tummy upsets. It is the lightest type of diet, designed to place as little strain as possible on the digestive tract.

It is not nutritionally adequate and should be followed only for a strictly limited time—ideally 2–3 days. If after 3 days on a clear fluid diet you can't keep anything down or food passes straight through your bowels, you need to seek medical advice.

Growing bodies
Dehydration can quickly become an issue with diarrhoea, particularly with children. Rehydration solutions and ice-blocks such as Gastrolyte or Hydralyte are excellent and can be purchased from pharmacies.

CLEAR FLUID DIET

FOODS TO INCLUDE:

- ✔ Clear broth
- ✔ Weak black tea with a slice of lemon (may be sweetened with a little sugar or honey)
- ✔ Flat lemonade (or other non-cola soft drink), diluted
- ✔ Diluted cordial
- ✔ Jelly.

FOODS TO AVOID:

- ✖ Milk—the lactose (sugar) of milk is poorly absorbed when the digestive system is damaged or upset; stay off milk and dairy products for 4–7 days after resuming food
- ✖ Fruit juice—the high content of fruit sugars can sometime worsen any diarrhoea and delay recovery, but if that's all you have, dilute it down with water
- ✖ Alcohol—avoid it completely; white wine is not a clear fluid!

CLEAR BEEF BROTH

A tried and true remedy for upset tummies and people recovering from an illness is beef tea.

500 g gravy beef or chuck steak
1 onion, chopped
2 sticks celery, chopped
1 parsnip, chopped
1 carrot, chopped
A few sprigs of parsley
2 ½ litres (10 cups) water
Whole black peppercorns
Salt (optional)

Trim any fat from the beef and dice into large chunks. Place in a large saucepan with the onion, celery, parsnip, carrot and parsley. Add water, pepper and salt. Increase the heat and skim off any scum that comes to the surface. When almost boiling, reduce heat, cover and simmer for one hour or until the beef is tender. Strain through a sieve over a large bowl or saucepan. Serve broth while hot, and discard drained ingredients. Store any remaining broth in the refrigerator and reheat as needed. Makes 4–6 serves.

TRANSITION TO YOUR NORMAL DIET

After 2–3 days on clear fluids, introduce light, bland food such as:

- ✔ Unbuttered toast (dip it in soup or weak tea)
- ✔ Plain crackers or rusks
- ✔ Boiled rice
- ✔ Steamed chicken or fish
- ✔ Soup (no cream)
- ✔ Stewed or canned apples or pears, or other soft fruit
- ✔ Jars of apple puree
- ✔ Boiled or mashed potato (no milk).

Dietary Guidelines

Dietary guidelines are designed to give consumers a set of 'rules' around which to build a varied and balanced diet. They highlight the groups of foods and lifestyle patterns that will foster good health, and are most likely to minimise your chances of diet-related illnesses such as heart disease, type 2 diabetes, certain cancers, obesity, gall bladder disease and dental caries. Dietary guidelines are one example of food selection guides that have been around since the 1950s. They vary in their complexity and purpose.

Most countries including Australia, New Zealand, the UK, the US and Japan have produced several editions of their own guidelines over the past 30 years that highlight the groups of foods unique to their own country. Updated as new evidence emerges, they are used by dietitians, teachers, doctors and governments as a reference base for teaching about nutrition.

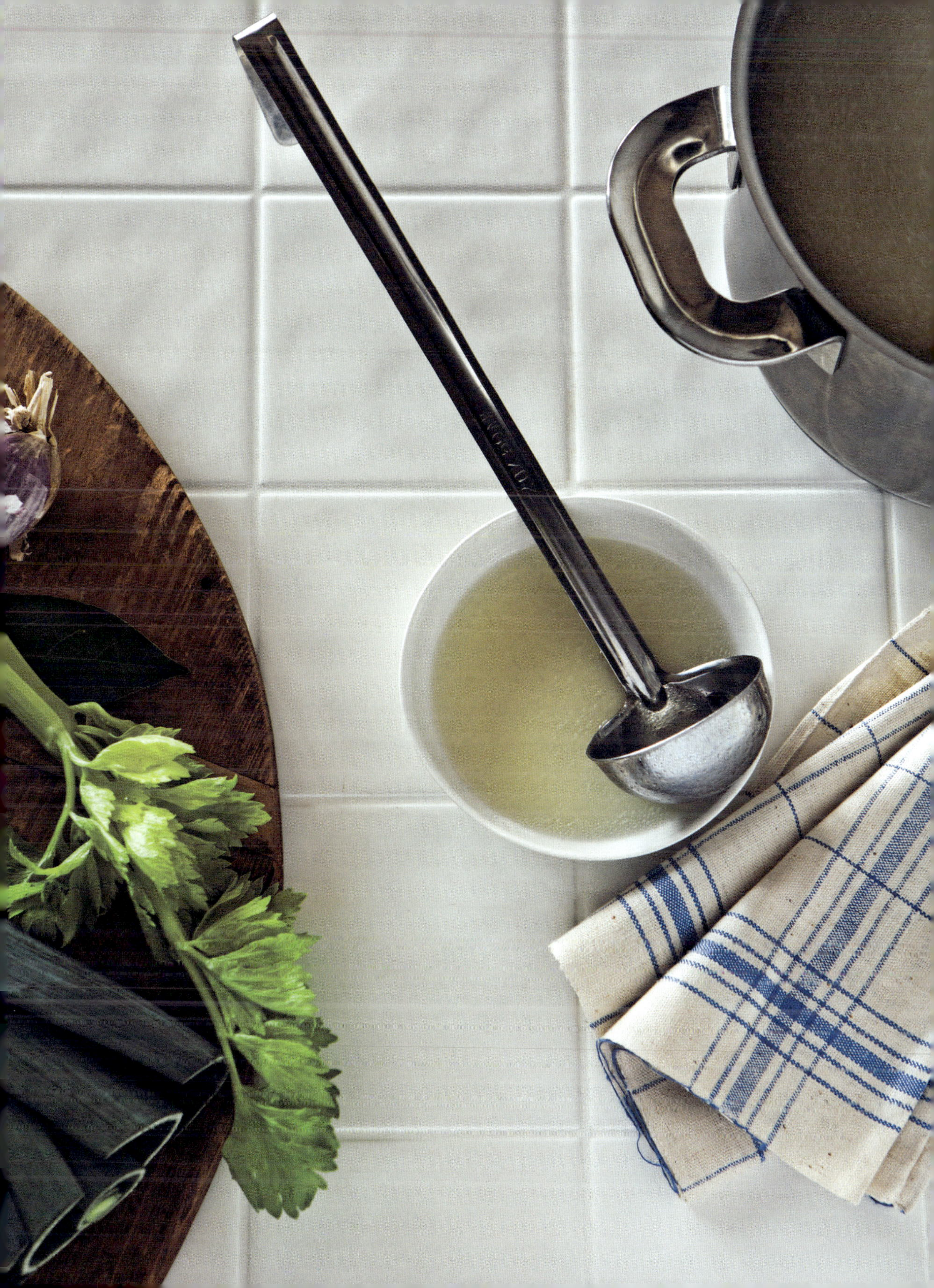

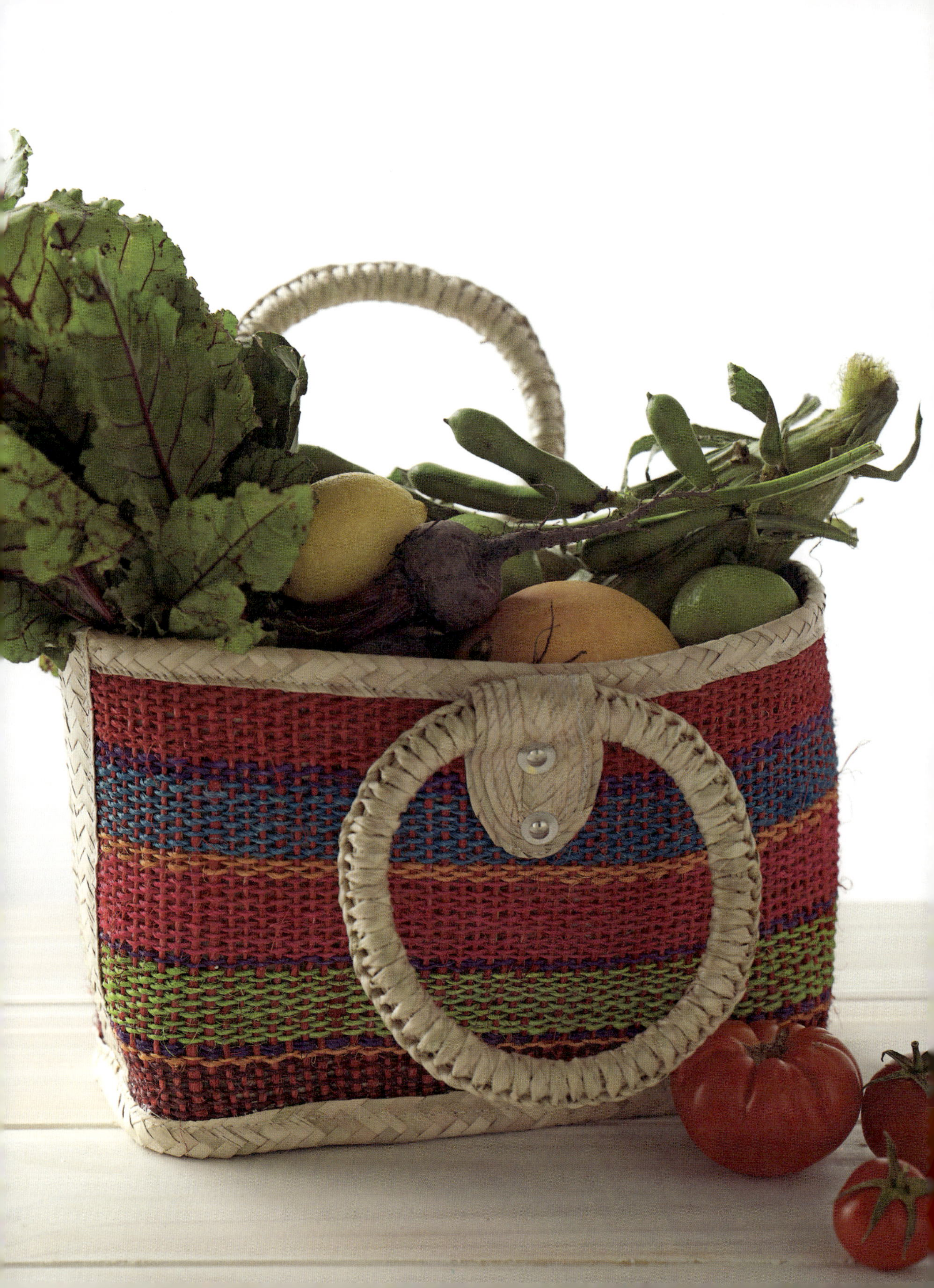

As a general rule, it is important to enjoy a wide variety of nutritious foods at all life stages, though children and adolescents in particular need sufficient nutritious foods to grow and develop normally. A healthy, long-term diet suitable for most people would contain:

- ✔ Plenty of vegetables, including a range of varieties and colours, and legumes
- ✔ Fruit
- ✔ Grain (cereal) foods, mostly wholegrain, including breads, cereals, rice, pasta, couscous, oats, quinoa and barley
- ✔ Lean meat, poultry, fish, eggs and/or alternatives like nuts, seeds and legumes
- ✔ Milk, yoghurt, cheese and/or alternatives, mostly reduced fat (note that reduced-fat milks are not suitable for children under the age of 2 years)
- ✔ Water as the main drink option.

Take care to avoid:

- ✖ Saturated and trans fats
- ✖ Added salt
- ✖ Added sugars, in particular sugar-sweetened drinks
- ✖ Alcohol.

And also:

- ✔ Achieve and maintain a healthy weight by being physically active and eating nutritious food to meet your energy needs.
- ✔ Encourage and support breastfeeding.
- ✔ Care for your food: be sure to prepare and store it safely.

LIMITATIONS

All such guidelines have their limitations. They are only broad principles—they can't help you to assess the proportions of your diet overall, plan healthy meals or see how much variety you're getting. They are based on basic foodstuffs like vegetables and meats with limited inclusion of treats, snack foods and alcohol which feature in many diets. If you are teaching people about nutrition, use them as a starting point for teaching but add in other teaching tools as well.

See also **Adolescents and Diet; Adults and Diet; Food Groups; Infants; Primary School–aged Children and Diet; Pyramid and Healthy Eating; Toddlers and Diet.**

Diets

See **Weight Loss.**

Digestive Disorders

Digestion is the mixing and breakdown of food by juices and enzymes from the stomach, pancreas, liver and intestine, to allow absorption of nutrients into the bloodstream. Carbohydrates are converted to glucose and fructose, protein to amino acids and fat to glycerol and fatty acids. Indigestion—that unpleasant feeling of discomfort or illness in your tummy region—results from an inability to digest or process food properly. It has a number of causes and it's worth listing these so you know what's what before you head to the doctor for a diagnosis.

CONSTIPATION

This makes it difficult for you to have a bowel movement. Not everyone has bowel movements once a day; a normal range can be anywhere between three times a day and three times a week. Eating enough fibre and drinking enough fluids are key to treating constipation. In addition, not going to the bathroom when you have the urge, lack of exercise and pregnancy can all aggravate this condition.

HEARTBURN OR GASTRO-OESOPHAGEAL REFLUX DISEASE

Despite its name, heartburn doesn't affect the heart. Heartburn is a burning feeling in the lower chest, along with a sour or bitter taste in the mouth. Acid from your stomach can get through the sphincter (muscle at the stomach opening) and into your oesophagus, irritating it and causing heartburn (this is known as reflux). Heartburn is most common after over-eating, or when bending over or lying down. Pregnancy, being overweight, stress, cigarette smoking, lack of exercise and spicy or rich foods can also make heartburn worse.

IRRITABLE BOWEL SYNDROME (IBS)

IBS is a chronic problem with the large intestine and is a common condition, with up to 30 per cent of the population having symptoms at some time in their life. In people who have IBS, food either moves too quickly or too slowly through the intestines. Symptoms include abdominal pain, bloating, diarrhoea, gas (wind), variable bowel habits (sometimes too frequent and runny, sometimes infrequent with constipation), or urgency of defecation. For some people, a low-FODMAP diet works well (see page 119).

INFLAMMATORY BOWEL DISEASE (IBD)

IBD is the name of a group of disorders that cause the intestines to become inflamed (red and swollen). Two kinds of inflammatory bowel disease are Crohn's disease and ulcerative colitis. The exact causes of IBD are unknown but the best treatment is eating a healthy diet as well as managing stress and getting enough rest.

GALLSTONES

The gall bladder is an internal organ just under your liver. It stores the digestive fluids that are made by the liver. Sometimes these fluids can solidify and form stones called gallstones. You're more likely to get gallstones if:

- You are a woman
- You are over 60 years old
- You have diabetes
- You have a family history of gallstones
- You are pregnant
- You are overweight or obese with most of your excess around your waist
- You are on a low-kilojoule diet and have recently lost weight rapidly.

DIVERTICULAR DISEASE

Diverticular disease may be caused by not eating enough fibre, leading to harder stools and constipation. This increases the pressure in the bowel walls which may create internal 'blow-outs', small pouches that can form along your digestive tract. Eat more fibre, drink plenty of fluids and exercise regularly to help prevent the pouches from becoming infected or inflamed.

COELIAC DISEASE

Coeliac disease is an inherited disorder where your body cannot process gluten, a protein found in wheat, rye and barley. When eaten, gluten 'damages' the small intestine, which prevents your body from taking in many of the nutrients from the foods you eat.

Q

My husband suffers from indigestion. A friend suggested he eat fresh pineapple before or after each meal. Since he's been on the pineapple he no longer has the problem. Is this an old wives' tale or is there a scientific reason for it?

A

Pineapple contains an enzyme called bromelain, which breaks down proteins in food and is the reason why fresh pineapple will not set in a jelly. Pawpaw and kiwi fruit have similar protein-dissolving enzymes, so these may be helpful if your husband tires of pineapple. But if you boil the pineapple first, this destroys the enzyme, so cooked or canned pineapple will not have the same effect. Another reason pineapple helps is simply because of its acidity.

FRUCTOSE MALABSORPTION

Fructose malabsorption is common in patients with symptoms of irritable bowel syndrome, and occurs when there is a problem with the absorption of fructose (fruit sugar) out of the small intestine. This results in an increased concentration of fructose in the entire intestine. Fructose malabsorption is found in up to 30 per cent of the population of Western countries.

Symptoms can range from bloating (from fermentation in the small and large intestine), flatulence, stomach pain (as a result of muscle spasms), loose motions and/or constipation. Like lactose intolerance, it is diagnosed with a breath hydrogen test. Dietary treatment involves avoiding food that contains high levels of fructose as well as dietary sources of fructans. Do not self-diagnose. Advice from an accredited practising dietitian is crucial.

See also **Irritable Bowel Syndrome; Gallstones; Heartburn; Coeliac Disease; Constipation; FODMAPs; Crohn's Disease.**

Dinner

For most of us, dinner is our main meal and a time to unwind and relax, whether it's a sit-down meal of meat and vegetables, or a frozen dinner in front of the TV. Ideally, dinner should not be too heavy or too late in the evening. Unfortunately with working families, the evening meal usually ends up being a big meal late at night, which is not good for digestion, nor is it conducive to weight loss. Most of us are sedentary at night; we sit and watch TV or do some reading and don't burn off the kilojoules from the dinner. These then go into fat stores.

While we all love to eat out, I've found that when you cook at home you have more control over the nutritional value of that meal. You can serve a larger portion of beans, carrots and other vegetables (you often have to pay extra for vegetables at restaurants). You can also go easy on the butter, cream or oil when you cook and hold back on the salt if you need to. These are all things you have no control over when a chef cooks for you.

BEEF IT UP WITH VEGETABLES

The evening meal is the perfect opportunity to take in more vegetables or salad, and get your recommended five serves for the day. Aim to serve lots of vegetables, either cooked or raw, and drizzled with a lemon-oil dressing or a splash of balsamic vinegar. It's easy to team vegetables with the main meat or fish, or vegetarian alternatives like lentils, tofu or beans.

Making vegetables the feature of the evening meal is also a good way to set up healthy eating habits for your children. Several US studies have reported that kids who eat dinner as a family are more likely to have a better nutritional intake compared with that of children who eat alone or in front of the TV. In addition, teenagers who regularly ate with the rest of their family performed better at school and were less likely to smoke, use drugs or drink alcohol. So if you have kids, try to have a sit-down dinner with them as often as you can—at least three times a week. Turn off the television, make conversation and ask them about their day.

Disaccharides

These are 'double sugars' such as lactose (glucose with galactose), sucrose (glucose with fructose) and maltose (glucose with glucose). They are mainly broken down to their component sugars in the upper intestine before being absorbed.

Diuretics

Diuretics are substances that force the kidneys to flush out more urine than normal ('water pills'). They are often prescribed for sick people who suffer from oedema, an intense accumulation of fluids in the body's tissues, and those who suffer from high blood pressure or heart-related diseases. Increasing the production of urine not only releases fluid, but also helps rid the body of excess electrolytes (sodium or potassium) and may reduce blood volume.

As with laxatives, using diuretics for weight loss is not recommended.

Some people take diuretics to lose weight. Yes, the scales show you're a few kilograms lighter but it's fluid—not fat—and it's temporary. The weight will be regained once your body adjusts and you drink normally again. As with laxatives, using diuretics for weight loss is not recommended. Taking them unnecessarily can be harmful, as it can lead to dehydration and electrolyte imbalance. This in turn can then lead to potassium deficiency, which can be dangerous.

Certain foods can have a natural diuretic effect, such as alcohol and caffeine; however, you need to consume quite large quantities before it causes concern. Foods high in potassium are often recommended if you're taking diuretics to counteract the loss of potassium that inevitably occurs.

See also Potassium.

Diverticular Disease *See* Digestive Disorders.

E

Ectomorph

A body build that is sharp and thin, with narrow shoulders and hips and little fat or muscle.

Eggs

Eggs are great to cook, and great for you. As one of nature's convenience foods, they are a true cradle-to-grave option. Babies love their soft texture as a weaning food; the yolk can be introduced after 6 months, while the white is usually held back until after 9 months to minimise the possibility of allergy. Older folk who need to eat a 'soft diet' appreciate their soft texture and easy cooking options. A dozen eggs stored in the refrigerator is one of the most convenient of the protein foods—it's so simple to create a quick omelette or frittata or whip up scrambled eggs on toast.

READ THE LABEL

If you or a member of your family have an allergy, you need to thoroughly scrutinise all food labels for any ingredient containing egg or derived from egg. Watch out for these terms on the ingredient list on the back of the label: powdered egg, dried egg, yolk, egg white, egg lecithin, albumin, ovalbumin, globulin, livetin, ovomucin, ovomucoid, silica albuminate, vitellin and ovovitellin. Remember that many popular recipes contain eggs, from meat loaf and burgers (where eggs are used to bind the mixture) to cakes, biscuits, custards and some types of pastry and ice-creams.

NUTRITIONAL VALUE

Eggs are a nutritional powerhouse, supplying high-quality protein, some fat and a host of essential minerals, including selenium (an antioxidant), iron, and zinc for the immune system. For a very modest 355 kilojoules, you also get 18 different vitamins—every kind, except vitamin C. Worth mentioning is vitamin B_{12}, which is hard to obtain on vegetarian diets, and folate, a B vitamin that can help minimise birth defects. There's also choline, a substance related to B vitamins that's important for our brain and liver metabolism.

Eggs are a surprising source of two carotenoids, lutein and zeaxanthin, natural compounds related to the beta-carotene of carrots and usually found only in vegetables and fruits. These two antioxidants are now under study for their role in preventing macular degeneration of the eye, a common cause of blindness in older folk.

Regardless of the type of egg you choose, they all offer similar amounts of protein, total fat and cholesterol.

NUMBER CRUNCH

One large egg (35–70 grams in the shell) gives us 6 grams of protein, 6 grams of fat, a trace of sugar, a trace of starch, no fibre and 355 kilojoules.

WHAT EGG IS THAT?

CAGED EGGS

Caged eggs come from hens that are continuously housed in cages within a large shed. Each cage houses between three and five hens that have access to food troughs and water drinkers, and have just enough space to stand up and turn.

SHOPPER'S GUIDE

Are you buying a true dozen? Beware of the 10-egg carton. Some large organic eggs (70 g) are sold in dozen-sized cartons, but contain only ten eggs.

BARN-LAID EGGS

These come from hens kept in a large barn or shed where they can move around, spread their wings, bathe in dust and scratch for food.

FREE-RANGE EGGS

Free-range hens are housed overnight in sheds, similar to those of barn-housed hens, but have access to the outdoors during the day.

VEGETARIAN EGGS

Vegetarian eggs are from hens fed grain and legume-based feed only. No feed is derived from meat or fish products.

OMEGA-3 EGGS

These come from hens fed canola, flaxseed and fishmeal. They have a higher proportion of omega-3 fats, which are important for a healthy heart, eyes and brain.

ORGANIC EGGS

These must be laid by free-range hens that are fed a diet with at least 95 per cent organically grown grain. There are no pesticides, herbicides or synthetic fertilisers used in the paddocks where the hens are kept, or in the production of the hens' feed. To be certain you're getting organic, look for a certification logo from one of the organic organisations.

LUTEIN-ENRICHED EGGS

These eggs are from hens fed marigold petals, which boosts the level of the natural antioxidants lutein and zeaxanthin. These two antioxidants are needed by the macula of the eye, a tiny part at the back of the eye that absorbs and neutralises damaging light rays. A high intake of lutein and zeaxanthin has been linked to lower risk of macular degeneration.

CHOLESTEROL AND EGGS

According to the Heart Foundation, healthy adults with normal cholesterol levels can enjoy six eggs a week without increasing their risk of heart disease. The dietary cholesterol in eggs has only a small effect on blood cholesterol levels, especially when compared with the much greater effects of saturated and trans fats. This means you can eat one egg for breakfast most days of the week or eat a serve of eggs (two eggs) a couple of meals a week. Boil, poach or scramble in a little olive oil—don't fry them in bacon fat or coddle them in cream.

EASY EGGS

- ✔ Serve poached egg with asparagus and chutney on toasted Turkish bread or crunchy, grainy toast.
- ✔ Add hard-boiled eggs to salads and rice dishes.
- ✔ Beat eggs with chopped green onions (shallots), parsley, grated cheese and a little ham and cook for a quick omelette dinner.
- ✔ A raw egg cracked into a smoothie will boost the protein and make a well-rounded breakfast-to-go (not for pregnant women though, due to the risk of listeria contamination, nor for the elderly due to salmonella).

Growing bodies

Allergy to egg is the most common food allergy in babies and young children, affecting about 1–2 per cent of preschool children. It generally becomes apparent between the ages of 6 and 15 months, when egg is given for the first time. Unlike peanut allergy, egg allergy is generally mild, resulting in symptoms such as hives or rashes. Allergy to both egg white and yolk can occur, though egg white is more likely to cause a reaction. The good news is that egg allergy is the most likely allergy to fade over time, with around 80 per cent of children being free of it by the time they start school.

See also Eye Health and Diet.

Eicosapentaenoic Acid (EPA)

See also Fish Oil.

A long-chain omega-3 fatty acid with 20 carbon atoms and 5 double bonds, made from the fatty acid alpha-linolenic acid in the body.

Electrolytes

These are mineral ions in solution in body fluids—sodium, potassium, calcium, magnesium, chloride, phosphates and sulphates, which control much of the body's biochemistry. Electrolyte balance can be disturbed through extreme fluid loss caused by illness, diarrhoea, vomiting and heavy sweating.

Elimination Diets

See also Allergy; Lactose Intolerance.

At present, a strict elimination diet remains the best way to diagnose which foods or chemical components are triggers of intolerance reactions. The Elimination Diet was developed by the Allergy Unit at Sydney's Royal Prince Alfred Hospital.

Emulsifiers and Stabilisers

Emulsifiers are substances that stabilise mixtures and prevent oil and water from separating. In a salad dressing, for instance, an emulsifier keeps the oil and vinegar mixed so they don't separate into two layers on standing. Emulsifiers are closely related to fats and so can be considered quite safe. Lecithin (code number 322) is one of the most common emulsifiers and you will find it in things like margarine, chocolate, ice-cream, salad creams, cake mixes, pastry and coffee whiteners. Other emulsifiers include sorbitan monostearate (491) and monoglycerides and diglycerides of fatty acids (471).

See also Additives.

Energy Measures

See the table on page 97 to compare kilojoule and calorie counts for dietary intake and some popular foods.

Energy is the ability to do work, which can be chemical energy (from food), mechanical energy (in muscular activity) or thermal energy (as body heat). The units used to measure the energy of food and diets are the kilojoules (kJ). In the metric system, the kilojoule has replaced the kilocalorie (commonly called just calorie) and 1 calorie equals 4.186 kilojoules (4.2 or 4 is close enough for a quick conversion). For example, a thin or sandwich slice of bread supplies 250 kilojoules or 63 calories (250 divided by 4).

Energy and Energy Foods

Do you want more energy? Would you like to jump out of bed in the morning and power through your inbox? Busy, overworked people want energy, and lots of it! As a nutritionist, I find that the term energy is a most misunderstood word. These days it's everywhere—on energy drinks, energy bars, B vitamin pills and even breakfast cereals claiming to contain 'carbs for energy' as if there was something magical about their cereal.

The problem is that the term energy has two meanings. Tired people see energy on food and think it will give them more vitality and vigour for a healthy lifestyle. To a science-based person, however, energy refers to the fuel value supplied by food and diets and burned by activities. This is what's meant when you spot energy on a food label.

ENERGY MEASURES: COMPARING KILOJOULE AND CALORIE COUNTS

DIETARY INTAKE	KJ	CALORIES
Typical intake of most teenagers	10,000	2400
Average intake figure used to calculate %DI on food labels	8700	2070
A typical weight-loss level for a moderately active man	7500	1800
A typical weight-loss level for a sedentary man	7000	1650
A typical weight-loss level for a moderately active woman	6000	1500
A typical weight-loss level for a sedentary woman	5000	1200
Supervised fast or meal replacement intake—too low for normal activity	4000	1000

POPULAR FOODS	KJ	CALORIES
1 slice (30 g) bread	250	63
1 egg (60 g)	335	80
1 small (105 g) can pink salmon	525	125
2 Tim Tam biscuits	840	200
2 Krispy Kreme doughnuts (original glazed)	1680	400
1 cup orange juice	400	95
1 apple (150 g)	310	75
1 serve (25 g, approx. 3 fruit jellies or snakes) lollies	355	85

A high-energy food (seemingly positive) simply means it's high in kilojoules (not so positive), something to avoid if you're sedentary or overweight.

Energy drinks and chocolate bars are often promoted as high energy, together with images of athletes sprinting, running a marathon or doing push-ups. If that's what you do with your day, then you need high kilojoules. If you're a tired office worker getting little or no exercise then you definitely don't!

MY TAKE
Vitality comes from a balanced lifestyle, which sounds like an impossible myth but is much more achievable than you realise. I take it to mean a happy compromise between feeling good about yourself and eating healthy meals, doing something physical that you enjoy, and finding ways to relax and de-stress. I like to think of being in balance as being made up of two parts, inner balance and outer balance, rather like body and soul.

ENERGY DRINKS

An energy drink is another misleading term for the processed, coloured, flavoured caffeinated drinks sold at nightclubs and workplaces. The boost to energy from these comes from their caffeine (added, or from guarana) and sugar—simple! Caffeine is an effective aid to both mental and physical performance. We love it because it decreases our perception of fatigue and increases alertness for 2–3 hours, but then we crash. And if you're not active, beware of all that sugar—if you're not burning if off, it slips into your fat stores.

Overdo the caffeine and it can have side effects ranging from insomnia to the very serious cardiac arrhythmia in caffeine-sensitive people. In 2009, *The Medical Journal of Australia* published a report of a healthy 28-year-old man who suffered a cardiac arrest after consuming seven to eight cans of energy drinks within 7 hours (up to 640 milligrams caffeine). Energy drinks make it easy to overshoot your caffeine intake without realising.

NUMBER CRUNCH

One 250 ml can of energy drink gives us 0 grams of protein, 0 grams of fat, 11 grams of carbohydrate (of which 11 grams are sugars), 0 grams of fibre, 80 milligrams of sodium and 192 kilojoules.

ENERGY BARS AND NUT AND SEED BARS

Chock-full of sesame seeds, sunflower seeds, coconut, nuts, oats and dried fruit, bars line the counters of many juice bars and gyms (and were the forerunner of the now-popular breakfast cereal bars). Compared with chocolate bars and lollies, they obviously offer more fibre, vitamins and minerals and thus are a more nutritious snack. But what binds these ingredients together is honey, glucose or some form of sugar, which usually makes up about half the weight of the bar. Even sugar-free bars that are sweetened with dried fruit are high in natural sugars. Drying fruit removes water and concentrates the remaining sugars—dates, raisins and sultanas are 75 per cent sugar. Often regarded as healthier than biscuits or cake, these single-serve bars are no longer the humble oats and dried fruit fingers of old. Today, many come with chocolate chips or a thick yoghurt topping to make them more interesting, or they're a high-sugar processed version of bestselling kid's cereals.

Back in 2006, a *Choice* magazine survey of 150 brands of muesli bars, cereal bars and breakfast bars found most of them are more than 20 per cent sugar, and some deliver more saturated fat than a packet of chips. Even the 'fruit' in them can be a sham—a laboratory creation of fruity flavours, gels and sugar.

See also **Energy Measures; Caffeine.**

Erucic Acid

Erucic acid is a mono-unsaturated fatty acid with 22 carbon atoms that is usually found in mustard, rapeseed oil, cabbage and other plants of the brassica family, and fatty fish. In high concentrations it is toxic. A variety of rapeseed oil was bred to be low in erucic acid in Canada in the 1970s and is now known as canola oil.

Exercise

Regular exercise not only helps you lose weight, it's also important for general health and wellbeing. The key benefits of being physically active include:

- ✔ Lower blood cholesterol, including a proportion of the dangerous LDL cholesterol fraction
- ✔ Reduced blood pressure in mildly hypertensive people
- ✔ Lower blood-glucose levels, making your muscles better able to recognise insulin, which helps avoid type 2 diabetes
- ✔ Improved muscle strength and joint flexibility, which helps fight osteoarthritis
- ✔ Reduced risk of bone fractures and development of osteoporosis in later life, especially with weight-bearing exercise
- ✔ Improved sleeping patterns
- ✔ Reduced mild depression and stress
- ✔ Prolonged life among middle-aged and older men, although there might be a period of 5–10 years before an effect is seen on total mortality.

GET MOVING

In the past, the recommendation for exercise was to do 30 minutes of vigorous, continuous aerobic activity (like jogging) at least three times a week. Today's modern conveniences mean there are fewer physical demands in our daily lives, and obesity and lifestyle illnesses such as diabetes and heart disease are on the rise.

As a result, Active Australia published the National Physical Activity Guidelines as a set of more achievable recommendations that will still benefit overall health. They provide four ways to add activity and exercise to your day.

OPPORTUNITY, NOT INCONVENIENCE

If you can't get the closest spot in the car park, view the extra walk as healthy for your waistline.

INCIDENTAL EXERCISE

Use the stairs instead of the lift, walk to work or the shops, walk to someone's office instead of emailing them, do the mowing yourself instead of paying for it, hire an exercise bike and pedal while watching television or reading, attack the housework with vigour and energy, and take regular short breaks at work to stretch and use inactive muscles.

THIRTY MINUTES A DAY

Small amounts of light to moderately intense activity (such as walking) accumulated over the course of the day may be all that's required to stay healthy—provided it is regular (at least every second day). Remember, you can exercise in two or three short spells during the day; it doesn't have to be done in one block to be useful.

SPORTS

Vigorous sports such as lap swimming, singles tennis, aerobics, rowing, cycling and dancing can get you puffing—they are great for your health if you can manage them.

EXERCISE MYTHS

IT'S BEST TO EXERCISE IN THE MORNING

There is no reliable evidence to suggest we burn more kilojoules when we exercise in the morning. However, many people find getting their exercise done in the morning easier as there are fewer distractions or unexpected events so you don't miss out. Any exercise is better than no exercise, so choose the time of day that suits you best.

WEIGHTS MAKE WOMEN TOO MUSCLED

Incorrect. Women have less muscle than men and not enough testosterone to create big, bulky muscles. Just aiming for general strength and conditioning of muscles will not make a woman look like a body builder—that requires a lot more effort. Strength training (weights) helps women strengthen their muscles and bones. It also improves balance and lessens the likelihood of osteoporosis later on in life.

MUSCLE REPLACES FAT SO YOU WON'T LOSE WEIGHT

When you exercise aerobically on a regular basis and follow a diet, you may find the scales show no weight loss at all, or sometimes even a weight gain. Don't become discouraged. Muscle is heavier than fat and, as you lose body fat, you are replacing it with heavier muscle as well as increasing your muscle-to-fat ratio. Rather than registering on the scales, it will show up in your measurements. It is best not to weigh yourself more than once a week; instead rely on the measuring tape and how your clothes fit.

TRIMMING TROUBLE SPOTS

It is impossible to remove fat from only one problem spot of the body like the stomach, bottom or thighs, by exercising that area alone. Fat is lost from all over the body, not just the fattest part, but exercise can tone individual muscles and tighten loose skin. Generally your overall proportions remain the same. One weight loss expert has commented that large pears often slim into smaller pears!

The best way to slim a flabby tummy or large hips is by eating less (reducing the kilojoules consumed) and/or by aerobic exercise (increasing the kilojoules burnt up). The exercise may not even involve those parts of the body where trouble exists—have you ever seen a marathon runner with a fat stomach? With 'spot' exercises, like sit-ups for the stomach, you may just end up with a tight, fat stomach. The muscles underneath become tight, but the fat over the top remains there! You may still need to watch what you eat and start your whole body moving to shed the excess fat first. But if you have little fat covering your muscles, spot exercises can improve the shape of a particular muscle, resulting in lost centimetres and a more contoured outline.

PASSIVE EXERCISE CAN BREAK UP FAT AND CELLULITE

See also **Weight Loss.**

Passive exercises such as massages, rubs, vibrator belts or muscle stimulation are of no benefit. They do not break up the fat or work your muscles without effort from you.

Eye Health and Diet

Just as there are optimum ways of eating for a healthy heart, liver, skin, brain and kidneys, there is also one for the eyes. The nutrients in orange, green and yellow produce are all phytochemicals (antioxidants) that belong to a large family of more than 600 carotenoids. These can slow the progression of age-related macular degeneration (AMD), as can leafy greens that are rich in lutein and zeaxanthin, and egg yolks.

AMD is a progressive eye disease that affects the central macula of the eye, leaving sufferers with only peripheral vision. AMD Alliance International estimates that 25–30 million people are affected worldwide. It's the macula (the central part of the retina where light-sensitive cells send signals to the brain) that lets us see fine detail and is critical to our central vision, helping us to recognise faces, drive a car, read a book or newspaper, or do close handiwork.

It is one is the most common causes of blindness in those over 50 in the Western world. As we age our risk increases—people in their fifties have around a 2 per cent chance of suffering AMD, which then leaps to 30 per cent by the age of seventy-five. Exactly what causes it is still not fully understood, but if you have a parent with AMD, you have a 50 per cent risk of suffering from it yourself. Smokers have a four times greater risk than non-smokers, and those with high blood pressure, obesity or high cholesterol are also more likely to suffer from it. Looking after yourself in your later years can have a significant impact on how long your eyesight lasts.

Omega-3 fats from oily fish like salmon are the ultimate anti-ageing nutrients.

LUTEIN AND ZEAXANTHIN

These are two dietary carotenoid pigments found in the eye, and in greatest concentration in the macula. Their function appears to be the absorption of damaging UV-blue light and as antioxidant scavengers of destructive-free radicals. Foods rich in lutein and zeaxanthin are mostly the dark-green leafy types such as kale, spinach, lettuce, Brussels sprouts and cabbage, as well as colourful fruits and vegetables like red/orange capsicum, corn, mandarins and oranges. They may also be found in eggs, but the amount depends on the diet of the bird they come from. Some research has shown that people with the lowest concentration of lutein and zeaxanthin in their eye are more likely to have AMD and that having more of these in your diet, either from food or supplements, will increase eye tissue levels.

OMEGA-3S

These fats from oily fish like salmon are the ultimate anti-ageing nutrient. They are an integral part of the structure of your brain and nerve tissues, so they work to keep you mentally sharp (fish truly is brain food!). They're also good for your eyesight—the lens of the eye is particularly sensitive to any nutrient deficiency. One omega-3 called DHA plays a key role in the development of babies' brains and eyesight. It is abundant in breast milk and many cultures have traditionally fed fish to new mothers to increase their milk levels.

HOW TO MAKE YOUR EYESIGHT LAST

- ✔ Avoid smoking.
- ✔ Maintain a healthy weight that's right for you—neither too fat nor too thin.
- ✔ Eat large serves of dark-green vegetables and salad leaves as often as you can.
- ✔ Enjoy different-coloured fruits and vegetables for natural phytochemicals.
- ✔ Make the switch to low-GI carbs.
- ✔ Use oils rich in mono-unsaturated fat (olive, canola) or polyunsaturated fat (sunflower, grape seed); limit intake of saturated fats (dairy, takeaway, deli meats).
- ✔ Enjoy fish twice a week.
- ✔ Stay active to help manage your blood pressure and cholesterol.

CAN CARROTS HELP YOU SEE IN THE DARK?

Deficiency of vitamin A results in night blindness, which is an inability to see in dim light. If prolonged and severe, it can eventually lead to total blindness. Carrots were issued to British pilots during World War II in the hope of improving their night vision, and this has perpetuated the belief that carrots help you see in the dark. They certainly can help your vitamin A status, but whether eating lots really helps you see significantly better is debatable. Nonetheless it's a handy line for parents to remember to entice their kids to eat their vegetables!

Nutritionally carrots contain beta-carotene, an orange-yellow pigment that is converted to vitamin A in the body and is required for eyesight. It—and related carotenoids like alpha-carotene and lutein—have antioxidant activity that research suggests may protect against eye problems in later life.

F

Fast Food

In Australia it's estimated we buy over two million fast-food meals and snacks each day. On average, we spend one-third of our total food bill on food we eat outside the home, and there's no sign of this trend abating with our increasingly busy lives and the decline in home cooking skills. Despite the visibility of the big franchise chains like McDonald's, Subway, Pizza Haven and KFC, we actually spend more money in small independent takeaway shops on fish and chips, rotisserie chickens, burgers, sushi, Thai curries, meat pies and donor kebabs. Food courts, train stations, quick-service cafés and petrol stations with food outlets are where we're increasingly buying a meal to go, while the old-fashioned, freshly made sandwich shop has all but disappeared.

Some chains have done a lot in recent years to improve their offerings. McDonald's, for example, has changed the type of oil that they use to make their fries to one that's lower in saturated fat with almost no trans fat—a huge shift from the beef tallow they stuck to for years. They've also reduced the salt level in many items, added salad boxes and offered meal deals that are healthier or lowest in kilojoules such as the Filet-O-Fish plus salad and water.

Subway advertises its healthier rolls, each containing only 6 grams of fat, such as their Subway Six Inch Tuna or Six Inch Roast Beef rolls. Others have introduced grilled burgers and chicken pieces in place of the fried offerings. In addition, new gourmet burger chains, such as Grill'd, have sprung up making healthier grilled burgers.

THE QUICK SERVICE FOOD INITIATIVE

This roundtable of all the major chains has convened to work out how to make fast food healthier as a whole. Ideas include re-thinking the toy that baits children to buy a Happy Meal, cutting back on advertising directly to children, introducing green marketing with better biodegradable packaging, removing trans fat, and using less artificial colouring and fewer preservatives.

THE PROBLEM WITH FAST FOOD

Fast food is often sky-high in kilojoules, saturated fat and salt, which can make us fatter, clog our arteries and send our blood pressure through the roof. On its own, fast food does not make for a balanced meal, lacking vitamins and minerals for the number of kilojoules eaten, although it is frequently advertised as a 'complete meal'. While nutritionists admit that an occasional fast-food meal does no harm, they certainly do not recommend it more than once a week.

Not all fast food can be labelled as 'junk'. Some items do make a nutrient contribution, but at a price. A plain hamburger, for example, can supply about 25 per cent of the recommended intake of protein, iron and zinc for an adult man. A hamburger with cheese supplies 20 per cent of his calcium requirement as well—but it will also give him 1590 kilojoules, 17 grams fat and a hefty dose of salt.

In Australia it's estimated that we buy over two million fast-food meals and snacks each day.

LARGE PORTION SIZES

A takeaway meal can provide over half the suggested daily intake of kilojoules for most women and children. It is certainly no between-meal snack. From cheese-crust pizzas to deluxe sumo burgers, fast-food portions are big. Everything is 'super', 'whopper' or 'jumbo', appearing to give customers maximum value (and unfortunately kilojoules). A

MY TAKE
I'm in favour of having highly visible kilojoule counts on fast-food (and other) menus. I believe it will help many people make better choices at least sometimes, if not every time. Kilojoule counts give us a way of comparing menu items. For example, if you can see that large fries have almost double the kilojoules of small fries, you can choose to opt for the small bag. Or seeing the kilojoules may help you downscale to a single burger instead of a double burger with extra cheese and a hash brown. Many people don't realise that they can easily consume almost 50 per cent of their daily kilojoule allowance just by eating a big hamburger with fries.

standard fast-food burger will pile on about 20 grams of fat (10 grams of it saturated) and 1800 kilojoules.

A standard serve size is now double or triple that of a few decades ago. When McDonald's first began in 1955, a serve of French fries weighed only 72 grams; today it's a fat-inducing 205 grams—almost three times as much. Coke was served in a 200 millilitre glass; now it comes in a whopping 950 millilitre bucket. Meal deals, two-for-one offers or 'free drink with your order' vouchers only encourage overconsumption. It is value for money, but it's a bargain our waistlines don't need. Fast food also promotes fast eating, which only contributes to the obesity problem.

> When McDonald's first began in 1955, a serve of French fries weighed only 72 g; today it's a fat-inducing 205 g—almost three times as much.

TOO MUCH 'BAD' FAT

Even if it's not deep fried, fast food has plenty of hidden fat. Fat keeps buns and pizza bases soft and moist, while making fries and chips crisp. And it's the worst type of fat, namely saturated or trans fats, which raise blood cholesterol and your risk of heart disease and diabetes. Until recently, the common commercial frying fats were either beef tallow or palm oil (often advertised as 'vegetable oil'), both of which are saturated and unhealthy. McDonald's switched to frying in a modified canola oil, which helped remove tonnes of saturated fat from the food supply.

TOO MUCH SALT

Just about everything in fast food contains salt—from the buns, pizza bases and chicken crumbing to pickles and sauce—because salt is a cheap way to add flavour. It's nearly impossible to get a low-sodium fast-food meal. With the upper limit of sodium intake pegged at 2300 milligrams a day, one fast-food meal alone gives you around half the day's intake.

LET'S COMPARE KILOJOULES, FAT AND SODIUM

	QUARTER POUNDER AND REGULAR FRIES	FRIED CHICKEN, 2 PIECES PLUS REGULAR CHIPS	SUPREME PIZZA, 3 SLICES FROM A LARGE PAN PIZZA	FISH AND CHIPS	STEAK SANDWICH
Kilojoules	3620	3671	2292	3760	1498
Fat (g)	47.6	45.2	25.5	53.2	17.3
Saturated fat (g)	16.7	11.0	14.7	24.9	4.6
Sodium (mg)	1330	1255	1311	1099	487

TOO MUCH SUGAR

Sugar isn't a problem with main-meal items, but the fizzy drinks, thick shakes, smoothies, sundaes, cookies and hotcakes that go with them contain lots of it.

NOT ENOUGH VEGETABLES AND SALAD

In the past, fast-food outlets offered few salads or vegetables and nothing wholemeal, as they would interfere with the soft texture of fast food. You were hard-pressed to get any fibre or wholegrains. New salad menus and take-home cartons of salads now being offered by the chains have made a big difference, but it's still not widespread enough.

TOO FEW VITAMINS OR MINERALS

Levels of vitamin C and folic acid can fall short, unless you drink orange juice or help yourself to the salad bar. Calcium is hard to obtain without a milkshake or cheese on your burger. Holding food at hot temperatures before sale will also affect the heat-sensitive B vitamins, like vitamin B_1 and folate.

FAST-FOOD SWEETS	SUGARS (g)
Cola, large 660 ml	53
Cola, medium 430 ml	35
Cola, small 300 ml	24
Strawberry shake, large 550 ml	75*
Strawberry shake, medium 410 ml	55*
Strawberry shake, small 300 ml	41*
Hot fudge sundae	47*
Choc chip cookie	16

* These figures also include natural sugars from milk and fruit.

KILOJOULES, THE IN-YOUR-FACE FACTS

From 2012, all major fast-food chains in NSW, Victoria and SA began displaying the kilojoule counts of their food with the same prominence as the price. It's not only the McDonald's, Pizza Huts, Pizza Havens, Eagle Boys and KFCs that have to comply—any food restaurant with 20 or more outlets in each state, or 50 or more nationwide, will have to display the average adult daily energy intake of 8700 kilojoules plus the kilojoule content of all their menu items.

KILOJOULE COUNTS ARE NOT A MAGIC BULLET

I am under no illusions that this will solve the obesity crisis. People who are in a hurry will still want to grab a quick meal on the road and pull over into the drive-through at a burger, pizza or chicken place. However, one reason many types of fast food are fattening is because you eat with your hands, not a knife and fork. You eat while you walk or drive, not seated at a table. Chowing down quickly makes it very easy to over-eat. For this reason, it's very important not to over-order in the first place, and this is where those kilojoule counts on the menu can help you reign in your eating and spending.

BETTER FAST-FOOD CHOICES

	ORDER THIS	NOT THAT
McDonald's	Grilled chicken burger with salad and small fries, yoghurt berry crumble.	Big Mac and large fries, strawberry sundae.
Pizza Hut, Pizza Haven, Dominos, Eagle Boys	Vegetarian or marinara on thin 'n' crispy crust.	Super supreme pan pizza with cheesy crust.
KFC	Roast chicken breast, mashed potato and gravy, corn cob.	KFC chicken pieces (with skin), potato wedges.
Hungry Jack's	Aussie burger with beetroot and onion.	Double whopper burger with cheese.
Subway	Turkey breast, ham, roast beef or any of the seven subs with fewer than 6 g of fat.	Meatball sub or Italian pepperoni sub.
Chinese/Asian	Stir-fried vegetables and beef or chicken, with steamed noodles or brown rice, or steamed or boiled noodles with vegetables.	Sweet and sour chicken or pork with fried noodles or fried rice.
Mexican	Soft wheat tortillas filled with lean beef, beans and tomato.	Nachos with melted cheese, guacamole and sour cream.

ADVERTISING

The problem with the fast-food chains is the vast amount they spend on television advertising, offering special deals, convenience, friendly service, hygiene and freedom from cooking. Before you realise it's happened, an occasional eating out treat becomes a daily habit. Motivating children and teenagers to eat at their local fast-food chain is a key aim of much advertising, and many parents worry about the effect this has on their children's eating habits. Children may come to like French fries instead of plain potatoes, thick shakes in place of milk and sweetened buns over regular bread.

THE SKINNY ON CHIPS

Whether straight-cut, fries or wedges, Australians consume a staggering 250 million serves of chips each year; they are the standard accompaniment to most fast food and to kids' meals at restaurants. But chips get the thumbs down from nutritionists due to their high fat content (an average bucket of hot chips packs a whopping 23 grams of fat), which is usually saturated, and the added salt.

The Heart Foundation and the University of Auckland surveyed 150 fast-food outlets and found that only 17 per cent cooked chips at the right temperature and that 39 per cent of fryer thermostats were inaccurate. If the temperature is too low, chips take longer to cook and tend to absorb more oil. If the temperature is too high, the chips turn out dark and the oil develops off-flavours and potential carcinogens (cancer-causing compounds).

Fasting

There are numerous reasons why people may need to fast for a short period of time, be it for a religious cause, for medical tests, or for an operation. That said, there are some people who should not fast. These include pregnant women, those who've had surgery recently, or anyone with diabetes, ulcers, heart conditions or kidney complaints. You will also need to seek your doctor's advice if you have been sick recently with the flu or gastro, if you are under 12 years old (going without food for charity is OK for up to eight hours), or if you are planning to play sport.

If you do fast, be sure to ease your way back to normal eating when you finish by having something light and healthy such as a salad, fruit or a soup. It's best to stay off fatty foods and milk for about eight hours, and stick to clear fluids like water, soft drink and weak black tea. Also avoid eating too much as your stomach will have shrunk and needs time to readjust.

FASTING FOR WEIGHT LOSS

Long-term fasting as a way to lose weight is unhealthy and can be dangerous. A short fast, say for 24 hours, to help rest and 'cleanse' your body may be beneficial. But fasting deprives your body of nutrients and does nothing to help you re-learn a healthier way of eating. Prolonged fasting can lead to loss of muscle tissue, headaches, low energy, weakness; light-headedness and constipation and can trigger an increase in food cravings.

When you fast, your body doesn't realise it's temporary—it thinks you're heading into a famine. So to conserve energy and fat-stores, it starts to slow down your metabolism, which burns kilojoules more slowly. Once you start eating again, it's easier to regain the lost weight and you'll find it more difficult to lose weight in the future.

RAMADAN

People of the Muslim faith must fast during daylight hours during the month of Ramadan. The elderly, chronically ill and mentally ill are exempt from fasting, although the first two groups must endeavour to feed the poor in place of their missed fasting. Pregnant women are also exempt if they believe it would be harmful to them or their unborn baby, as are women during their menstruation. Anyone who is travelling (*musaafir*) is exempt, but must make up the days they miss.

A recent Moroccan study found that most people with type 2 diabetes, which was well controlled before Ramadan, could safely observe Ramadan fasting. However, it's wise to seek the advice of your healthcare team before starting and at the end of the fast, since they may advise you to change the times or amount of medication you take.

Tips to follow if you have diabetes:

- Do not stop taking your medication.
- Avoid eating lots of unhealthy foods as a reward. Try to maintain a healthy eating pattern after you break the fast. Make sure that you have lots of non-starchy vegetables and dhal as these are slowly digested and help your blood glucose to rise more slowly too. Remember to drink plenty of fluids.
- Divide your daily food intake into two equal portions, one to be taken at *Sehri* and one at *Iftar*.
- Remember to check your glucose level regularly, at least once a day at different times of the day.

TIPS WHEN FASTING FOR A CAUSE

- ✔ Drink plenty of water, mineral or soda water, weak black tea, green tea, herbal teas or well-diluted fruit juice (one part juice to four parts water).
- ✔ Suck a boiled sweet (e.g. barley sugar). Have one every four hours or so to keep your blood glucose up, but check with your doctor first if you are fasting prior to a medical test or procedure.
- ✔ Conserve energy. You may not really feel hungry, but you will feel lethargic. This is the main problem, so try to keep your activities as stationary as possible.

See also Detox Diets.

Fat-burning Foods and Drinks

It sounds like a dieter's dream: you eat certain foods and they magically speed up your metabolism, burn off your body fat, 'dissolve' it away or put you in 'kilojoules deficit'. They don't exist or if they do, the effect is so small it is insignificant. Here are the products that pop up time and again.

CHINESE DIET TEAS

Advertised as miracle slimming products (but often with little description of their ingredients), there's scant proof that slimming teas work. Most have only a minor effect on metabolic rate or insulin sensitivity. Some contain natural diuretics, which force your body to flush more water, while some contain herbs with laxative properties, which encourage diarrhoea.

CHILLI AND HOT SPICES

Extracts of chilli (capsaicin) and hot spices such as black pepper (piperine), ginger (zingerone) and turmeric (curcumin) have been shown to raise the metabolic rate and/or increase the feeling of fullness (satiety) in a number of studies. In combination with caffeine, they contributed to minor weight loss and a slight increase of metabolism.

While promising, remember that these trials did not look at chilli consumed as a regular part of the diet, but as capsules or liquid extracts. It may be hard to get the dose up high enough from the spice alone.

CELERY

This is one of several foods pushed by negative kilojoule promoters. The list usually includes the same low-kilojoule 'free vegetables' that you eat to quell hunger pangs such as asparagus, broccoli, cabbage, cauliflower, carrot, cucumber, green beans and zucchini. Tough, fibrous, water-filled celery is the favourite. When you eat a stick of it raw (theoretically containing 15 kilojoules), you expend more than 15 kilojoules chewing and digesting it. Your body has to get the energy from somewhere, so it's forced to draw the kilojoules it needs from your body fat—or so the theory goes.

Even if this theory was correct (which it isn't), you'd only save at most 15 kilojoules from each stick of celery, hardly enough to combat the daily load of over 8700 kilojoules most of us consume. However, if your mouth is busy chewing celery, there's no room for chips or chocolate!

CAFFEINE

Black coffee and energy drinks are often used by models, ballet dancers and others trying to remain thin and quiet the hunger pangs of a strict diet. Caffeine triggers the release of fatty acids into the bloodstream, which provides an alternative fuel to glycogen. Coffee is also high in fibre, which could also help. The downside is caffeine's well-known side effects of insomnia and stomach upsets.

GRAPEFRUIT

Often regarded as a slimming food with the power to 'dissolve' unwanted flab, grapefruit has appeared on breakfast menus for dieters ever since the 1960s, when grapefruit diets first rose to popularity. The fruit's sour taste has no doubt contributed to this impression, but it has no special slimming powers. Half a grapefruit supplies around 125 kilojoules, the same as from half an orange. It is also rich in vitamin C and fibre. And don't believe all you read on the internet—pineapple isn't a slimming food either.

CIDER VINEGAR

Often promoted as a slimming aid by the health-food industry, cider vinegar has no magical weight-dissolving properties. It is sometimes marketed in combination with kelp, vitamin B_6 and lecithin as a diet supplement, but none of these have been scientifically proven to speed up weight loss.

FIBRE SUPPLEMENTS

Fibre supplements (powders, granules or tablets) are designed to be taken with water before a meal to swell up in the stomach and create a feeling of fullness. Made of psyllium, cellulose, guar gum or citrus fibre, they are helpful for people who tune in to their body's signals of satiety and cease eating when full. But for dieters who binge, they are of limited benefit. Fibre pills are expensive and are no substitute for food fibre if your diet is deficient. It would be cheaper and better for you to switch to more high-fibre foods instead.

CHITOSAN

Chitosan and its precursor chitan have been hailed as 'fat binders' with the power to soak up any fat eaten and then excrete it. Advertisements often show a beaker of oil with chitosan being mixed in and then forming clumps of fat. The idea is that it does the same thing in your digestive tract. A 2005 trial of the weight-loss supplement on 24 men and women in the USA was the fifth study to reach the conclusion that chitosan does not work. The volunteers were fed 2.5 grams of chitosan a day (10 capsules) and the researchers detected a mere 1.8 grams of extra fat excreted in the men and no difference in the women. The researchers concluded that chitosan was a waste of money.

Even if it did work, chitosan could only mop up so much fat. In the laboratory, a gram of chitosan can bind around 3 grams of fat. But with average fat intake somewhere between 80 and 100 grams a day, the amount of fat trapped would be too small to make any difference to fat excretion. The bottom line is that you will still need to cut back on fat.

CHROMIUM PICOLINATE

Promoters of the supplement chromium picolinate say that it lowers blood glucose and insulin levels, which stops any fat from being stored. It's been heavily hyped as a weight-loss aid and a means to improve sports performance, but proof that it helps burn fat is scant. Chromium is an essential mineral and is involved in the metabolism of carbohydrate, protein and fat, and it also helps insulin transfer glucose into cells. Picolinate supposedly increases chromium absorption.

WEIGHT-LOSS PILLS

Pills containing the Chinese herb *ma huang* (also known as ephedra) have been sold for weight loss. A medicinal plant cultivated for thousands of years in China, it has been used there to help asthma and bronchial conditions. But *ma huang* has been removed from sale in the US because its two active alkaloids, ephedrine and pseudoephedrine, can increase blood pressure and heart rate and may be dangerous for anyone with a heart condition, diabetes, hypertension or thyroid disease.

See also **Weight Loss.**

Fat and Fatty Acids

Cholesterol. Saturated fats. Trans fats. Mono-unsaturated fats. Omega-3s. Fish oils. Olive oil. Good fats. Bad fats. Over the past few years, no other nutrient has had as much attention as fat. However, we often forget that fat is an essential nutrient, needed for good health, just like protein and vitamins. It would be difficult, and undesirable, to avoid all fat. Children in particular need some fat in their meals, in order to grow and develop correctly—a low-fat diet is not recommended for young children under the age of 2 years.

FAT IS IMPORTANT

- ✔ It supplies two essential fatty acids (linoleic acid and alpha-linolenic acid), which our bodies cannot manufacture.
- ✔ It provides insulation and 'cushioning' for internal organs and reproductive organs.
- ✔ Fat spares protein for its primary role of building.
- ✔ It serves as a carrier of fat-soluble vitamins (vitamins A, D, E and K) and phytochemicals such as beta-carotene and lycopene.
- ✔ Fat is the most concentrated supplier of kilojoules, having twice as many per gram as carbohydrate or protein.

GOOD AND BAD FATS

Not only the amount of fat you consume, but also the type of fat you consume, can make a big difference to your health. When it comes to things like blood cholesterol levels or diabetes, not all fats are 'bad'. Most saturated and trans fats are the culprits, but mono- and polyunsaturated fats are beneficial and can be consumed in reasonable amounts, as they are in the Mediterranean Diet. Remember that all fats, regardless of type, supply the same amount of fat and kilojoules per gram.

Fats are oily or waxy substances made up of fatty acids attached to a glycerol 'backbone'. It's these fatty acids that determine whether a food is more saturated or more mono-unsaturated or polyunsaturated. No fat is completely saturated or completely polyunsaturated. The predominant fat gives the food its classification. For example, olive oil is classed as mono-unsaturated, yet contains 70 per cent mono-unsaturated fats plus 15 per cent polyunsaturated and 15 per cent saturated.

ESSENTIAL FATTY ACIDS

Two essential fatty acids—linoleic acid, which belongs to the omega-6 family, and alpha-linolenic acid, of the omega-3 family—cannot be made in the body and must be provided by our diet. They are necessary for growth and development and for maintaining health. Once in the body, they are elongated and converted to longer-chain versions eicosapentaenoic acid (EPA), docosahexaenoic acid (DHA) and arachidonic acid (AA). These provide the building blocks for compounds known as eicosanoids, which are precursors for prostaglandins. These hormone-like substances are important in the formation of cell membranes and are involved in blood clotting, wound healing and inflammation. Although the body is able to convert some alpha-linolenic acid into the long-chain versions, the conversion is quite limited, usually estimated at around 15 per cent. For this reason we also need direct sources of the long-chain omega-3 fats from food.

SATURATED FATS

These tend to be solid and are found mainly in animal foods such as butter, cream, meat fat, cheese, milk fat, lard and dripping. However, two vegetable oils are saturated and are used in the food industry. Palm oil (50 per cent saturated) is derived from a tropical palm and is widely used for deep-frying in fast-food outlets and to make snack foods, pastries and biscuits. It is commonplace because it is cheap and readily available and has good storing qualities. Coconut oil (90 per cent saturated) is a fat with unique characteristics necessary to make certain types of biscuits, pies, confectionery and fillings for chocolates.

Both of these products are often listed as 'vegetable oil' on food packs, so there is no way of knowing they are present. Saturated fats (not all) tend to raise the 'bad' LDL cholesterol, which increases your risk of heart problems. Both palm oil and coconut oil have been linked to type 2 diabetes and certain types of cancer, notably bowel, prostate and breast. We need to eat less of these types of fats.

MONO-UNSATURATED FATS

These fats are found predominantly in olives, olive oil, canola oil, avocados, peanuts, peanut oil, and most other nuts. All oils contain some mono-unsaturates, as do lean meats, chicken, eggs and fish. Mono-unsaturates reduce levels of LDL cholesterol in the blood, although not as effectively as the polyunsaturates. But they tend to be more stable and less likely to oxidise, so draw less on antioxidants.

POLYUNSATURATED FATS

Polyunsaturates occur in the germ of all grains (e.g. wheatgerm) and are extracted from seeds such as sunflower, safflower, soy beans, cottonseed, maize, sesame and grape seed to make cooking oils. Polyunsaturated fats are good for reducing total cholesterol, which has made them an important component in diets for the heart.

OMEGA-3 FATS

Omega-3s are a sub-group of polyunsaturates with a slightly different chemical structure from other polyunsaturates (which chemically are known as omega-6s). Fish (especially oily fish such as herring, salmon, tuna, mackerel and sardines) and seafood contain EPA and DHA, two highly polyunsaturated fats that can reduce the tendency for the blood to clot and so lessen its 'stickiness'. The Inuit people, Japanese villagers living by the sea and other fish-eating groups are known to have a low rate of heart disease. This is attributed largely to their high intake of fish.

TRANS FATS

Trans fatty acids are polyunsaturated or mono-unsaturated fatty acids that can raise LDL cholesterol to the same degree as saturated fats. Although chemically they are unsaturated, trans fats have a different configuration of atoms and so behave biologically as if they were saturated.

Humans have been consuming trans fatty acids for centuries, as they occur naturally in butter, milk, beef and lamb. But the industrial trans fats are the ones to worry about. They are formed during the manufacture of commercial fats, when liquid vegetable oils are hydrogenated (hardened) to turn them into semi-solid spreads. In Australia and New Zealand, the intake of trans fats is lower than in the US or the UK. Most margarines (the soft types for spreading) have been free of trans fats since the 1990s.

CHOLESTEROL AND FAT

Cholesterol, a waxy, fat-like compound found in the blood, is different from fat. Researchers now consider cholesterol from food less of a concern to heart health than saturated fats, as the body manufactures its own cholesterol and can cut back on production when there is a lot eaten, such as after a meal of several eggs or brains. For most people, reducing the saturated fats they consume is of greater benefit than restricting the cholesterol from eggs, organ meats, seafood or other animal foods.

HOW MUCH IS HEALTHY?

This is not a simple issue. You have to take into consideration not only how much, but what type of fat to eat, as well as whether you're at risk of high cholesterol, heart disease or type 2 diabetes. One or 2 tablespoons of a good oil or some nuts, avocado, wheatgerm, salad dressing or mayonnaise per day is enough to supply good nutrition. The trouble is most of us exceed this intake many times over.

Nutritionists recommend that our fat intake should be 30 per cent or less of the total kilojoules consumed, with the emphasis on mono- and polyunsaturated in preference to saturated fats. Most of us should aim to reduce the fat we eat by a third or even half. The table shows how many grams of fat you can eat if you reduce your fat intake to 30 per cent of total kilojoules a day.

	KILOJOULE INTAKE	30 % KJ FROM FAT (g)
Moderately active woman	8400	65 g
Sedentary woman	6300	50 g
Aiming for fat loss, woman	5000	40 g
Moderately active man	10,500	85 g
Sedentary man	8400	65 g
Aiming for fat loss, man	6300	50 g

Here's how a typical daily fat intake adds up for adult men and women.

85 GRAMS FAT FOR A MODERATELY ACTIVE MAN

Oil, 1 tbsp for cooking	20
Margarine or mayonnaise, 2 tsp	10
Avocado, ½	20
Milk, low-fat, 1 glass	6
Yoghurt, low-fat, 200 g tub	4
Almonds or walnuts, 30g	15
From fish, meat or chicken	10
TOTAL	85 g

40 GRAMS FAT FOR A WOMAN AIMING FOR FAT LOSS

Oil, ½ tbsp for cooking	10
Low-fat spread or light mayonnaise, 2 tsp	6
Egg, 1	6
Milk, skim, 300 ml	0
Yoghurt, low-fat, 200 g tub	4
Cottage cheese, 200 g tub	6
From fish, meat or chicken	8
TOTAL	40 g

WAYS TO CUT BACK ON SATURATED FATS

- Trim away visible fat from meat and skin from chicken.
- Use cooking methods that require minimal fat or oil like grilling, stir-frying, steaming, poaching, microwaving, boiling and baking.
- When roasting, place meat or chicken on a rack to allow the fat to drain away.
- Roast vegetables in a separate pan sprayed or brushed with a little oil.
- Leave soups, curries and casseroles to cool overnight in the refrigerator and skim off all surface fat the next day.
- Forget about frying; instead sauté in a little olive or canola oil or use an oil spray.
- Switch to low-fat milks, low-fat yoghurts and reduced-fat cheeses instead of full-fat types.
- Use ricotta and cottage cheese more often.
- Replace some saturated fats with unsaturated fats.
- Use mono- or polyunsaturated oil for cooking and salads.
- Use soft margarine or reduced-fat spreads in place of butter.
- Avoid creamy salad dressings and use a simple oil and vinegar dressing or buy a light mayonnaise.

> Over the past few years, no other nutrient has had as much attention as fat. However, we often forget that fat is an essential nutrient, needed for good health, just like protein and vitamins.

WEIGHT LOSS AND FAT

Gram for gram, fat packs in more kilojoules than either carbohydrate or protein. For example, 10 grams of pure fat supplies 370 kilojoules, while 10 grams of pure carbohydrate provides only 160 kilojoules and 10 grams of protein supplies 170 kilojoules. This means a low-fat diet is a more painless way to keep the kilojoules low. In addition, excess dietary fat is not readily oxidised (burnt up) but is quite efficiently stored as body fat around the stomach, hips and thighs. With the abundant supply of food in our society, that famine never arrives!

Eating fat also appears to give you less satisfaction than eating carbohydrate or protein, so your stomach doesn't feel as full after a high-fat meal nor is your appetite as adequately suppressed. These are all sound reasons to minimise the fat you eat when trying to shed excess weight. But cutting back on fat doesn't mean cutting it out. We need some mono- and polyunsaturated fats for good health, just like we need protein, vitamins and minerals. On a typical weight-loss diet, women should eat no less than 40 grams a day and men no less than 50 grams a day.

See also **Fast Food; Weight Loss.**

Fatty Liver and Diet

Our liver, one of the key organs of metabolism in the body, is susceptible to the excesses of modern life. And as our waistlines are burgeoning and the obesity crisis grows bigger, it's suffering. Non-alcoholic fatty liver (or NAFL as doctors call it) now affects around 25 per cent of the Australian population. As the name suggests, fatty liver disease is the accumulation of fat within the cells of the liver because it is unable to break down the fats at the rate at which it usually does. If left untreated, this liver can become inflamed and scar gradually which may progress to liver failure, cirrhosis and liver cancer.

Fatty liver disease is thought to be aggravated by carrying too much weight, uncontrolled diabetes, the influence of certain chemicals and medications and sometimes by a form of weight loss that is too rapid, such as gastric bypass, overzealous fad diets or fasting.

The good news is that a healthy diet and lifestyle can reverse this—as long as you don't leave it too late. Losing weight is essential. Start by cutting out snacks and rich food and eating smaller portions. Enjoy your dinner out, but go for fish or a lean steak and order double serves of vegetables or salad. Give up white bread and swap to low-GI carbs such as grainy bread, porridge oats, lentils and yoghurt. These 'slow carbs' will help you lose weight and call for less insulin. And try to exercise every day; it can make a big difference. Finally, it's best to abstain completely from alcohol for 6 months or until your liver is better. If your liver is labouring to cope with its load, it's wise to abstain completely to get your liver working at peak performance again.

Fibre

Eating more fibre is one of the best and easiest ways to improve your daily diet. In fact, fibre was probably responsible for the old saying 'an apple a day keeps the doctor away'! Fibre is now recognised as a food factor that can help prevent many of the illnesses of affluent countries.

Once known as roughage or bulk, fibre is what's left over after our body has finished digestion. It consists of a number of carbohydrate compounds plus lignin and gums. Most of these are not digested in the small intestine because, unlike grazing animals, humans do not possess the enzymes to break them down. Bacteria living in our large intestines, however, make use of this waste residue and partially reduce it to volatile fatty acids, which we occasionally pass as wind. Fibre is divided into two major categories.

INSOLUBLE FIBRE

This is made up of mostly cellulose, lignin (a 'woody' component) and hemicelluloses. Insoluble fibre does not dissolve in water; as it travels through your intestinal tract, its form stays relatively the same. It aids bowel function by increasing the weight of the faeces (providing bulk) and by speeding the transit of material through the bowel, both of which are important for preventing constipation. It also helps to create a friendly environment for 'good' bacteria. Good sources of insoluble fibre are wheat bran, bran cereals, wholegrain cereals and wholemeal breads, carrots and cabbage.

SOLUBLE FIBRE

Soluble fibre encompasses pectin, gums and mucilages as well as some hemicelluloses. It partially dissolves in water and so, once consumed, starts to form a gel in your intestines, and this gel is what slows the flow of material through your digestive tract and gives you a feeling of fullness, also known as satiety. This gel also removes cholesterol from the body. Good are oats, oat bran, barley, apples, prunes and legumes.

SHOPPER'S GUIDE

Legumes (dried beans, peas and lentils), vegetables, grains, nuts and fruit are all good sources of fibre. Next time you are in the supermarket, add some of these fibre foods to your shopping trolley. Try wheat bran, bran breakfast cereal, rice bran, oat bran, dried figs, passionfruit, muesli, wheat biscuit cereals, brown rice, wholemeal pasta, wholemeal flour, dried dates, dried apricots, prunes, wholemeal bread, nuts, green peas, canned beans and lentils, Brussel sprouts, broccoli and mixed grain bread.

CHOOSE THIS	NOT THAT
Whole oranges or pears cut into quarters	Juice
Sprinkle 1 tablespoon wheat bran or oat bran over Weet-Bix or Vita Brits. Rolled oats or muesli	Rice Bubbles, Corn Flakes
Wholemeal bread, grainy bread, rye bread, pumpernickel or rye crispbread	White bread
Bran and apple muffin Replace ¼ cup of flour in your recipes with oat bran or psyllium	Butter cake
Brown rice Baked jacket potato Corn on the cob Add ½ cup peas to your rice	White rice
Ice-cream with fruit salad	Ice-cream and flavouring
Oatmeal biscuits Fruitcake Dried fruit and nut snack pack	Sweet biscuits
Peanuts, Corn chips	Chips

FIVE REASONS TO EAT MORE FIBRE

MAINTAINS HEALTH

Eating a fibre-rich diet can help prevent many of the illnesses of later life like gallstones, bowel (colon) cancer, haemorrhoids and diverticulitis. Fibre helps prevent cancer in a number of ways. It dilutes the bowel contents and shortens the time for the food residue to pass through, thus minimising contact with any carcinogens (cancer-causing substances) ingested. It has also the ability to bind possible cancer agents and excrete them.

ENCOURAGES THE GROWTH OF FRIENDLY BACTERIA

Scientists have discovered that the bacteria living normally in the bowel can ferment fibre to produce gases and short-chain fatty acids, which prevent tumours and polyps forming.

KEEPS YOU REGULAR

Fibre offers the safest, simplest solution to relieve constipation. It increases the bulk of the stool, giving the faeces the correct soft consistency so they can be eliminated without effort. Bowel motions are passed more easily and more frequently and you won't need to resort to laxatives and enemas. You also need to drink six to eight glasses of water a day and do some regular exercise.

FLUSHES OUT CHOLESTEROL

Soluble types of fibre (oat bran, barley bran, rice bran, pectin, guar gum and dried beans) bind and hold bile acids and sterols, end products of cholesterol metabolism, and sweep them out in the faeces. This prevents them from re-entering the bloodstream and lowers blood cholesterol levels.

HELPS MANAGE BLOOD-GLUCOSE LEVELS

Soluble-fibre foods also slow down the absorption of glucose during digestion so it trickles into the bloodstream, making less demand on insulin production. Many high-fibre foods such as fruit and grainy bread are also low GI.

WHAT FIBRE IS THAT?

Just as we need different vitamins, a number of fibre components are essential to good health.

CELLULOSE

Cellulose is found in all plant foods, but especially in wholegrains, brans, wholemeal bread, dried fruit and vegetables from the cabbage family. It helps produce bulkier, softer stools.

A DAY ON A HIGH-FIBRE DIET

This menu plan offers plenty of fibre from wholegrains, beans, fruit and vegetables. Enjoy large serves of these to reach a goal of 30–40 g or more of fibre a day.

- BREAKFAST—Bran cereal or muesli with low-fat milk and soft prunes, or wholegrain breakfast biscuits with low-fat milk and a sliced banana (sprinkle a tablespoon of bran or psyllium husks over your usual cereal).
- LUNCH—Wholemeal pocket bread filled with sliced, lean cold meat, lettuce, grated carrot and sprouts and a fresh pear or apple.
- DINNER—Grilled or pan-fried whiting fillet served on wilted spinach with pumpkin and lentil risotto, and stewed soft apricots and prunes with custard for dessert.
- SNACKS to choose from—Two rye or grainy crispbreads with peanut butter, an apple or pear, celery and carrot sticks, a small handful of unsalted nuts, a small handful of dried fruit.

LIGNIN

Lignin escapes digestion, even by bacteria in the bowel. It literally goes 'in one end and out the other'. It's mainly found in wheat bran and bran cereals.

HEMICELLULOSES

These are found in grains, vegetables, fruit and beans and are not related to cellulose. They have a high water-binding capacity, which, like cellulose, helps produce bulkier, softer stools.

PECTIN

Pectin's ability to form a gel is crucial in making jam, and it is this very action that helps us stay healthy. In the intestine, it creates a thick gelatinous mass which traps nutrients and slows down their absorption—important for preventing diabetes and lowering cholesterol. The richest sources are apples, citrus fruit and sugar beet, although all fruits are high.

Q

Is fibre OK for irritable bowel syndrome (IBS)?

A

IBS is a common digestive complaint characterised by abdominal pain, bloating, wind, diarrhoea and/or constipation. While high-fibre foods were once routinely prescribed, they may make things worse in a percentage of cases. They're helpful if you're constipated, but avoid specific foods if they cause pain or distension. The best approach is personal trial and error, bearing in mind that food intolerances also may co-exist and it would be worth having a chat to an accredited practising dietitian for an eating plan that will help you.

See also **Irritable Bowel Syndrome.**

GUMS AND MUCILAGES

These form a thick viscous mass in water and some, such as guar gum, have been extensively studied for their ability to lower cholesterol. Natural gums include gum arabic, and extracts from seaweed like agar, carrageenan (Irish moss) and alginate. Seeds such as slippery elm, carob seeds (locust beans), okra and quince seeds yield mucilages. Psyllium is a mucilage from the seeds of the *plantago* plant.

Q
Which bran is best?
A
All brans are useful but act in different ways in the body. At over 40 per cent fibre, wheat bran has the highest fibre content and is rich in insoluble fibre. It is the best choice for your bowel. Oat and barley bran contain some 17 per cent fibre, mostly soluble, so they help lower cholesterol. Rice bran, with 26 per cent fibre, lies in between and has a mix of both sorts of fibre.

See also **Bran.**

DAILY REQUIREMENTS

Most adults consume only about two-thirds of the fibre they should be eating, which is about 30 grams a day. For children, you should use the 'age+5' rule—simply add 5 to their age to come up with the quantity of fibre they should eat in grams. For example, a 10 year old would need 10+5=15 grams of fibre a day.

FIBRE SUPPLEMENTS

You're better off eating high-fibre food than taking supplements. The quantity of fibre contained in tablets is quite small (generally less than 3 grams), and they're expensive. They're an easy pre-meal filler; supplements like methylcellulose, psyllium or guar gum taken with water before a meal absorb water and swell in the stomach, creating a feeling of fullness, so you eat less. They also create a soft bulky stool, and act as a laxative and so prevent some kilojoules being fully absorbed.

Fibre powders, granules and sprinkles usually contain some form of soluble fibre such as psyllium or sterculia (brand names include Metamucil, Fybogel, Nucolox, Normafibre and Fibyrax). However, like fibre tablets, the quantity of fibre they provide is quite small and they are also expensive. Still, they are a convenient and quick way to boost fibre intake and help overcome constipation. They are particularly handy when you're travelling or can't eat your regular food.

WHAT YOU CAN DO ABOUT WIND

Wind is produced by the fermentation of fibre and other undigested carbohydrates (oligosaccharides) by bacteria, which break them down to gases, notably hydrogen, methane and carbon dioxide. Legumes, certain vegetables (cabbage, cauliflower, broccoli, onions and Jerusalem artichoke), dried fruit and seeds tend to be the culprits. Problem foods should be introduced into your diet gradually, starting with small portions. If you are cooking beans from scratch, soak them overnight, discard the water and add fresh water for cooking. Digestion enzymes in products such as Beano or De-gas can also help.

Fish

Fish is light, nutritious and cooks quickly, making it a wonderful food for busy people and dieters alike. If fresh fish is not readily available, use frozen or canned, which are convenient and easy to prepare. Nutritionally, frozen fish is similar to fresh—there are small losses of vitamins during the freezing process but levels of omega-3, protein and minerals are the same. Buy plain frozen fillets and steer clear of battered, crumbed types and also flavoured types, which tend to be high in added salt.

NUTRITIONAL VALUE

Fish is high in protein and packed with minerals from the sea including prostate-protecting zinc, iodine, iron and potassium. Canned salmon and sardines, with their small, softened bones, are a surprisingly good source of calcium. Fish is important for a number of B vitamins, notably niacin and vitamin B_{12}, and it is lower in cholesterol and total fat than meat or chicken. It is also very low in saturated fat, the type of fat that raises blood cholesterol levels.

> **Omega-3 is so important to our health that we are urged to eat oily fish at least twice a week.**

All types of fish carry some omega-3, but the oily, cold-water varieties are highest, including gemfish, tuna, ocean trout, sea perch, trevally, blue eye cod, silver bream, herring, mackerel, mullet and sardines. They have around double that of temperate-water fish. Omega-3 is so important to our health that we are urged to eat oily fish at least twice a week, particularly if we have any inkling of heart problems, blood pressure or diabetes. Fish has often been called 'brain food' thanks to the omega-3s, which are crucial for our brain function.

'Super fish' sources of omega-3 include: Atlantic salmon, New Zealand king salmon, canned sardines, canned salmon (pink and red), rainbow trout, canned mackerel, barramundi, swordfish. Excellent sources include: blue-eye trevalla, silver perch, Australian bass, john dory, snapper, frozen fish fillets, canned tuna and herrings. Seafood such as oysters, squid, green- and blue-lipped mussels, scallops, prawns and baby octopus are also good sources.

NUMBER CRUNCH

A serve of fresh or frozen fish (175–200 grams raw or 150 grams cooked weight) or a 120 gram can of fish (drain any brine to reduce the salt level) supplies 36 grams of protein, 13 grams of fat (including 4 grams of saturated fat), and 1090 kilojoules.

COOKING FISH

The healthiest way to cook fish is to cook it quickly without adding lots of butter or oil. My favourite ways include:

- Barbecuing on the grill
- Steaming
- Baking it with herbs, especially wrapped in baking paper to keep it moist
- Dry-frying in a pan sprayed with oil.

MERCURY IN FISH

Mercury is used in thermometers, blood pressure devices, batteries and some dental fillings (amalgam), but it's fish—one of our healthiest foods—that is the major source. Its toxic form, methyl mercury, has been in the news after surveys from the US reported that approximately 8 per cent of women had blood levels of mercury over the US's safe reference level. What's worse, women who regularly ate lots of fish had the highest blood levels.

WOMEN WHO ARE PREGNANT, PLANNING TO BECOME PREGNANT OR BREASTFEEDING

- Limit your intake of fish with the highest levels of mercury, which are those that are long-lived or large, e.g. shark (flake) or billfish (broadbill, swordfish and marlin). Eat no more than one serve per fortnight and eat no other fish that fortnight. One serve is equal to 150 g.
- Limit orange roughy (deep sea perch) or catfish to one serve per week and have no other fish that week.
- All other fish species are safe to eat at the recommended levels of two to three times per week.
- Eat a variety of different fish species, not always the same type of fish.

Our food authorities have responded by reviewing their guidelines on fish consumption, and they have stressed that there has never been a documented case of mercury poisoning from fish in Australia. We are comparatively low consumers of fish, eating on average only one fish or seafood meal a week. The majority of fish has such low levels of mercury that they're undetectable. In the Seychelles, where 12 times more fish is eaten, there have been no adverse reports. However, just because there have been no 'documented' cases doesn't mean mercury poisoning hasn't happened or that you shouldn't take care if you eat a lot of fish.

See also **Omega-3s, Seafood.**

Fish Oil

Fish oil is extracted from the flesh and skin of oily fish such as anchovy, salmon, tuna, herring, cod and menhaden (a Northern Hemisphere fish species) and encased in clear gelatin capsules. They're recommended as an easy way to boost your intake of omega-3 fatty acids for anyone who doesn't eat much fish (two fish meals a week is generally recommended), those who have macular degeneration of the eyes and those with high triglycerides, high blood pressure, rheumatoid arthritis and other inflammatory conditions. During pregnancy and breastfeeding, fish oil is often suggested to nourish the new baby's brain, eyes and nerve tissues.

Regardless of the marketing hype, you'll find little difference between brands of fish oil supplements. Almost all have 1 gram (equal to 1000 milligrams) of fish oil, which contains 180 milligrams of EPA plus 120 milligrams of DHA. You may see this expressed as 300 milligrams of omega-3s in total. Whichever you buy, remember to store your capsules in a cool dark place away from sun and heat. I recommend the fridge in hot weather.

Q

I have an allergy to fish. Are fish oil capsules safe for me?

A

Fish oil capsules are quite refined, undergoing purification and deodorisation steps to remove metals and virtually all protein (the compound that triggers the allergic reaction). Theoretically they should be safe, but it's wise to be extra cautious. The Allergy Unit of the Royal Prince Alfred Hospital in Sydney suggests you test your reaction by having your doctor do a skin prick test with the contents of a fish oil capsule. Have your emergency adrenalin on hand and make sure there is resuscitation equipment, just in case.

BURP-FREE CAPSULES

You'll pay more for the enteric-coated 'burpless' capsules, which don't cause reflux or leave a sardine-like aftertaste. They dissolve only when past the stomach. Not everyone is bothered by the aftertaste so if it doesn't worry you, just buy the standard capsules.

SUPER-STRENGTH CAPSULES

You'll also pay more for 'super strength' or high-dose capsules, which contain 600 milligrams or so of omega-3 per capsule—double the standard amount. This means you get more omega-3 from fewer capsules, which is a help if you need to swallow a lot.

LIQUID FISH OIL

Liquid oil is less expensive and allows you to ingest a higher dose in one go without having to swallow capsules. For example, 1 teaspoon (5 millilitres) of liquid fish oil is equivalent to five regular capsules. If you need to swallow 14 fish oil capsules each day, you'd find it easier and quicker to swallow a tablespoon of the liquid oil. Pour it into a small glass of juice or milk and swallow in one go like a shot.

COD LIVER OIL

Fish oil is not equivalent to cod liver oil. Cod liver oil contains less EPA and DHA but is rich in two fat-soluble vitamins, A and D, which is why it's dispensed these days. You get some omega-3, but not as much as from fish oil.

Flatulence (Wind) and Diet

Flatulence, often known as wind or farting, is caused by gases in the bowel like methane, nitrogen, hydrogen sulphide and carbon dioxide. The smell depends on the ratio of gases, which is influenced by the foods we eat. The gas can be generated by swallowed air, the process of digestion, high-fibre foods and bacteria in the intestine, which convert fibre and other indigestible carbohydrates (e.g. raffinose or stachyose). Some digestive disorders, such as lactose intolerance and irritable bowel syndrome, can produce excess gas.

Foods that commonly cause excessive flatulence are legumes (beans, peas, chickpeas, soy beans), dairy products such as milk if lactose intolerance is present, dried fruit like raisins and prunes, fresh fruit, foods high in insoluble fibre (particularly bran, corn kernels, seeds and husks) and windy vegetables (cabbage, Brussels sprouts, cauliflower, onion, cucumber).

See also **Fibre.**

Flavonoids (Bioflavonoids)

This is a large group of natural plant compounds being researched for their action as antioxidants including flavones, flavonols, catechins and anthocyanidins. They are found in all vegetables and fruit. The richest sources are tea, wine, grapes, apples, onions, berries, cocoa powder and soybeans. Research shows they help reduce the risk of heart disease by maintaining the flexibility of the inner lining of the blood vessels and keeping the blood free-flowing.

See also **Phytochemicals.**

Flavour Enhancers

These are compounds which bring out the flavour or aroma of a food but contribute no flavour of their own. They are used in many savoury foods including cracker biscuits, gravy powders, stock powders, sauce mixes and instant noodle sachets.

See also **Additives.**

Fluoride

Fluoride is required during early years for building strong tooth enamel that is resistant to decay. Fluoridation of public water supplies (one part per million) reduces dental caries. Today, over-fluoridation may be a problem as fluoride now comes from many sources such as toothpaste, food, medicines and pesticides as well as water. However, the fluoride level must be over three parts per million before mottling of the teeth (or other side effects) occurs.

The recommended daily intake is 3 milligrams for women and 4 milligrams for men. Rich sources: fluoridated drinking water, fish (especially if eaten with the bones) and tea.

FODMAPs

If you have abdominal bloating and cramping, you may be one of a group of people thought to have undiagnosed intolerance to common foods such as fruit, vegetables, dairy products and artificial sweeteners. Many of the foods we eat contain short-chain carbohydrates (saccharides) that most of us can easily digest. However, for a small number of people, these carbohydrate components may not be digested well in the small intestine. They end up in the large intestine along with water, where they undergo bacterial fermentation into hydrogen, carbon dioxide and short-chain fatty acids. These gases can cause the bloating, cramping and pain so often associated with irritable bowel syndrome (IBS).

The term FODMAPs was coined by researchers from Monash University and is the acronym to describe these fermentable, short-chain carbohydrates: fermentable oligosaccharides, disaccharides, monosaccharides and polyols. Common examples include:

Fructose—a monosaccharide found in fruits such as grapes and pears, honey, sucrose (table sugar) and high-fructose corn syrup (more commonly used in the US).

Lactose—a disaccharide found in dairy foods containing cow, goat and sheep milk, including soft cheeses. Lactose intolerance is common in people from Asia and the Mediterranean.

Fructans—chains of fructose molecules linked together, found in wheat, rye, garlic, onion, cruciferous vegetables and some fruits such as melon and peach. This also includes inulin, which is often added to processed foods.

Galactans—chains of different monosaccharides joined together, such as raffinose, found in legumes (baked beans, kidney beans, chickpeas and lentils). They can be reduced by cooking.

Polyols—sugar alcohols including sorbitol, xylitol, mannitol and maltitol, these are often found in artificially sweetened gums and lollies but also occur naturally in apples, stone fruit and mushrooms. If you see the words 'excessive consumption may have a laxative effect' on a pack, the product probably contains polyols.

The research team at Monash University found a low-FODMAP diet, particularly avoiding fructose and fructans, relieved the symptoms of IBS in 75 per cent of their patients. Reducing excessive gas production can lessen nerve-ending stimuli in a hypersensitive gut and so may lessen the bloating, wind, pain and unpredictable bowel habits so common with IBS.

DIAGNOSING FODMAP INTOLERANCES

A hydrogen breath test, which can identify both fructose and lactose malabsorption, is used for diagnosis. Not everyone will react to every FODMAP type; those with one FODMAP intolerance may be able to tolerate others.

To relieve symptoms, sufferers may not need to remove all FODMAPs from their diet, but rather reduce the quantity or frequency of consuming foods high in multiple FODMAPs, or avoid those foods that are particularly high in an offending FODMAP. For instance, those with a fructose intolerance may be able to tolerate lactose and small amounts of fruits and vegetables lower in fructose. Fruits and vegetables that contain several FODMAPs include apple, pear, stone fruit (nectarine, peach), watermelon, beetroot, green beans, cruciferous vegetables (broccoli, Brussels sprouts, cabbage), chickpeas, onion and mushrooms. Removing or reducing these from the diet first may help. But don't self-diagnose; talk to your doctor or an accredited practising dietitian and ask them to arrange for a hydrogen breath test first.

Folate

Now widely regarded as a 'miracle cure' for spina bifida and other birth defects, folate (also known as folic acid or folacin) takes its name from the Latin word for foliage, as high concentrations of this superstar vitamin are found in leafy green vegetables. Thus the folate story provides still another good reason to heed the advice of nutritionists (and mothers everywhere) and eat a healthy balanced diet with lots of vegetables.

Folate was first discovered in the 1940s and was recognised then as important in keeping red blood cells strong and preventing a certain form of anaemia. We now know it plays a key role in the growth and reproduction of all body cells and is essential for the healthy development of the brain, spinal cord and skeleton of the foetus. Folate is one of eight vitamins of the B group. It is crucial for several steps in the synthesis of the genetic material DNA, so when it is in short supply, the nuclei of cells cannot make new DNA and cells cannot divide and multiply. Thus growth stops or is distorted.

DAILY REQUIREMENTS (mcg)	
Adults	400
Children 1–3	150
Children 4–8	200
Children 9–13	300
Children 14 and over	400
Women planning pregnancy	600

Rapidly dividing cells, such as those that make up the neural tube, need folate in plentiful supply. The anti-cancer drug methotrexate has a similar structure to folate, but interferes with its biochemistry and is used in chemotherapy to block rapidly dividing cells (mostly cancer cells) from multiplying.

FOLATE SOURCES

Folate is found in all dark-green vegetables such as silverbeet, spinach, broccoli, bok choy, asparagus, herbs and dark lettuces e.g. mignonette, rocket and watercress. Other important sources are lean meat, particularly liver and kidney, wholegrain cereals, wheat germ, yeast extract, citrus fruit, berries, nuts (particularly peanuts) and tea. It is extremely sensitive to light, heat and air and is easily destroyed during cooking, so eating some of your vegetables and fruit raw each day makes good sense.

Many breakfast cereals are now fortified with added folate and a bowl (usually 30 grams) provides between 25 and 50 per cent of the recommended intake of folate. Bread, flour, pasta, fruit juice, vegetable juice and yeast spread are also permitted to carry extra folate.

FOOD	FOLATE (mcg)
GRAIN FOODS	
2 tbsp wheatgerm	40
2 tbsp wheat bran	52
1 slice wholemeal bread	10
45 g fortified cereal	100
VEGETABLES	
1 cup (15 g) lettuce	7
55 g tomato	7
3 slices beetroot	30
5 canned asparagus spears	100
3 cooked Brussels sprouts	66
½ cup cooked English spinach	65
½ cup cooked broccoli florets	80
½ cup cooked green beans	35
½ cup cooked cabbage	20
1 medium boiled potato	24
½ cup cooked green peas	15
½ cup sliced raw mushrooms	20
1 small cooked carrot	15

FOOD	FOLATE (mcg)
FRUIT	
1 orange	43
200 ml orange juice (fortified)	40
1 medium banana	15
½ cup strawberries	10
½ medium avocado	80
UNSALTED NUTS (40 g)	
¼ cup peanuts	43
¼ cup cashews	25
¼ cup hazelnuts	25
LEGUMES	
⅓ cup baked beans	45
½ cup cooked lentils	24
½ cup cooked chickpeas	40
OTHERS	
2 sliced lamb's liver, fried	190
1 medium boiled egg	20
1 small can salmon	12
200 g tub skim plain yoghurt	35

FOLATE FIGHTS BIRTH DEFECTS

> **DID YOU KNOW?**
> One bowl of folate-fortified cereal will provide 100 mcg of folate. That's 25 per cent of the daily recommended intake for adults.

Each year around 500 pregnancies in Australia occur with a neural tube defect, such as spina bifida (where the spinal cord is not completely formed) or anencephaly (a fatal defect in which a major part of the brain never develops). Half of these pregnancies eventually end up as babies that are stillborn or die within the first month of life, while many foetuses are aborted after identification in early pregnancy.

Evidence from several large, well-designed trials in the 1990s revealed that seven out of 10 cases of neural tube defects can be prevented by increasing folate intake prior to conception or, more specifically, at least 1 month before and during the first 3 months of pregnancy. Around 400 micrograms per day of folate was recommended. This critical period in early pregnancy, when the neural tube closes over, occurs often before a woman knows she is pregnant. The neural tube, a row of cells from which the baby's brain and spinal cord form, grows rapidly in the first 6 weeks after conception and needs folate in plentiful supply. But, because 30–40 per cent of pregnancies are unplanned, most women are not thinking about eating for a healthy baby at that critical time.

It is for this reason that health authorities looked at ways to ensure that all women obtain adequate folate. One of the strategies was targeting women of child-bearing age with awareness programs of the importance of adequate folate from foods and the use of a supplement if necessary. The other was allowing food manufacturers to voluntarily fortify foods with folate. In 2000, an evaluation of the effect of fortification concluded that it was still too early to assess. However, Food Standards Australia New Zealand (FSANZ) is considering the need for mandatory food fortification, particularly as it has been in place in the US since 1996. Studies have shown that the path taken by the US has led to a 19 per cent reduction in neural tube defects. This contrasts with the situation in Europe, which has relied upon public health messages alone and shown no change in rates of neural tube defects since the early 1990s. Folate may also have a role to play in preventing other birth defects such as cleft palate and heart and urinary tract defects.

> Seven out of 10 cases of neural tube defects can be prevented by increasing folate intake prior to conception or, more specifically, at least 1 month before and during the first 3 months of pregnancy.

SUPPLEMENTS

Folate supplements (folic acid) are sold in doses of 0.6 milligrams (600 micrograms). If you have already had a baby with a birth defect or have a relative who has had a baby with one, you are at greater risk and will require a higher-dose supplement. Check with your local dietitian or doctor.

Food Colours

You've probably seen claims of 'no colours' on all sorts of food packs, because colours are one of those things in food that gets parents' hackles up. They're regarded as unnecessary cosmetic additions for eye appeal only. And the urban myths abound: red cordial sends kids into hyperactive overdrive, while green lollies can give them eczema and hives. Parties that are helped along by cakes with coloured icing, sweets, ice-blocks and sugary drinks are destined to be a nightmare.

Yet it seems we can't live without it. Colour reflects flavour, and we can all relate to the sentiment of 'eating with our eyes'. No child would be happy with lollies that were flavoured but colourless, or fizzy drinks that all looked clear. Homemade lemonade, with its subtle lemon yellow tinge, looks different from store-bought lemonade.

It's a controversial issue. Fortunately, the list of permitted colours in Australia and New Zealand is more restricted than that overseas. Like other additives, the safety of food colours is evaluated by Food Standards Australia New Zealand and its expert advisory groups. Approved colours can be either natural or artificial, and they can be identified on food labels by their chemical name, such as Brilliant Blue FCF, or their code number (133). Natural colours are part of a worldwide trend away from processed foods and towards 'all natural', cleaner ingredients. It's spurring food manufacturers to source their colours from pure juice concentrates or natural sources.

The result of this shift can be seen on the labels of our favourite foods. Kids' lollies are now made red with carmines derived from cochineal (120), annatto extracts (160b), beet red (162) or cherry juice extract, instead of the more suspect red number 122 (azorubine), or number 129 (Allura Red AC). Yellow and orange hues are derived from the beta-carotene of carrots or pumpkin, curcumin (100) from turmeric or paprika. Purple tones come from anthocyanins (163) found in grape skin extract, elderberry or red cabbage, and browns from a number of caramels (150a–d). This trend parallels the general rise of farmers' markets, organic fare and less-processed products. It's part of the huge swing to healthier options, identified as one of the top ten global food trends. And with the trend taking such a broad scope, it's safe to assume that what's good for the kids is probably good for the parents too.

See also **Additives.**

Food-combining Diets

Don't mix proteins with carbs? Eat fruit separately from everything else? The theory behind food combining goes back to the beginning of the 1900s but pops up every so often in another form including *The Hay Diet* in the 1920s, *The Alkaline Diet* by Gary A Martin in the 1970s and *Fit for Life* by Harvey and Marilyn Diamond in the 1990s. All chase the same notions of proper digestion with rules like carbohydrates and proteins should never be put in the stomach at the same time as they start to 'rot'; water should never be drunk at meals; and dairy foods should never be eaten. The supposed basis for this is that your digestive enzymes get confused when you eat. To my thinking, two main lines of evidence bust this myth: what takes place in digestion and what is actually in food.

WHAT GOES ON INSIDE

Our body contains all the necessary mechanisms to break down protein, carbohydrate and fat at the same time. An enzyme called amylase is present in the saliva in our mouth and also in our upper intestine. It breaks down any starchy carbohydrate into smaller sub units and ultimately into single sugar units such as glucose and fructose, which are absorbed into the bloodstream. At the same time, our stomach contains pepsin and trypsin, which cut the protein down into shorter peptides and eventually into single amino acids. These enzymes can and do work happily together—otherwise you would never be able to digest a meal like steak with mash and peas or fish and chips or spaghetti with Bolognese meat sauce.

	PROTEIN (%)	CARBOHYDRATE (%)
Soy beans, dried	31	13
Peanuts, raw	25	9
Lentils, dried	24	35
Buckwheat, raw	12	66
Oats, raw	11	58
Bread, wholemeal	9	40
Brown rice, raw	7	77

WHAT IS ACTUALLY IN FOOD

Many foods contain protein and carbohydrate in the same food. You automatically ingest both at the same time when you eat rice, oats, bread, beans or cereal with milk. In fact many so-called starchy foods are a mixture of protein with carbohydrate so you can't avoid consuming them together. Many cultures have lived on such staples for countless years and survived in good health. Take a look at the comparison at left.

FOOD-COMBINING DIETS AND WEIGHT LOSS

Many people swear they shed weight on a food-combining diet but I suspect it's simply because there are so many rules about what and when to eat that many people end up being too scared to eat much at all. For instance, you can only eat fruit for breakfast and nothing else until noon; you have to wait four hours after consuming fruit before you can eat anything else after; melons must be eaten in isolation!

MY TAKE

There's scant research on food combining as a diet, with only one clinical trial, which reported no difference for weight loss when compared with a standard, balanced low-kilojoule diet. Food combining doesn't make sense from a digestive point of view, or from a food point of view. Your body can handle protein and carbs at the same time, like chicken with noodles or cheese on toast. In fact, they make a balanced meal—along with a heap of vegetables.

Food Groups

Nutritionists generally divide foods into basic food groups (sometimes called foundation or core foods) based on their nutritional profile. Eating from all the food groups each day is the goal; this should ensure you get your full quota of vitamins, minerals, protein, fibre and various phytochemicals to result in good health in adults and growth in children. It's easy, makes good sense and saves money too.

Here are my eight basic foods listed with the minimum number adults need to eat for health and energy.

VEGETABLES AND SALADS

You need five or more serves a day. Fresh, frozen or canned—vegetables have almost no fat and are good sources of fibre, vitamins and antioxidants. This is the food group you can eat up on! Choose types that are in season as they will be the cheapest and at their peak nutritionally. Aim for a mixture of different colours so you receive a variety of different vitamins and antioxidants. For example, beta-carotene is found in yellow/orange vegetables such as pumpkin, carrots, rockmelon and mangoes, while lycopene occurs in red produce like tomatoes and ruby grapefruit. Lutein occurs in green leafy vegetables like silverbeet and spinach.

Buy at farmers' markets or grow a few of your own. Lettuce, baby tomatoes, silverbeet, parsley, basil and other herbs are easy to grow in a sunny spot. Frozen are a good alternative to fresh, provided you cook them quickly. Canned vegetables have lost more nutrients and carry added salt; they are not as good as frozen but are a convenient stand-by.

- One serve is ½ cup cooked vegetables (broccoli, beans, peas etc.), 1 small carrot, 1 tomato, 1 cup salad leaves.

FRUIT

You need two or more serves a day, which will boost fibre, vitamin C, beta-carotene and antioxidant intakes. Buy what's cheap and in season and, as with vegetables, variety is important. Whole fresh fruit is always the best choice but canned, juice or dried can be convenient when fresh is expensive. Both fruit juices and dried fruits are much higher in kilojoules (calories) and sugars and juice is also expensive and doesn't have the benefit of fibre. Dilute any juice down with water.

- One serve is 1 medium apple, banana, orange or pear; 2 plums, apricots or kiwifruit; 1 cup fruit salad or canned fruit; 2 tablespoons sultanas; 4 dried apricot halves.

LEGUMES

You need three serves or more of legumes per week. Also known as pulses, they are valuable for their soluble fibre, protein, B vitamins, minerals and heart-friendly phytonutrients. Many varieties are available in canned form and make a great addition to soups, one-pot meals and pasta sauces.

- One serve is ½ cup (75 grams) cooked or canned beans, ½ cup (75 grams) cooked lentils or split peas, 1 small can (100 grams) baked beans, ½ can (100 grams) mixed bean salad.

DID YOU KNOW?

To round off a healthy diet, drink plenty of water, be moderate with sugar and sweet foods, and shake the salt habit.

MEAT, FISH, CHICKEN OR EGGS

You need two serves of these per day. These high-quality protein foods contain many nutrients essential to health including iron, zinc, B vitamins and omega-3s. They are filling and satisfying for the kilojoules they provide. Choose lean cuts of red meat and remove skin from chicken to reduce the saturated fat. Fish doesn't have to be fresh; you can include frozen and canned fish such as salmon, tuna or sardines. Use cooking methods such as grilling or dry-frying, which allow fat to drain away and don't contribute any extra fat.

- One serve is 125 grams cooked meat such as 2 slices roast meat, 2 medium chops, 1 small steak, ¾ cup mince; 150 grams cooked fish or seafood, e.g. 1 large fish fillet or 120 gram can tuna or salmon; 125 grams cooked chicken, e.g. 1 small chicken breast, 2–3 drumsticks; 2 eggs.
- For vegetarians, one serve is 125 grams tofu or tempeh; 125–150 grams soy 'steaks' or rissoles; ½ cup cooked or canned beans, lentils or split peas; 1 small can (100 grams) baked beans.

DAIRY FOODS

You need three serves per day. Rich in bone-building calcium, low-fat dairy also has a role to play in keeping blood pressure down and helping with weight loss. In addition, dairy foods are good sources of protein, phosphorus, vitamin B_2 as well as many bioactive ingredients. Most are now available in a low-fat version, but children under 2 years should be given full fat products.

- One serve is 1 cup milk or soy milk; 1 tub (200 grams) yoghurt; 1 cup custard; 2 slices (40 grams) cheese; ½ cup evaporated milk.

If you cannot tolerate dairy products, look for soy or rice beverages, but make sure they are fortified with calcium so they're equivalent to milk.

NUTS AND SEEDS

You need one serve per day. Nuts and seeds are concentrated sources of kilojoules and fat but, apart from coconut, their fat is in the form of 'good' fat, which is accompanied by vitamin E, fibre and many minerals like magnesium, copper, potassium and selenium. A handful of nuts (30–50 grams) a day is now recommended for a healthy heart. Choose unsalted nuts rather than salted.

- One serve is ¼ cup (30 grams) almonds, walnuts, cashews, macadamias, pecans or peanuts, or 2 tablespoons (50 grams) peanut butter or tahini.

GRAINS AND CEREALS

You need four or more serves per day. Go for wholegrain, wholemeal, bran or high-fibre types to give you B vitamins, minerals, antioxidants, polyunsaturated fats and fibre. Include different grains like rye, barley, oats, maize, triticale, millet and buckwheat. Avoid over-processed breakfast cereals, refined flour products or crackers—they're low on nutrition and not as filling.

- One serve is 1 thick slice bread, ½ bread roll, ¼ cup (90 grams) cooked rice, ½ cup (90 grams) cooked pasta or noodles, ¾ cup (30–40 grams) breakfast cereal, ½ cup cooked porridge, ¼ cup muesli.

FATS

It's OK to eat two or three serves of high-quality fats for your skin, hair and heart. Fats add essential fatty acids and vitamin E to your diet so don't go fat free. Choose the 'good fats', polyunsaturated or mono-unsaturated, as you need a little fat in a healthy diet.

- One serve is 1 tablespoon of any mono- or polyunsaturated oil (olive, canola, peanut, sunflower, grape seed), 2 tablespoons margarine, 4 tablespoons light spread (reduced-fat), ½ small avocado, ⅓ cup hummus.

Food Processing

Our ancestors relied on drying, smoking, salting and fermentation (the underlying biological process responsible for making cheese, yoghurt, bread and beer) to preserve their food for lean times or long winters. Today, consumers have frozen, canned, chilled, dried and pasteurised products at their disposal, as well as many novel forms of minimal processing.

In days gone by, we did our own processing at home. We bottled our own fruit, made jam and chutney, dried grapes to make sultanas or stale bread to make breadcrumbs, home-smoked fish, pickled meat in brine and cooked tomatoes for sauces. Some of us even prepared our own wine or mead, preserved lemons in salt, made our own yoghurt, baked bread or rolled out pasta, as many gourmets do today.

Home cooking has similar effects on food as processing as virtually every step in food preparation is a form of processing. Apart from the food we eat raw—such as fresh fruit, salad, vegetables, raw fish or meat—all food has something done to it to make it edible. Light processing is not all negative; there are actually benefits, which we tend to forget. It enables food to keep longer and ensures a reliable food supply; that way, if there is one bad season, we won't all starve.

Processing also adds variety and interest. At certain times of the year, it is often said that the choice is between frozen, canned or dried peas—or none at all! It makes food attractive and also offers convenience and less work in the kitchen—think of the time saved because of canned tomatoes, canned corn niblets, frozen peas, and bottled pasta sauce and baby food.

However, there are also unwanted effects of processing. Processing can soften the texture and change the flavour of food in varying levels, which is obvious when you compare fresh and canned asparagus or fresh and frozen peas. It can decrease nutrients, and add unwanted salt, sugar and additives (colours and preservatives) to your meals. The bottom line is to combine the best of minimally processed food with fresh ingredients when available.

PROCESSING METHODS

Freezing is the best form of processing for retaining nutrition, flavour and texture. Disadvantages include thawing time and the large inputs of energy.

Canning is handy as canned foods need no special storage and have a long shelf life. Disadvantages include some loss of flavour and texture and leaching of nutrients into surrounding liquid.

Drying allows food to keep without refrigeration and creates 'new' flavours and textures. Disadvantages include the loss of water-soluble vitamins and food texture can become tough.

Curing/pickling allows meat and vegetables to keep for a long period of time, often without refrigeration, and creates new flavours and textures. The problem is that cured foods are high in salt and nitrites.

Food Safety

Many people get food poisoning each year, costing governments a great deal through visits to doctors, prescriptions for antibiotics, days of lost work and occasionally, sadly, deaths. The risk of food poisoning is almost entirely eliminated if food is handled correctly and cooked and stored properly. Here are some tips for handling food correctly to avoid food poisoning:

THE BASICS

- ✔ Always wash your hands before preparing or eating food.
- ✔ Keep food out of the temperature danger zone, which is 4°C to 60°C; this is the 'warm' temperature at which bacteria love to grow and multiply.
- ✔ Cook foods until they're steaming hot at 60°C or above.
- ✔ Reheat foods until they're steaming hot.
- ✔ Make sure there's no pink left in cooked meats such as mince or sausages.
- ✔ Look for clear juices when you're roasting chicken or pork.
- ✔ Heat marinades to boiling point.

The risk of food poisoning is almost entirely eliminated if food is handled correctly and cooked and stored properly.

TEMPERATURE

- ✔ Put any food that needs to be kept cold in the fridge straight away.
- ✔ Defrost and marinate food, especially meat, in the fridge.
- ✔ Shop with a cooler bag; picnic with an esky.
- ✔ If the food is not to be eaten immediately after cooking, it should be cooled in the refrigerator to below 4°C.
- ✔ Place hot food directly in the refrigerator to cool (you may be reluctant to do this but modern refrigerators can cope with the load; provided the dish is covered, you will not frost up the refrigerator).
- ✔ Divide large amounts into smaller portions in shallow dishes to increase the rate of cooling.

- ✔ Serve food to be eaten cold direct from the refrigerator; this applies particularly to seafoods, meat and vegetable salads, rice salads, desserts and cakes containing cream.

CROSS-CONTAMINATION

Cooked meats eaten cold are a common cause of food poisoning because organisms have been transferred back to the cooked product via knives, cooking boards and hands contaminated by fresh meat. To avoid transferring bacteria from the raw to the cooked meat:

- ✖ Never handle cooked and uncooked meats together.
- ✖ Don't let raw meat juices drip onto other foods, and use different cutting boards and knives for both.
- ✖ Do not cut up raw and cooked foods with the same utensils or use the same boards without thoroughly washing the board and the utensils and, of course, your hands.
- ✖ Avoid excessive handling of food because bacteria are always on our bodies; use utensils such as tongs or spoons to serve food.

STORING THEN REHEATING

- ✔ Reheating should ensure that the centre of the food reaches 75°C.
- ✔ Thoroughly reheat fried and barbecued meats, particularly chicken bought from takeaway food shops; if this type of food is not to be eaten straight away, it should be kept either below 4°C or above 60°C to avoid growth of any harmful bacteria.

Freezing Food

If stored correctly (at –18°C for no more than 6 months), freezing is the most nutritious and efficient way to preserve food. Make sure you label and date any foods or meals you freeze yourself. A freezer can help you eat more healthily—a frozen dinner thawed and heated with the addition of your own vegetables or fresh herbs makes for a more balanced meal than just cheese on toast or reheating food that's been in the fridge for days. A freezer saves you time too. You can make up a large pot of soup at the weekend and freeze portions to heat during the week when you're pressed for time, adding a handful of fresh parsley or baby spinach leaves before you serve. Curries, casseroles and 'wet' dishes are ideal to freeze. And you can pack diced lamb, chicken breasts, steaks and salmon cutlets in family-friendly portions.

FREEZING TIME

FOOD	TIME (MONTHS)
SEAFOOD	
Raw fatty fish (tuna, salmon)	4
Lean fish (whiting, snapper)	6
Cooked and shelled prawns	3
MEAT	
Mince	1
Chops and sausages	3–4
Other red meat, raw cuts	6–9
Poultry, raw cuts	6–9
FRUIT AND VEGETABLES	
Fruit	6–12
Vegetables	6–12
CAKES, BISCUITS, MUFFINS	
Sponge cake	6
Butter cakes and cheesecakes	4
Muffins and biscuits	8
Pancakes	2

REFREEZING

Don't refreeze meals once they've thawed out, although it is OK to put them back if they're still frozen and firm to touch. If you're using the microwave, make sure you heat them thoroughly.

Fructans

This is a type of storage carbohydrate that occurs naturally in a broad range of vegetables. Chemically it is composed of long or short chains of the sugar fructose, linked by unusual beta 2–1 bonds. It is not digested in the small intestine but is fermented in the large bowel where it promotes the growth of 'friendly bacteria', specifically bifidobacteria. This health promoting benefit is termed prebiotic. Rich sources include Jerusalem artichoke, chicory root, onion, garlic, asparagus, rye and banana.

Fructo-oligosaccharides (FOS)

This is a group of carbohydrates of the fructans group. It consists of chains of up to 10 fructose units often, but not always, terminated by a glucose molecule. Commercially they are synthesised from sucrose and often added to foods as a prebiotic, designed to stimulate the growth of 'friendly bacteria' in the large bowel.

Fructose

A monosaccharide (simple sugar) that's abundant in nature, fructose is found mostly in fruit and honey and there are also small amounts in most vegetables and grains. It's also one of two sugar units that make up sucrose or table sugar (50 per cent fructose and 50 per cent glucose from sugar cane). Fructose has a low GI (19) because it is absorbed and taken directly to the liver, where it is immediately metabolised and only a small proportion is converted to glucose. Don't confuse fructose with high-fructose corn syrup, which is a mix of 50 per cent fructose and 50 per cent glucose with a high GI (89).

Adding fructose to foods and drinks has been a controversial topic in nutrition for many years. There are concerns it is doing something else in our bodies besides adding kilojoules (calories). A 2008 study in the *American Journal of Clinical Nutrition* reported that consuming more than 50 grams of pure fructose in a single hit raised post-meal triglycerides (blood fats)—a known risk factor for cardiovascular disease. However, it's worth keeping in mind that studies where people (or rats) are given high doses of fructose don't actually reflect what happens out here in the real world. People rarely consume pure crystalline fructose just for fun, let alone 10 teaspoons (50 grams) of it in a single sitting.

Fructose malabsorption can occur when the small intestine loses some or all of its ability to absorb fructose, although we don't yet fully understand the actual mechanism. When fructose is not absorbed properly in the small intestine, it can travel through to the large intestine where bacterial fermentation can cause symptoms such as bloating, wind, pain, nausea, diarrhoea and/or constipation.

MY TAKE

Despite numerous plausible theories, there is no convincing experimental evidence that dietary fructose actually does increase food consumption in humans in the long term. We need more studies with realistic amounts of fructose to determine if it truly is a unique and dangerous form of energy. In nutrition, just about everything (including all the fat-soluble vitamins and many minerals) are toxic when consumed to excess. That shouldn't be the basis for excluding them from our diet.

FRUCTOSE AND OBESITY

Consumption of high-fructose corn syrup has increased significantly in the US since the 1970s, and this increase has run parallel to the increase in obesity. However, while fructose may be one factor associated with the US obesity epidemic (think of all those extra kilojoules for starters), it is unlikely that it is a major factor elsewhere. For example, Australians and Brits are also getting fatter while total and added fructose intakes have actually decreased in both those countries.

One theory as to why fructose may be less satiating than other carbohydrates, potentially increasing the risk of weight gain, is that it stimulates insulin secretion much less than other sugars such as glucose. Because insulin increases leptin release, consuming fructose may inhibit appetite less than the consumption of other carbohydrates, possibly leading to an increased energy (kilojoule) intake. Another possible theory is that, unlike glucose, fructose bypasses the rate-limiting step of glycolysis and uses a rapid energy-requiring reaction that abruptly depletes our cells' energy stores—potentially stimulating appetite.

See also **Sugar.**

Fructose Malabsorption

See **Digestive Disorders.**

Fruit

The word fruit comes from the Latin verb *frui*, which means 'to enjoy' or 'take pleasure in'. From what we know of our hunter-gatherer ancestors, humans quickly discovered that sweet fruit and berries were safer to eat than plant foods with a bitter taste—a giveaway for the presence of toxins. Our innate sweet tooth seems to have had a very practical purpose. Not only were fruits and berries a delicious form of food that nourished us, we and other animals and insects played our part too and helped disperse their seeds. It was a two-way street.

The sugars in fruit and berries have provided energy in human diets for millions of years. Today we know that these foods not only provide glucose, our brain's essential fuel, but are important sources of dietary fibre, vitamins and minerals. They also contain nature's bodyguards—phytochemicals such as carotenoids and anthocyanins—which help protect cells from damage caused by pollutants and the natural ageing process. The message from health authorities around the world is clear: eat more fruit (and vegetables).

THE DEFINITION OF FRUIT

To a botanist, a 'true fruit' is simply a mature ovary, a home for the seed or seeds inside. So in their scientific fruit basket, along with what are normally regarded as fruits and berries, you will find nuts and many foods we traditionally think of as vegetables, e.g. tomatoes, eggplant (aubergine), capsicum, cucumber, pumpkin and squash.

Cooks are different. In the kitchen, taste rules, and how a food is served tends to define the difference between fruit and vegies. Certainly that's the approach the US Supreme Court took in 1893, when it ruled that a vegetable refers to a plant grown for an edible part that is generally eaten as part of the main course, while a fruit refers to a plant part generally eaten as an appetizer or dessert or out of your hand.

CITRUS FRUITS

Citrus fruits share a unique structure—a tough skin dotted with aromatic oil glands encloses a white pith of varying thickness, inside which are the segments with seeds embedded in large juicy cells.

- Citron
- Grapefruit
- Kumquat (or cumquat)
- Lemon
- Lime
- Mandarin, clementine and tangerine (they are all varieties of *Citrus reticulata*)
- Orange
- Pummelo (or pomelo)
- Tangelo

SHOPPER'S GUIDE

Keep an eye out for the Australian lime finger (Dooja lime or Gympie lime). This traditional bush food is now being cultivated commercially.

NUTRITIONAL VALUE

Citrus are nutrition all-rounders. They are rich in vitamin C, minerals and vitamin B_1 and are a good source of folate and potassium. They contain a number of phytochemicals such as carotenoids and flavonoids, plus the soluble type of fibre, which can help to lower cholesterol. Even the peel contains nutritional 'goodies' that lower cholesterol or ward off cancer. Oranges and grapefruit have low-GI values.

STONE AND DRUPE FRUITS

These are fleshy fruits that contain a single stone or pit. This group includes those seasonal summer favourites such as plums, peaches, nectarines, apricots and cherries along with avocados and dates. All are good for fibre and certain vitamins.

POME FRUITS

Named after the French word *pomme* for apple, these fruits are all members of the rose (*Rosaceae*) family. They have a core of several small seeds, surrounded by a tough membrane that's encased in an edible layer of flesh.

- Apple
- Pear
- Nashi
- Quince
- Persimmon
- Loquat

NUTRITIONAL VALUE

Pome fruits are rich in carbohydrate and a good source of vitamin C and fibre. Apples are important for soluble fibre, which can help to lower cholesterol. Pears are a useful source of folate, and persimmons contain beta-carotene. Apples and pears are low GI.

AN APPLE A DAY KEEPS THE DOCTOR AWAY

It's an old adage, but seemingly still relevant according to research released over the last couple of years by Horticulture Australia. Apples have one of the highest antioxidant capacities of all fruits, with an average-sized apple offering more antioxidants than half a punnet of blueberries. When it comes to keeping you healthy, apples and their antioxidants have been shown to reduce the risk of cancer (particularly lung and bowel), improve lung function and protect against asthma and ward off the flu under stressful circumstances such as extreme exercise.

TROPICAL FRUITS

These include drupes, pomes, berries and more from the tropical areas of the world, which lie between the Tropics of Cancer and Capricorn.

- Banana
- Custard apple

- Mango
- Lychee
- Longan
- Papaya (pawpaw)
- Passionfruit
- Pineapple

NUTRITIONAL VALUE

There are such a variety of tropical fruits, it's impossible to generalise on their nutritional content. Most are good sources of vitamin C and fibre. The orange and yellow fruits such as mango and papaya are good sources of beta-carotene. Of the tropical fruits that have been GI tested, bananas, custard apples and mangoes have low GI values, while papaya and pineapple have moderate GI values.

DID YOU KNOW?

Back in the 1980s the Beverly Hills Pineapple Diet made headlines with claims that eating pineapple after meals helped burn off body fat. The theory was that papaya softens body fat, pineapple burns it off and watermelon flushes it out of your body. There's no science behind this at all—but a serving of tropical fruit salad is a delicious and nutritious way to finish a meal, just hold the cream!

WILD ABOUT BANANAS

Bananas are one the world's most popular fruits—especially with children—and a fixture in the family fruit bowl in many homes. They are also a nutritional goldmine: high in fibre, folate and vitamin C, and rich in potassium. Sportspeople consume them in great numbers after intense exercise to replace nutrients and help maintain peak performance. But however easy it makes your life getting healthy food into your kids, don't just stick to bananas for their daily serves of fruit. Offer them a variety of different fruits as they come into season—try apples, pears, apricots, strawberries, rockmelon, grapes and mandarins. This helps to establish healthy eating habits, and minimises the chance that either too little or too much of any one nutrient will be consumed.

BERRIES

Berries have their seeds embedded in their juicy flesh making them easy to eat; there's no core, pit or stone.

- Blackberries
- Blueberries
- Cranberries
- Feijoa
- Figs
- Mulberries
- Pomegranate
- Raspberries
- Strawberries

NUTRITIONAL VALUE

Nutritionally, berries are in a class of their own. As a group, they are all good to excellent sources of vitamin C, and supply smaller amounts of potassium, fibre and folate. Their blue and red pigments (anthocyanins) are powerful antioxidants that can neutralise 'bad' bacteria and fight off cancer. They have one of the lowest kilojoule counts of any fruit.

VINE FRUITS

These come from climbing plants that need a supporting structure to grow on such as a wall, trellis, pergola, or another plant. Some have tendrils to attach themselves to the structure; others twine up and around it. Compared with the large number of tree and bush fruit plants, there are comparatively few vine fruits.

- Grapes
- Kiwifruit

- Melons (rockmelon, honeydew and watermelon)
- Passionfruit

NUTRITIONAL VALUE

Grapes are a source of vitamin C, provide some fibre and have a low GI value. Red-skinned grapes also contain protective antioxidants called anthocyanins. The furry kiwi fruit provides plenty of vitamin C—just one will meet your daily requirements. They are also rich in fibre, a good source of both vitamin E and potassium and a moderate source of iron. Melons are good sources of vitamin C and are low in kilojoules, making them popular with weight watchers. Rockmelon and watermelon have high GI values; however, a normal serving of these watery melons won't have much effect on blood-glucose levels as they are relatively diluted sources of carbohydrate. In fact they only have about 5 per cent available carbohydrate, which makes their glycemic load very low per serving.

SHOPPER'S GUIDE

Keep an eye out for more exotic Australian-grown tropical fruits in season such as carambola (star fruit), dragonfruit (pitaya), mangosteen and rambutan. For tips on buying and storing, preparing and serving tropical and exotic fruits, check out the Australian Tropical Fruits website, www.australiantropicalfruits.org.au.

HOW MUCH FRUIT TO EAT PER DAY?

It is recommended you eat at least two serves of fruit a day—ideally fresh, but a serve can also be canned or dried fruit. This will boost your fibre, vitamin C, beta-carotene and antioxidant intakes. Fresh juice has all these nutrients, minus the fibre.

One serve is a medium apple, banana, orange or pear, two plums apricots or kiwifruits, a cup of fruit salad or canned fruit, 2 tablespoons sultanas, four dried apricot halves or 200 millilitres of juice.

See also **Berries; Citrus Fruit.**

Fruitarian

Fruitarians subsist only on fruit and nuts. This style of eating is considered too limited and leads to nutrient deficiencies.

Functional Foods

Functional foods are similar in appearance to conventional foods but have been modified to offer a health benefit in addition to their nutritional value. Also called medical foods, prescription foods, nutraceuticals or foodaceuticals, these foods are at the interface between foods and therapeutic goods. They have blurred the division between what is food and what is medicine. Functional foods can work in a number of ways. They can:

- Slow down ageing
- Prevent or control disease (e.g. heart disease, cancer)
- Improve recovery from illness, injury or surgery
- Boost the body's immune defence
- Enhance sporting performance.

Foods fortified with vitamins, minerals and fibre have become popular because they are widely perceived as an easy way to get nutrients while still eating 'normal' food like white bread or regular margarine. Examples of foods made functional include:

- Breakfast cereal fortified with folate to prevent birth defects
- Breakfast cereal with added psyllium to lower cholesterol
- White bread with added resistant starch to add fibre without changing the look or texture
- Bread with added iodine to prevent iodine deficiency and goitre
- Omega-enriched eggs to improve blood flow and heart health
- Margarine with added plant sterols to lower LDL cholesterol
- Iodised salt to prevent iodine deficiency and goiter
- Flavoured milk supplemented with vitamins A, B_1, B_2, niacin, C and D (to improve dietary intake)
- Yoghurts with added probiotic organisms or live cultures of bifidus and acidophilus to balance bowel bacteria
- Bread or muffins with oat bran to help lower cholesterol
- Sweets with xylitol, isomalt, or aspartame instead of sugar to prevent dental caries, to lose weight
- Carrots bred to have five times the concentration of beta-carotene to prevent cancer.

While functional foods offer great promise, their efficacy and safety need to be tested especially as they could be consumed in large quantities and are not dosage controlled. Precise wording of any health claim on the label must also be regulated to prevent misleading or over-enthusiastic suggestions. These products are also more expensive.

Many everyday foods are functional in their own right and can be properly called functional foods. For example, cranberries have made headlines for their natural anthocyanins, with biological activity that works to prevent urinary tract infections and cystitis. Wheat bran and bran cereal, with their high levels of insoluble fibre, have solid research behind them to show they can prevent constipation and reduce the risk of bowel cancer.

G

Gallstones

Gallstones are small, hard rocks of cholesterol and calcium that can block the tubes that drain the gallbladder. This blockage causes inflammation of the gallbladder or of the bile drainage tubes. Once this happens you experience terrible pain or colic, fever, and even jaundice (where your skin turns yellow).

Bile is made in the liver and stored in the gallbladder until ready to be used to help in the process of digestion. When we eat, this signals the gallbladder that bile is needed. The gallbladder contracts and pushes the bile down into a duct that carries it to the small intestine, where it breaks down any fats eaten. If the bile becomes too concentrated or 'supersaturated', substances in the bile can harden and form small stones that look like gravel. They can range in size from a tiny seed to as large as a golf ball. Generally they are made up of cholesterol (a type of blood fat) but can include calcium and/or bile pigments. Gallstones take years to form.

SYMPTOMS AND TREATMENT

People with gallstones may experience indigestion or an upset stomach, which they often notice after a rich or heavy meal. Many people, however, have gallstones without experiencing any symptoms at all. In fact gallstones can exist for years without causing any problems. It's only when gallstones block the tubes that drain the gallbladder that the problems begin. Symptoms are usually treated by surgery to remove the gallbladder (cholecystectomy), often done by keyhole surgery to minimise major abdominal work.

BEFORE THE OPERATION

There are a few measures you can take to make yourself more comfortable while you are waiting for your operation. Drinking plenty of water (eight to 10 glasses a day) helps, and avoiding particular foods will certainly lessen your pain, though it won't make gallstones disappear. If in doubt, make an appointment to see a dietitian. Avoid:

- ✖ Fatty, oily or fried foods, which are most likely to cause pain or feelings of sickness; they activate the gallbladder to release bile (needed to digest the fat) and so make your symptoms worse
- ✖ Concentrated fats like oil, butter and margarine, fat on meat or avocado, but you don't have to eat completely fat-free; often it's a case of trial and error while you work out how low in fat you need to go
- ✖ Alcohol until after you have had your operation.

AFTER THE OPERATION

The gallbladder is an organ that people can easily live without. Once it's been removed, bile that was formerly stored in the gallbladder will now flow directly from the liver (where it is made) to the small intestine.

This means you can return to your usual diet. Restricting fat is no longer necessary; however, it is healthier to avoid saturated and trans fats as much as possible, and eat plenty of fibre. Check with your doctor about when you can drink alcohol again.

PREVENTING GALLSTONES

Gallstones are estimated to effect around 10 per cent of people in Western countries. The classic gallstone patient is commonly female, overweight and older. In fact, women between 40 and 60 years of age are twice as likely to develop gallstones as men. There are six main factors that can increase your likelihood of developing gallstones.

OBESITY

Being even moderately overweight increases the likelihood of developing gallstones because overweight people create more cholesterol and secrete more of it into their bile, which is stored in the gallbladder. They also appear to empty their gallbladders less efficiently, which causes problems.

FAMILY HISTORY

Having close family members with gallstones also increases the chance of developing them, as does having large numbers of children.

TOO LITTLE FIBRE AND VEGETABLES

Slow transit time (the time taken for food to pass through the digestive tract) and constipation encourage the formation of gallstones. Eating more fibre and vegetables is the easiest way to improve your daily diet. This also brings with it a lower risk of bowel cancer, breast cancer and being overweight.

DIABETES

People with diabetes generally have high levels of triglycerides (a type of fat in the blood). These increase the risk of gallstones.

FEMALE HORMONES

Too much of the female hormone oestrogen from hormone replacement therapy or contraceptive pills alters the composition of the bile and decreases gallbladder movement, both of which can make you more prone to gallstones.

RAPID WEIGHT LOSS AND/OR FASTING

During rapid weight loss the body burns fat, causing the liver to secrete extra cholesterol into bile. Fasting slows down the movement of the gallbladder, which further concentrates the bile that can lead to gallstones.

REDUCING THE RISK

If you are a woman you are already at reasonable risk—make it your priority to address the risk factors you can change.

- ✔ Maintain a healthy weight by following a balanced diet and keeping up an achievable exercise plan. Make sure you eat plenty of fibre (bran cereals, grains, wholemeal bread) and vegetables.
- ✔ Try to keep your cholesterol under control with diet, rather than resorting to medication.
- ✔ Avoid cleansing fasts, detoxes or crash diets that cause rapid weight loss—it is impossible to maintain the weight loss in any case.

See also Digestive Disorders.

Gamma-linolenic Acid (GLA)

See also Fats; Omega-3 and Omega-6 Essential Fatty Acids.

GLA is an omega-6 fatty acid that can be made in the body, to a limited extent, from linoleic acid (LA).

Garlic

Long hailed as nature's penicillin, garlic is a folk medicine revered by the ancient Egyptian, Chinese and Greek civilisations as long ago as 3000 BC. The slaves who toiled to build the great pyramids are said to have kept their strength up with a daily ration of garlic and onion. Today, garlic is also sold as tablets, dried garlic powder, capsules and aged extract, as well as fresh cloves. It's one of my top superfoods and favourite ingredients for cooking.

NUTRITIONAL VALUE

Much has been written about the humble garlic clove, with claims for it curing everything from warts to tuberculosis (as well as warding off vampires and witches). Traditional Chinese medicine used garlic for the treatment of coughs, bronchitis, tuberculosis, diarrhoea, dysentery and many other diseases. Many naturopaths believe it is good for the heart and circulation.

Garlic contains a variety of antioxidants that protect against the formation of dangerous free radicals. Preliminary studies report that it may help in the prevention of cancer of the stomach and colon cancers. Although about 200 compounds have been identified in garlic, the most intensively studied have been the sulphur-containing compounds alliin, allicin and diallyl sulphide. Allicin is responsible for much of garlic's renowned aroma and flavour. Once formed, however, allicin gradually deteriorates to become diallyl sulphide together with ammonia and pyruvic acid.

Only in recent times have garlic's powers been supported by scientific and medical research. Pasteur first documented its broad-spectrum antibacterial activity in 1858. Today, research has proven that garlic can slow the growth of harmful bacteria, yeasts and fungi. But it is yet to be proven that garlic can keep vampires at bay!

Garlic's powers seem to extend to cardiac benefits, as it not only lowers high blood pressure and the harmful LDL cholesterol, but it can also keep your blood free-flowing and help dissolve clots. In both humans and animals, garlic has been shown to reduce the build-up of fats in the bloodstream after a fatty meal. The dose required, however, is reported to be quite large: 10–20 grams of fresh garlic (2–4 cloves) or 600–900 milligrams of powdered garlic daily.

EASY WAYS TO ENJOY GARLIC

Fresh garlic is always the best choice and must be used if you are seeking its antibacterial or antiviral properties. Many garlic devotees finely chop one or two cloves and simply swallow them with the help of a glass of juice. Others prefer to add the raw garlic to salads and enjoy it with a meal. You could try the pungent garlic paste that is often served with chicken in Lebanese cuisine, or:

- ✔ Slice the top off a whole head of garlic and roast for 30 minutes or until soft. Squeeze the soft, thick garlic puree out of each clove and spread over toast or use in cooking. It's much milder than fresh, crushed garlic.
- ✔ Use plenty of chopped or sliced garlic in your stir-fries and curries.
- ✔ Roast baby potatoes in olive oil, garlic cloves and rosemary sprigs.
- ✔ Add a couple of crushed cloves of garlic to enliven any salad dressing.

SUPPLEMENTS

Look for a brand that lists the amount of allicin it will produce in the body. Manufacturers have agreed to standardise different preparations in terms of their potential to produce allicin, which is being considered the best marker compound.

Steer clear of odourless garlic tablets as they have lost most of garlic's health properties—it seems that whatever is in the smell is also part of garlic's health-giving process. If you're taking large doses, heartburn, nausea and flatulence may be a problem.

Gastroenteritis

Gastroenteritis is an illness triggered by the infection and inflammation of the digestive system. Typical symptoms include abdominal cramps, diarrhoea and vomiting. In many cases, the condition heals itself within a few days. Some of the causes of gastroenteritis include viruses (rotavirus), bacteria (*E. coli*, campylobacter, giardia), bacterial toxins, parasites, particular chemicals and some drugs. Treatment depends on the cause but may include:

- Plenty of fluids
- Oral rehydration drinks (such as Gastrolyte, Hydralyte), available from your chemist
- Admission to hospital and intravenous fluid replacement, in severe cases
- Antibiotics, if bacteria are the cause
- Drugs to kill the parasites, if parasites are the cause
- Avoiding anti-vomiting or anti-diarrhoea drugs unless prescribed or recommended by your doctor, because these medications will keep the infection inside your body.

A clear fluid diet can help recovery from gastro and tummy upsets. It is the lightest type of diet, designed to place as little strain as possible on the digestive tract. It is not nutritionally adequate and should be followed for a strictly limited time only, ideally two or three days, but sometimes up to a week.

See also **Diarrhoea, for details of the clear fluid diet.**

Genetically Modified (GM) Food

Genetically modified (GM) foods have been altered via a process that involves taking genes from the cells of one plant, animal or microbe and inserting them into another cell to give a desired characteristic or function. This process has been used in the pharmaceutical industry to produce synthetic insulin and commercial quantities of other drugs.

In agriculture, it has been used to produce resistance to insect attack in corn, potato and cotton, and herbicide resistance in soybeans, corn, cotton and canola. Genetic modifications to food allow producers to use plant varieties with resistance to insects and herbicides. Farmers don't have to spray their crops as much, which results in fewer chemicals that could otherwise end up in our food.

GM yeasts and bacteria in the cheese and wine industry have been used for some years, and more recently, GM cottonseed oil, soy beans, canola, corn, potatoes and sugar beet have also been approved in Australia and New Zealand. Currently no GM fresh fruit, vegetables or meat are permitted.

Gestational Diabetes

Gestational diabetes is the type of diabetes women can develop during pregnancy. In any pregnancy, some insulin resistance develops, as a pregnant woman's insulin needs are two to three times her normal requirements. If you are overweight at the same time, it's worse, and if your body can't produce enough insulin to overcome the insulin resistance, your blood-glucose levels increase above normal. If gestational diabetes is undetected and untreated, the baby is at risk of growing too big in the womb, which can make the birth difficult. The baby is also at risk of other complications and is more likely to be overweight as a child, potentially developing health problems such as high blood pressure, heart disease and diabetes later in life.

No-one knows exactly what causes gestational diabetes, but it's possible that hormones from the placenta block the action of the mother's insulin. Without enough insulin, glucose cannot enter cells and instead, it builds up in the bloodstream, causing hyperglycaemia. The excess glucose and other nutrients flow through the placenta, causing the baby's insulin to rise, thereby encouraging faster growth. This produces significant problems such as a very large baby, an increased risk of the shoulder getting stuck during birth and injury to the mother during birth. There is also an increased risk of spontaneous labour and premature birth.

TREATMENT

About 16 per cent, or 1 in 6 pregnant women, will develop gestational diabetes and those numbers are increasing. Most women can manage their gestational diabetes with healthy eating, exercise and regular blood-glucose monitoring. Strategies include:

- ✔ Eating regular meals and mid-meal snacks, and avoiding getting overly hungry
- ✔ Limiting sugary foods and drinks including soft drinks, cordials, confectionery and desserts
- ✔ Limiting fatty foods, especially foods high in saturated fats such as fried food, fast food, crisps, pastries, butter, cream, cheese, biscuits and muffins
- ✔ Including low-GI (slow-release) carbohydrate foods at each meal and snack; there is evidence that a low-GI diet reduces the need for insulin injections during pregnancy
- ✔ Eating a wide variety of nutritious foods
- ✔ Being active in as many ways as you can each day.

Ghee

Ghee is made from unsalted butter, which is heated to separate and remove the milk solids. It is used in traditional Indian cuisine, and also for shallow frying, roasting potatoes and pan-frying meat. It has a very high smoke point, so doesn't burn or smoke easily. It has a nutty flavour, contains vitamins A and D, and keeps for longer than butter. It is very high in saturated fat. At 66 per cent, a little goes a very long way.

Ginger

Ginger is a rhizome or underground stem, which adds a wonderful fragrance and pungency to your cooking. I love it fresh—grated or sliced—but it can also be consumed as crystalline ginger pieces or as a tea or dried spice. In capsule or tablet form, it is a key component of traditional Chinese medicine, having been used for more than 2500 years as a digestive aid.

Ginger is often taken as a stomach settler to overcome nausea, settle motion sickness or reduce morning sickness during pregnancy. In Asian medicine, ginger has a reputation as an anti-vomiting agent as well as a digestive aid and diuretic. Claims have also been made, albeit unproven, that ginger can alleviate migraines, hangovers and peptic ulcers, and lower cholesterol.

Store fresh, unpeeled ginger in your fridge's vegetable crisper for 1–2 weeks. Alternatively, peel and chop it into pieces and freeze. Ground ginger, like other spices, should be stored in a sealed container away from heat and light.

NUTRITIONAL VALUE

Ginger is rich in hundreds of phytochemicals, including gingerols as well as eucalyptol, citral, some phenols, beta-carotene, capsaicin, caffeic acid, curcumin and salicylates.

These chemicals are the ones that scientists believe are responsible for ginger's therapeutic actions.

With very few kilojoules and virtually no fat, a tablespoon of grated fresh ginger (around 13 grams) adds its pungent flavour and aroma without adding to your waistline. It's 90 per cent water with a small quantity of the essential mineral potassium, needed for fluid balance, but only tiny amounts of other nutrients. In contrast, a couple of squares (10 grams) of glace or crystalline ginger will contribute around 130 kilojoules due to the 8 grams of sugar they contain.

Today, many of ginger's folklore benefits are being backed by Western research. Ginger's medical uses include the treatment of morning sickness, motion sickness and nausea caused by some cancer treatments. Early work in the 1980s showed ginger to be more effective than standard anti-nausea medicine in overcoming motion sickness in 36 college students who were highly susceptible to nausea. More recent studies have also had positive outcomes, while others showed no effect. Overall scientific evidence remains hopeful but inconclusive.

Ginger can also help reduce the pain and inflammation of osteoarthritis, the most common form of arthritis. Some sufferers have been able to reduce their arthritis medication with a daily dose of ginger extract.

EASY WAYS TO ENJOY GINGER

- ✔ Enjoy fresh ginger in cooking where it lends flavour and vibrancy to stir-fries and curries; peel a chunk of the ginger root and then grate, finely chop, slice or crush it in a garlic crusher.
- ✔ Fresh ginger teams well with garlic, fish, pork, chicken, beef, shellfish, beans, pumpkin and Chinese green vegetables.
- ✔ Make a homemade ginger tea by placing two or three slices of fresh ginger in a cup and pouring over boiling water; leave for a couple of minutes and then drink (the longer you leave it, the hotter it gets!); add lemon juice and honey to taste.
- ✔ Dried or ground ginger has a long history as a flavouring in cakes, biscuits and puddings,
- ✔ Pep up a Japanese meal with pickled ginger on the side.
- ✔ Indulge in a few squares of crystalline ginger as an after-dinner treat instead of chocolate.
- ✔ Add half a teaspoon of dried ginger to 2 cups of flour in your favourite fruitcake, cookies or muffins.

Ginseng

Ginseng is a root that has been valued for 5000 years in China, Korea and Russia. Korean ginseng is the most sought after and, if you can purchase the authentic thing, you will pay a high price for it. It's renowned as a tonic for physical and mental disorders and is said to overcome tiredness, stimulate vitality, build stamina and boost immunity. But what makes it such a popular medicinal substance is its alleged ability to increase sexual potency and work as an aphrodisiac (the root, with its unusual lumps and twists, often resembles the human shape).

> **SHOPPER'S GUIDE**
>
> If you buy ginseng, make sure you are buying the authentic product and check how much of it you are getting.

Ginseng is classed as an adaptogen, meaning that it will affect each individual according to their needs. So, it can both raise and lower blood pressure or white blood cell counts if needed. Any evidence as to its efficacy comes from animal studies or anecdotal evidence; few human studies have been carried out.

NUTRITIONAL VALUE

Scientific research into ginseng's properties began in the 1950s and revealed that it contains complex mixtures of medically active compounds known as ginsenosides. Different ginsengs vary greatly in their concentration of these, depending on where it was grown, the age of the root and the season when it was harvested.

Glucose

See also **Carbohydrates.**

Glucose (dextrose) is simple sugar, which is the building block of starch and a constituent of sugar.

Glutamates and *Umami*, Natural

Glutamic acid is an amino acid (a component of protein) most famous as its sodium salt, which is monosodium glutamate (MSG). It can exist in a free form or be bound to protein. It is the free form of glutamate that has the flavour-enhancing properties. It is believed to stimulate the tastebuds and increase the flow of saliva, adding a savoury quality known as *umami*.

See also **Allergies, Intolerances and Diet; MSG; Mushrooms.**

Glutamate occurs naturally in virtually all foods, including aged and cured foods (ham, parmesan, smoked fish), yeast extracts, fermented sauces such as soy sauce and miso, tomatoes, mushrooms and aged cheeses—foods recognised by cooks for their ability to make any dish more flavoursome.

Gluten

Gluten is part of a protein found in wheat, rye, barley and triticale (a cereal which is a cross between wheat and rye). When mixed with water, gluten forms an elastic-like substance, which expands when dough rises. It provides the structure to a risen loaf of bread or a well-made cake, so it's difficult to bake well without these gluten-containing grains. You'll see gluten declared on food labels, whether as an ingredient or thickener, no matter how small the amount.

WHO SHOULD AVOID IT?

People with coeliac disease cannot tolerate gluten and must avoid all foods made from these grains such as flour, bread, cereals, pasta, cakes, biscuits and porridge—all basic foods in our daily diet. Rice, potato, legumes and corn are gluten-free and can be substituted for gluten-containing grains.

Many people swear they get an upset tummy, bloating or loose bowels if they eat gluten and so avoid it. Research is ongoing, but a 2011 study showed

SHOPPER'S GUIDE

The presence of gluten in any food ingredient or component of an ingredient (including additives) must now be declared on the label, no matter how small the amount. Foods labelled as 'gluten free' must not contain any detectable gluten (less than 0.003 per cent). Foods labelled as 'low gluten' must not contain more than 0.02 per cent gluten. In addition, it's wise to double-check labels for ingredients that could be sources of gluten including wheat meal, bran, semolina, malt and cereal filler. It's also important to check for additives like starch or thickener (additives ranging from 1400 to1450). Many manufacturers have moved to thickeners derived from maize or potato. If it doesn't tell you, there should be a warning on the label. Some people can also react to the flavour enhancers 620–625, and the enzyme or flour treatment agent 1100.

evidence that gluten itself may trigger symptoms such as bloating, wind, pain and fatigue in individuals who do not have coeliac disease. It is important not to self-diagnose and exclude foods from your diet before seeing your doctor or an accredited practising dietitian.

GOING GLUTEN-FREE

Gluten-free foods have risen in popularity in recent times, thanks to better diagnosis of people with genuine coeliac disease as well as a belief that gluten-free is somehow healthier for you. But many gluten-free substitute foods like breads, bars, cookies and muffins require the addition of many additives (gums, fibres, cellulose) to give the structure that gluten normally provides. Many are refined, low in fibre and expensive. So you have to ask yourself if using these will really benefit your overall health if you don't have a diagnosed condition. You might be better off eliminating the main sources of gluten (bread, wheat cereals, pasta) and replacing them with rice and corn, and not worrying about the small amounts.

TIPS FOR GLUTEN-FREE COOKING

- Keep rice flour, arrowroot, soy flour or potato flour for thickening sauces, soups, casseroles and making gravy.
- Make sauces and dressings from ingredients you are sure are free of wheat, e.g. oil, vinegar, garlic, pure herbs, grated lemon rind.
- Substitute soy, rice, potato or corn flours for the wheat flour in your favourite cake or biscuit recipes; a blend of one-third of each is a good mix, but remember that you will need to vary the quantity of liquid needed in some recipes (you can also use a commercial gluten-free pre-mix).
- Cook Asian-style dishes like stir-fries and curries, based on rice, rather than wheat (such as pasta and bread).
- Keep a stock of rice breads, muffins and cakes in your fridge or freezer.
- Stock up on rice, rice noodles, buckwheat and alternative grains.
- Always remember, if in doubt, leave it out!

DEFICIENCIES

Avoiding most grains can leave you short on fibre and some of the B vitamins, so try to include brown rice or rice bran (or psyllium or guar fibre) and make sure you eat plenty of vegetables and fruit. Talk to your doctor about a calcium or iron supplement, particularly if you have had diarrhoea for some time.

BREAD

Gluten gives the structure to bread and cakes and enables pastry and biscuits to 'hold together'. Without gluten, most baked goods do not rise as well and so are flatter and less aerated. Bread is the food most missed and it's hard for children who like sandwiches for school lunch. There are now some gluten-free breads on supermarket shelves, but they aren't widely available. Puffed rice cakes, corn thins and rice crackers can help. Or if you have a bread machine, you can bake your own at home using a gluten-free bread mix.

WHAT ABOUT OATS?

Theoretically, oats don't contain gluten but because they're frequently grown, harvested, milled and processed alongside gluten-containing grains, they may be contaminated with gluten. They also contain a gluten like protein, which some people with coeliac disease react to. To recommend that people with coeliac disease avoid oats is controversial because some have been able to eat certain amounts of oats without any damage to their intestinal wall. Scientists are currently studying whether people with coeliac disease can tolerate oats and until the studies are complete, you should follow your doctor or dietitian's advice.

See also Coeliac Disease and Diet.

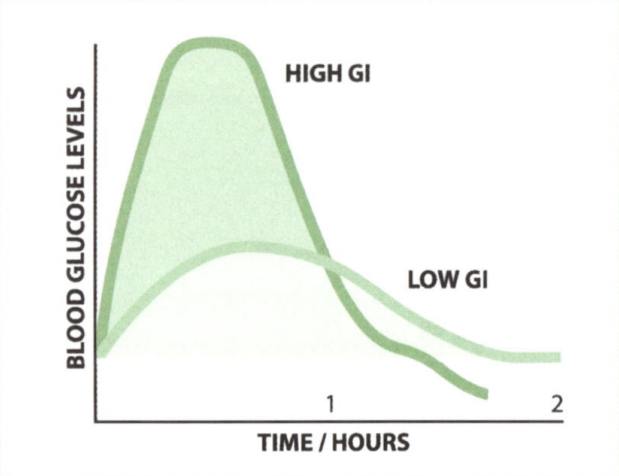

'Making healthy choices easier' reproduced with permission from the Glycemic Index Foundation Ltd.

Glycemic Index or GI

The glycemic index (or GI) is a physiologically based ranking of foods from 0 to 100, that tells us whether a carbohydrate food will raise blood glucose (sugar) levels dramatically, moderately or just a little. In the past, nutritionists believed that starchy carbohydrates like bread and potatoes were 'complex', and therefore took longer to be digested and absorbed than 'simple' sugars. It was reasoned that these 'complex' carbohydrates would produce smaller rises in blood-glucose levels than 'simple' carbohydrates like sugar, which was thought to cause a surge of blood glucose. As a result, sugar was banned from the diets of people with diabetes, and sugar-free recipes for desserts, cakes and biscuits, even though they may have been high in fat, became a part of diabetes therapy.

After more than 30 years of research around the world, studies have turned this notion on its head. After testing hundreds of foods around the world, scientists have found that foods with a low GI will have less effect on blood glucose levels than foods with a high GI. Their studies have shown that many starchy foods like white bread, potato and many types of rice are digested and absorbed very quickly while foods containing sugars have only moderate effects on blood glucose.

THE GI RATING

During digestion, carbohydrate foods (starch and sugars) are broken down into their simpler components, which are absorbed into the blood-stream to become glucose. Not all carbohydrates are digested and absorbed at the same rate. Carbohydrates that break down quickly during digestion have the highest GI values and they cause a sharp, steep rise in blood-glucose levels. Examples are pure glucose, baked potato, puffed crispbread and rice bubbles. Most of our modern starchy foods (white bread, refined breakfast cereals, snack foods and biscuits) are also digested and absorbed quickly.

LOW-GI BENEFITS

We now know that managing our blood-glucose levels is one of the keys to lifelong good health. Choosing low-GI carbohydrates—the ones that produce smaller fluctuations in your blood glucose and insulin levels—reduces your risk of type 2 diabetes and cardiovascular disease and is also one of the keys to sustainable weight loss. It can also delay or prevent age-related vision problems including age-related macular degeneration and cataracts. Studies around the world have now shown that a low-GI diet helps people with:

- ✔ Diabetes, pre-diabetes and gestational diabetes
- ✔ Hypoglycaemia or low blood glucose
- ✔ High levels of triglycerides
- ✔ Metabolic syndrome
- ✔ Polycystic ovarian syndrome
- ✔ Non-fatty liver disease or non-alcoholic steatohepatitis.

At the opposite end of the GI scale are foods that are slowly digested and therefore have a low-GI rating. These help delay hunger pangs, satisfy for longer and make weight loss easier. For people with diabetes, they mean better blood-glucose control. Examples of low-GI foods include pasta, kidney beans, All-Bran, traditional rolled oats, apples, pears, bananas, grapefruit, milk, yoghurt and dense grainy breads.

There is no way to estimate what GI rating a food will have, as many factors influence the GI including:

- The type of starch in the carbohydrate (amylose is more slowly digested than amylopectin)
- The type of sugar (glucose is rapidly absorbed, whereas sucrose moderately raises blood-glucose levels)
- How the food is processed or cooked
- Whether there is any fat accompanying the carbohydrate, as fat slows the rate of stomach emptying and so slows digestion
- The presence of any viscous fibre accompanying the carbohydrate; this increases the viscosity of the contents of the intestines, slowing down the interaction between digestive enzymes and starch and so slowing digestion
- The acidity of the food; acidic foods like vinegar, lemon juice, vinaigrette dressing and acidic fruit slow digestion.

SWITCHING TO LOW-GI MEALS

Check where most of your carbohydrates come from—they're usually from bread, breakfast cereals, potatoes or pasta as well as soft drink and juices. Swap the high-GI foods for low-GI foods at every meal. Here's how:

- Choose a breakfast cereal that's made from oats or bran, or sprinkle rice bran or oat bran over your usual cereal.
- Cook pasta more often than rice or potato, and cook it al dente, not soft and mushy.
- Eat a large salad with a vinaigrette dressing.
- Swap your bread for a low GI one with visible seeds or dark rye.
- Add butter beans, chickpeas or lentils to meat dishes.
- Serve starchy vegetables with a low GI at dinner; for example, peas, carrots, corn, parsnips, butternut pumpkin or the new low-GI Carisma potato.

Breakfast – choose traditional porridge or muesli instead of corn flakes

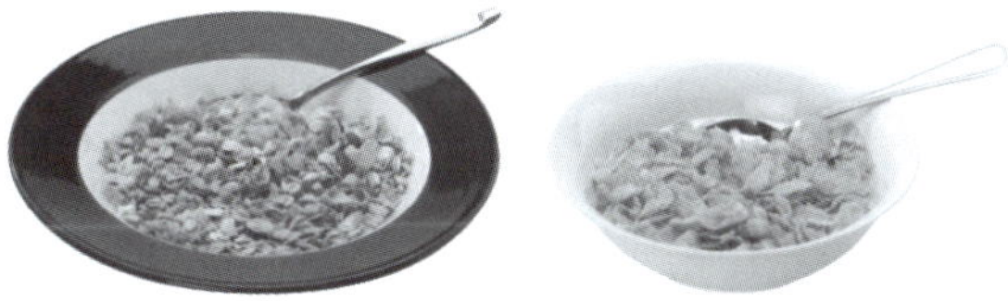

LOW HIGH

Lunch – choose a wholegrain bread instead of wholemeal or white breads*

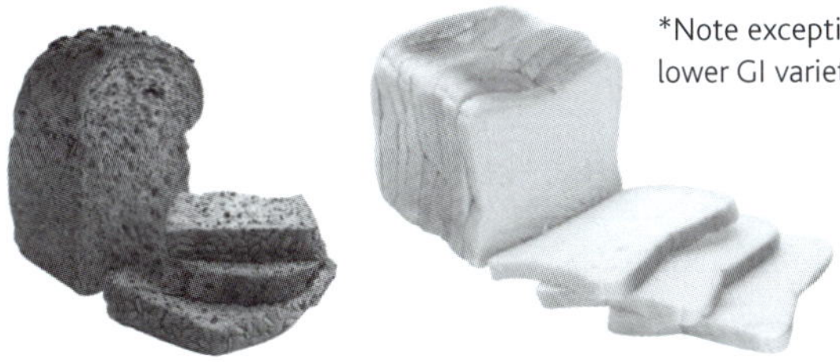

*Note exception: lower GI varieties

LOW HIGH

Dinner – choose Moolgiri, Doongara or Basmati rice instead of Jasmine rice

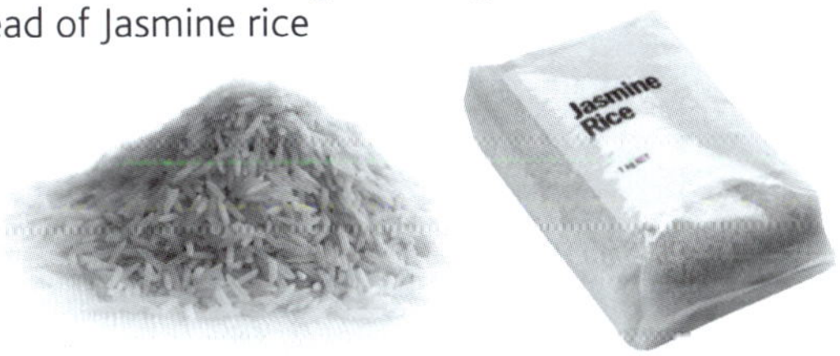

LOW HIGH

'Making healthy choices easier' reproduced with permission from the Glycemic Index Foundation Ltd.

- Cut back on the quantity of potato you serve at dinner or combine potato with legumes to produce a moderate-GI dish (as in potato and chickpea salad or half potato mash, half green pea mash).
- Finish your meals with low-GI fruit such as strawberries, oranges, peaches, apricots, apples, pears or plums.

A DAY ON A HEALTHY LOW-GI DIET

- BREAKFAST—Porridge, All-Bran or muesli with low-fat milk or yoghurt, toasted multigrain bread with margarine and cheese.
- MORNING TEA—Toasted fruit loaf with cream cheese or ricotta.
- LUNCH—Ham salad pita bread, fresh fruit salad, low-fat flavoured milk.
- AFTERNOON TEA—Fruit yoghurt.
- DINNER—Lean grilled steak or skinless chicken fillet, three-bean mix and pasta salad, green salad with oil-vinegar dressing.
- SUPPER—Scoop low-fat vanilla ice-cream with canned sliced peaches or apricots.

GLYCEMIC LOAD OR GL

The effect of a carbohydrate food on blood-glucose levels is determined not only by its GI or carbohydrate 'quality', but also by the quantity or amount of available carbohydrate in the food eaten. You can think of the glycemic load as the amount of carbohydrate adjusted for its glycemic impact. The GL of a food is calculated by multiplying the GI of a food by its available carbohydrate content (that means its carbohydrate minus fibre) in the serving (expressed in grams) divided by 100. The actual formula looks like this: GL = (GI x amount of available carbohydrate) ÷ 100. The GL is widely used in research, but there's no need to do maths every time you have something to eat; just keep your carbohydrate portions moderate.

THE GI SYMBOL PROGRAM

The GI Symbol Program helps consumers make nutritious carbohydrate choices. It is run by the Glycemic (also known as Glycaemic) Index Foundation, a not-for-profit organisation supported by the University of Sydney, the Juvenile Diabetes Research Foundation and Diabetes Australia. Manufacturers pay a licence fee to use the GI Symbol on their products and the income is channelled back into education and further research.

You will find the GI Symbol on a range of fresh produce and products including breads, breakfast cereals and sweeteners.

To find out the GI value of your favourite foods, go to www.glycemicindex.com.

Goji

Goji are usually marketed as superfood berries, but they actually belong to the same botanic family as tomato and capsicum.

To date, there have been no human clinical trials performed on goji and no scientific evidence published under peer review. Despite this, many producers make amazing claims that can't be backed up by research, and fail to comply with regulatory guidelines for marketing natural food products, often displaying incorrect labels. Don't believe all you read on the goji label—here are some claims I have investigated.

'Goji juice contains four polysaccharides that are unique to the goji fruit.'

Polysaccharides are a major constituent of goji, but also of other fruit and vegetables, so there's nothing remarkable about this. They may be different from what's in other produce but they're nothing extraordinary.

'Goji is rich in trace minerals, protein, vitamin C and B vitamins.'

These claims are often exaggerated or do not have a solid independent analysis to back them up.

MY TAKE

You can meet your daily vitamin and mineral intake by enjoying a wide range of fruit and vegetables. You don't need goji at $80 a kilo!

'Goji juice contains more protein than whole wheat.'

Depending on its type, whole wheat contains between 12–15 grams of protein per 100 grams, which is not much when you compare that to high-protein foods such as red meat (27 grams/100 grams) or chicken (28 grams/100 grams). From an analysis of dried goji berries, we found they contain only 10–12 per cent of protein, which is lower, not higher, than whole wheat.

'Goji contains vitamin C at levels 500 times higher than orange juice.'

The vitamin C content of goji can range anywhere from 29 to 148 milligrams per 100 grams. Oranges typically contain 53 milligrams of vitamin C per 100 grams, so goji are definitely not 500 times higher than oranges—on a par, or maybe double, but not 500!

GORD (Gastro-Oesophageal Reflux Disease)

See **Digestive Disorders.**

Grains and Cereals

Cereal grains are the edible grains or seeds of grasses. They have been the main source of food for humans for centuries, and have often been called the 'seeds of civilisation' thanks to their small bulk and excellent keeping qualities; true civilisation only arose when nomadic hunter-gatherer tribes were able to cultivate cereal crops and settle permanently. Wheat and barley were the staple foods of ancient Egypt and later Greece and Rome; rice predominated in Asia, maize (or corn) in the Americas; oats and rye in the colder regions of Europe; and millet in Africa and parts of Asia.

NUTRITIONAL VALUE

All grains are nutritious and are similar in food value. Their major nutrient is starchy carbohydrate, present at 65–75 per cent by weight, which helps make grains filling and sustaining foods. Their protein content ranges from 7 to 15 per cent and is often overlooked, despite the fact that they are the main source of protein for people in developing countries.

In Australia, bread and cereals supply 25 per cent of the total protein we consume, second only to meat. Generally millet, rice and maize fall to the lower end of the protein range, whereas rye and barley are intermediate and wheat and oats are the highest.

Cereal protein is not classified as 'first class' protein, like that of eggs or milk, as it is low in lysine and, to a lesser extent, threonine—two limiting amino acids. But combining grains with foods that are rich in lysine, such as legumes, nuts, dairy foods or meat, at the same meal improves the overall quality of the protein. Such complementary protein patterns have evolved over the years with traditional dishes such as pea soup with bread, rice and lentils, maize tortillas with beans and noodles with cheese sauce.

Wheat, barley and rye stand out among grains because they contain gluten, a unique protein complex with elastic properties essential to baking. Without gluten, it is impossible to knead dough or produce well-risen bread. Only these three grains can produce bread or cakes—wheat and rye being better sources of gluten (and making lighter, more risen loaves) than barley.

Grains are low in fat (2–4 per cent) except for oats, which contain double that of the others. Almost all the fat is located in the germ (seed embryo) and is high in polyunsaturated fat. Grains are low in sugars and sodium and are noted for their B vitamins, especially thiamin (vitamin B_1), riboflavin and niacin, with lesser amounts of vitamins B_6 and folic acid. They contain no vitamin A, C or D, while vitamin E is found in the germ and is present only in wholegrains and wholemeal flours. Grain foods supply one-third of the iron in the Australian diet, plus small amounts of potassium, calcium, zinc, magnesium, manganese and copper, although these vary depending on the soil in which the grain is grown. Research has uncovered many protective factors in wholegrains such as lignans in wheat, which can influence oestrogen levels and beta-glucans in barley and oats, for which there is solid evidence demonstrating their cholesterol-lowering ability.

DAILY REQUIREMENTS

There are no official daily requirements for grains, but for good health you should aim to eat at least 4–6 serves of grain foods a day, with the emphasis on wholegrain, wholemeal or bran types to give you more B vitamins, minerals, antioxidants, polyunsaturated fats and fibre. Include a variety of different grains and avoid over-processed breakfast cereals, refined flour products or crackers—they're low on nutrition and not as filling. Watch out for the added sodium content in those tasty-sounding, quick-cooking prepacked rice, risotto and couscous meals. Save money and salt and buy the plain variety and add the flavour yourself with a teaspoon or two of a spice blend. One serve is:

- 1 thick slice of bread (40 g)
- ½ bread roll (40 g)
- ¼ cup (90 g) cooked rice or pearl barley
- ½ cup (90 g) cooked pasta or noodles
- ¾ cup (30–40 g) breakfast flake–type cereal
- ½ cup cooked porridge (100 g)
- ¼ cup muesli (40 g).

Don't cut out grain foods to lose weight, but stick to smaller quantities of the healthier options.

YOUR GUIDE TO GRAINS

Check out the 9 most popular grains you will find on supermarket shelves. Whatever grain you choose, remember that ideally, minimally processed wholegrain versions are the best choice and should be chosen over more refined products wherever possible. And, most importantly, try and include a wide variety of grains in your diet.

CEREAL GRAINS

BARLEY

Pearl barley and other barley products are rich in beta-glucan fibre, which helps sweep 'bad' LDL cholesterol out of the body. They contain tocotrienol, compounds that are converted into vitamin E in the body, and pearl barley also has a very low GI, which means it's good at staving off hunger pangs. If you want more bang for your buck, watch out for BARLEYmax, a variety of barley developed by the CSIRO. It ticks more boxes, being wholegrain, high in fibre (two to three times more than other grains), with loads of soluble fibre as well as resistant starch.

MY TAKE

When choosing between ancient and modern, why not add variety to your diet and enjoy both? Try spelt bread or kamut pasta for a change. Ancient grains tend to have more fibre and protein than modern wheats with a lower (but not zero) gluten content, but they can't replace modern breads or cereals and they aren't available in every supermarket. If you really want a grain variety that is better for you, my tip is to serve brown rice or pearl barley more often. These staple foods are inexpensive and widely available, and there are a number of quick-cook brown rice products on the market these days too.

OATS

In my book, oats are a winner among all the grains. Their fibre is the soluble type that prevents breakdown products of cholesterol from re-entering the system via the intestine. The result is less cholesterol being made in the body. They have small amounts of good fats, more than wheat or rice, and also give you B vitamins and vitamin E, as well as protein and minerals. Compared with quick cooking or instant oats, traditional rolled oats or steel cut oats have a lower GI.

RICE

One of the world's oldest and most cultivated grains (there are some 2000 varieties worldwide), rice is a staple food for over half the world's population. White rice has been milled and polished and the husk, bran and germ removed—this process removes important nutrients. One way to add some back is to serve white rice with legumes—rice and lentils make a great combination in terms of flavour and nutrition.

Brown rice not only has a deliciously nutty flavour, it has three times the fibre of white rice along with those important B vitamins. And at 350 kilojoules for half a cup (cooked) it has a place in any weight-loss plan. Because it's gluten free and relatively non-allergenic, it's a godsend for anyone with food intolerances or allergies. Brown rice also contains an unusual antioxidant, oryzanol (found in the natural oil in the outer bran layer), which may help keep cholesterol low.

RYE

Rye contains plant oestrogens called lignans, which can help lower the risk of heart disease and may help protect against breast and prostate cancer. Whole kernel rye is used to make bread, including pumpernickel and some crispbreads. It's an excellent source of fibre and also a good source of vitamins and minerals. It is more commonly sold as rye flakes, which are the hulled, steamed and rolled rye grains. Like rolled oats, you can eat the flakes as a porridge or sprinkle them over bread before you bake it.

WHEAT

Among the first food plants to be cultivated in the early days of agriculture, today wheat production is second only to maize among the world's cereal crops. Its high gluten content is a key reason why it has become so popular, producing a range of staple foods including breads, breakfast cereals, pasta and noodles. Wheat provides us with carbohydrate, protein, fibre, B vitamins and iron—but how much you get depends on milling and other processing.

My advice is to choose the wholegrain versions of wheat products—wholemeal or wholegrain breads and wholemeal pasta, for example, so you get all the nutritional goodies from the seed's bran, endosperm and germ. Some wholesome options for enjoying wheat products include bulgur, cracked wheat, wheatgerm and whole wheat kernels (also called 'groats' or wheat berries).

GLUTEN-FREE GRAINS FROM HERBACEOUS PLANTS

BUCKWHEAT

Belonging to the *Polygonaceae* family, buckwheat (kasha) is traditional in eastern European cuisines. It is a good source of carbohydrate, protein, B group vitamins, magnesium and iron, and is gluten-free. It contains an unusual antioxidant called rutin (related to the quercetin in wine) that can strengthen capillaries (fine blood vessels).

CHIA

A member of the mint family, chia was a highly valued crop and its seeds a staple food for Mayans, Aztecs and south-west Native Americans. It is fussy about where it grows and the past five years have seen Australia's Kimberley region become the world's largest producer, thanks to being spot on when it comes to latitude and climate. Like all seeds, chia seeds are high in fat, especially the good fats. They are also big on fibre, low in carbohydrate and contain 15 per cent protein—as much as from wheat—along with a variety of vitamins, minerals and trace elements including folate, phosphorus, iron, manganese, copper and potassium.

> Cereal grains have often been called the 'seeds of civilisation' thanks to their small bulk and excellent keeping qualities; true civilisation only arose when nomadic hunter-gatherer tribes were able to cultivate cereal crops and settle permanently.

QUINOA

This is a small, round, quick-cooking grain similar in colour to sesame seeds. It's a nutritional power-pack—an excellent source of low-GI carbohydrates, fibre and protein, and rich in B vitamins and minerals including iron, phosphorus, magnesium and zinc. You can also buy quinoa flakes and quinoa flour.

WILD RICE

These are the seeds of an aquatic grass native to North America. It is brown to black in colour with a pleasant nutty flavour. As it is hard to cultivate and has to be harvested by hand, it carries a high price tag so is generally sold blended with white rice. It has a similar nutrition profile to brown rice.

See also **Coeliac Disease; Gluten; Oats; Rice; Wheat.**

Grapefruit

Grapefruit gets the thumbs up from every nutritionist. Like other citrus fruits, they are packed full of vitamin C, providing an entire day's needs from just half a grapefruit.

NUTRITIONAL VALUE

They offer a lot of potassium, smaller amounts of other minerals as well as vitamin B_1, making them a nutritional all-rounder. Few other fruit can match this overall nutrition profile. Containing little in the way of fat, sugar or protein, grapefruits are high in water (over 85 per cent of their flesh is water) with natural fruit sugars. They give us sizable quantities of a type of fibre that's rich in soluble fibre, including the gelling fibre pectin and several gums which are well known to home marmalade makers.

Pink, ruby and red grapefruit contain lycopene, which gives them their red blush and may help protect against prostate cancer. Fresh grapefruit has the lowest GI value (25) of all fruit tested so far. It's not just the acid that has a blood glucose–lowering effect; it's also the pectin. Best of all, I find the tang of fresh grapefruit helps me start my day with zest.

NUMBER CRUNCH

One grapefruit provides 1 gram of protein, a trace of fat, 13 grams of sugar, no starch, 4 grams of fibre and 265 kilojoules.

GRAPEFRUIT AND MEDICATIONS

Grapefruit and grapefruit juice can interact with a number of medications, either making them work too strongly or causing unpleasant side effects. Grapefruit inhibits two key enzymes in the inner lining of the intestine (a cytochrome P450 enzyme and P-glycoprotein). These enzymes usually slow and limit the absorption of the drugs into the body. Once they are 'inactivated', there is an increase in the amount of parent drug available for absorption. This may result in an exaggeration in its effect. For the calcium channel blockers, it's usually low blood pressure (hypotension) and related symptoms such as feeling dizzy or weak. For the statins, it's usually muscle weakness (myalgia) and associated effects. Drugs enhanced by grapefruit juice include:

- Some heart and blood pressure medicines like amiodarone (Cordarone X) and felodipine (Felodur, Plendil)
- Many of the cholesterol-lowering medicines, known as statins, particularly atorvastatin (Lipitor) or simvastatin (e.g. Lipex, Zimstat, Zocor) as well as cyclosporin, saquinavir and cisapride
- Some drugs that suppress the immune system
- Minor tranquillisers (benzodiazepines) such as midazolam and triazolam
- Anti-anxiety drugs.

THE LATEST ADVICE

If you are taking medication, avoid grapefruit and the juice altogether, or have grapefruit each and every day but tell your doctor and ask them to adjust the dose if necessary. You can't just take your medication and the grapefruit juice separately; there's evidence the effect can last 24 hours or longer, though it trails off.

Fresh grapefruit has the lowest GI value (25) of all fruit tested so far.

Guarana

Derived from the seeds of a climbing vine native to South America, guarana has become an ingredient in trendy carbonated 'energy' beverages as well as being sold in capsules to sports people and stressed executives.

It is claimed to boost stamina and mental-energy levels. What gives guarana its kick is simply caffeine, which, like caffeine in coffee, increases heart rate, overcomes tiredness and raises alertness and the ability to concentrate. A 1 gram dose of guarana will provide about 80 milligrams of caffeine—as much as from a medium-strength cup of coffee.

Gums

Gums are a diverse group of polysaccharides, most of which are not digested. They are used to set and thicken foods such as salad dressings, desserts and confectionery or to aerate gluten-free bread. Examples include guar, pectin, gum arabic, tragacanth, carboxymethylcellulose, agar-agar and carrageenan.

Guar gum

Guar gum is a vegetable gum and source of dietary fibre obtained from the cluster bean of India. Not palatable in large amounts, guar is useful in the food industry as a thickener, emulsifier and stabiliser in many foods including salad dressings and ice-cream. Its additive code is 412.

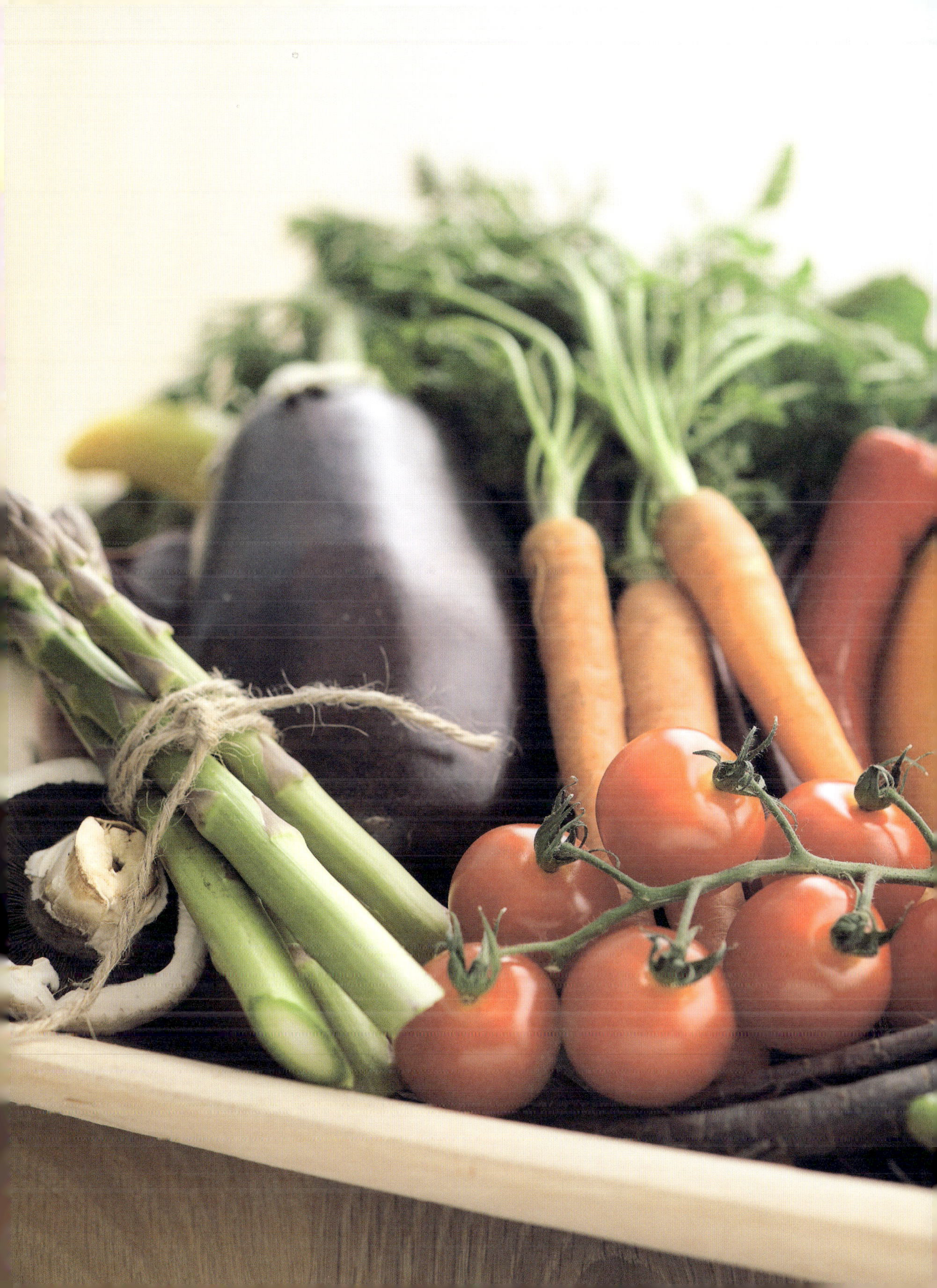

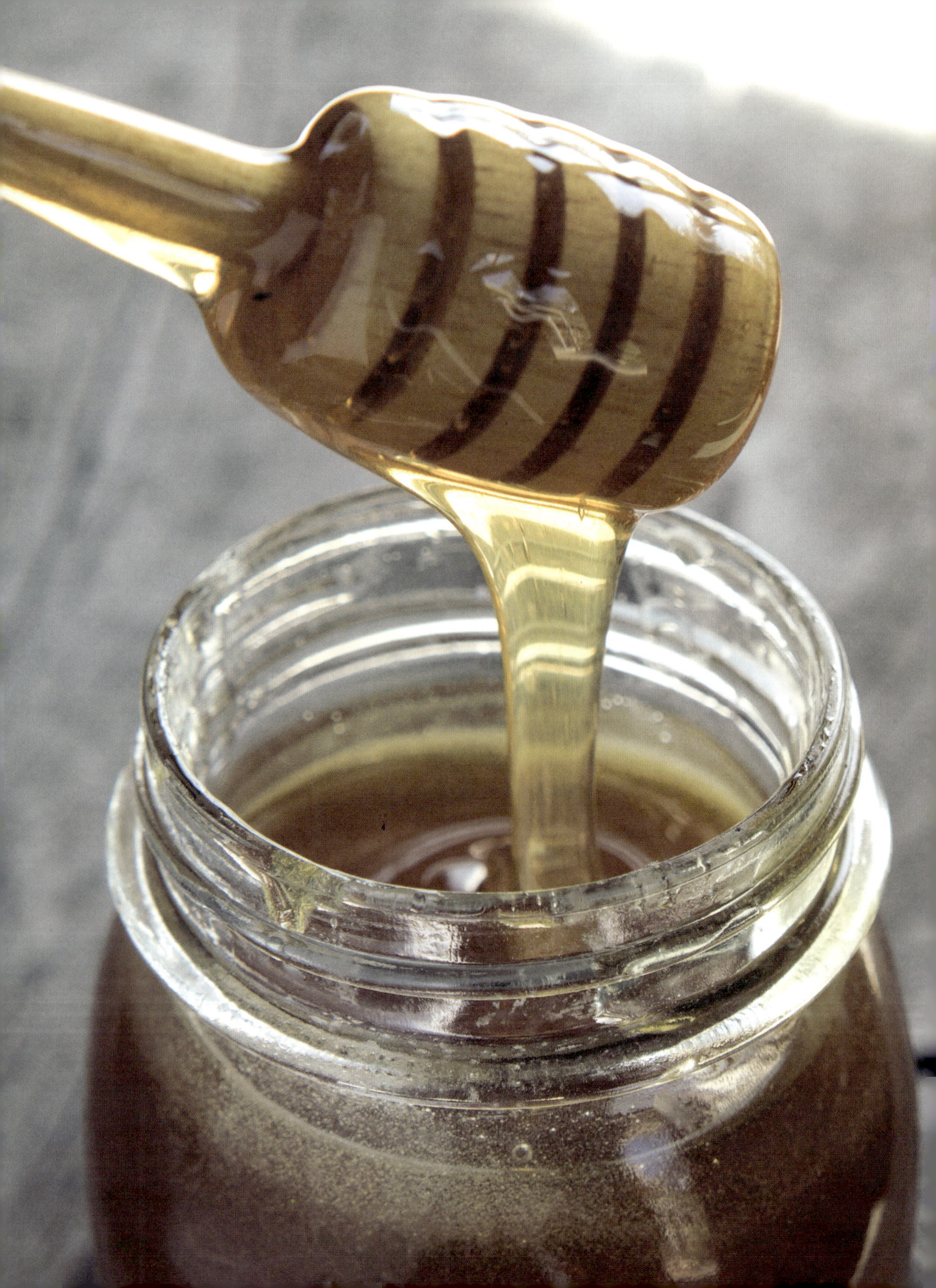

H

Hangovers

Many people suffer from hangovers after too much alcohol, waking up with a pounding headache, drier-than-dry mouth, loss of balance, nausea, fatigue, sweating, tremors and remorse.

Excessive alcohol consumption can cause dehydration, loss of electrolytes and low blood-glucose levels. It is also a diuretic, which means it speeds the loss of water from the body, causing the thirst, headache and dizziness. Nausea and vomiting are the result of the direct action of alcohol irritating the lining of the digestive tract. You need to drink plenty of water and replenish sugar and mineral levels.

BEFORE YOU START DRINKING

Have something to eat something with fat (cheese, for example) or drink a glass of milk. Don't drink alcohol on an empty stomach.

WHILE OUT DRINKING

Intersperse your drinks with a glass of water, mineral water with a twist of lime or lemon or a soft drink to reduce your alcohol intake and keep you hydrated.

BEFORE YOU GO TO BED

Drink a large glass of water.

THE MORNING AFTER

Everyone has their own hangover remedy but there is little research to prove any actually work. If you wake with a hangover, keep up your fluids with:

- Diluted fruit juice
- Lemonade
- Rehydration solution (such as Hydralite or Gastrolyte)
- Weak black tea with a teaspoon of sugar and a squeeze of lemon
- Clear soup or broth.

If you can manage to eat, have a small serve of light, bland food such as:

- Dry toast
- Plain boiled rice
- Crackers
- Canned pears or other fruit
- Plain yoghurt
- Stewed apple.

Eat a little and wait to see if you keep it down. If you have a pounding headache and vertigo, take some paracetamol as long as you know you can keep the food down first. B vitamins may also help.

> **Everyone has their own hangover remedy but there is little research to prove any actually work.**

See also **Alcohol.**

HANGOVER 'CURES'

HANGOVER 'CURES'	CLAIMED USE	MY TAKE
Fizzy vitamins	Effervescent tablets such as Berocca and Hairy Lemon have long been marketed as hangover remedies best taken at the end of a big night before you go to bed. The theory is that alcohol depletes the body of B vitamins (which are all water soluble), so adding them back helps top up your supply.	*Effervescent tablets are not hangover cures. They're basically multivitamins that claim to increase energy, but years of urban myths have given them 'celebrity hangover cure' status. Unless you're deficient in vitamin B, your daily diet should be ample. Some do contain herbal ingredients like ginseng or gingko, but these don't generally act quickly or are in such small quantities they don't do much. If anything, the bicarb of soda that creates the fizz loads you up on salt! A multi-B vitamin would be better for you.* *There are some small positives—the vitamin C is handy as it can speed up metabolism of alcohol by the liver, and some contain guarana (touted as 'natural', but really just another form of caffeine), which can be helpful to pick you up the morning after—but not before you go to bed. If they do help, it's most likely it's the water that is responsible—prevent dehydration and you stave off the worst of a hangover. Dehydration is responsible for most of the nastier effects of a hangover.*
Sports drinks	Drinking a Gatorade gives you a nice big glass of water and the fluid is absorbed better thanks to the electrolytes like sodium and potassium and their light sugar content (around 6 per cent rather than 11 per cent in juice or soft drink). The sugar is good as it helps counteract the blood glucose–lowering effect of alcohol and will settle your stomach.	*You could just as well have a piece of toast and a glass of diluted fruit juice. Nothing mystical about this!*
Over-the-counter tablets	Over-the-counter hangover remedies such as Alcodol, Onedose, Chaser, Sob'r-K Hangover Stopper, Russia Party, RU-21 and Rebound usually contain some type of sugar (fructose, glucose) along with vitamins B or C, minerals or herbal liver tonics such as milk thistle, artichoke, taurine or dandelion. You pop a couple before you start drinking, before you go to bed and the next morning 'if required'. Some are based on charcoal granules or clays such as Bentonite, which claim to 'filter' out any impurities while passing out undigested.	*Don't believe the hype about these so-called 'miracle cures'; the herbals are not there in sufficient quantity to do much, while the charcoal and clay claims are unproven. In 2005, the British Medical Journal published a study of eight trials assessing eight different hangover products. It reported there was 'no compelling evidence to suggest that any conventional or complementary intervention is effective for preventing or treating alcohol hangovers'. Again, it's the water you drink with them that does the job.*
Breakfast fry-up	Greasy eggs and bacon are a popular hangover cure. They fix the 'munchies', particularly if you've been dancing or have otherwise burned off heaps of energy. But it's wise to hold off on the greasies if the nausea and vomiting are bad. Light fare goes down better on a delicate stomach.	*There may be some evidence to support the virtues of eggs—both cooked and raw, with or without Tabasco. Egg yolks are rich in cysteine, a component amino acid of protein that scientists believe can break down acetaldehyde, one of the major end products of alcohol metabolism. Cysteine supplements are sold at pharmacies for this reason.*
Hair of the dog	This does work, but it's only a temporary relief that will delay your hangover until later in the day—sometimes worse than before. Why? Hangovers are partly caused by a toxic by-product of alcohol metabolism called methanol. When you down another beer or a chaser of vodka the next day, the body's enzymes that break down methanol prefer to work on the fresh ethanol first so they switch to that. The breakdown of methanol is left until last. The extra alcohol may dull the pain but it soon wears off.	*Don't fall for the myth that drinking more alcohol the morning after will fix your symptoms.*

Health Food

Health food shops were formerly frequented by a few vegetarian hippies and alternative cranks. Today, the industry is huge, encompassing independent and franchise 'health' restaurants, resorts, spas and shops. Stroll through any supermarket and you'll find mainstream products made popular by devotees—vitamins, muesli bars, herbal teas, organic vegetables, soy milks, gluten-free breads and yoghurts with acidophilus.

WHAT IS HEALTH FOOD?

The term is virtually impossible to define. Nearly all foods can be regarded as 'health foods' because they contribute nutrients and, when eaten as part of a balanced diet, promote health and wellbeing. Through general usage, many people apply the term 'health food' to those foods which have been grown organically or biodynamically, are natural (processed as little as possible) and contain no added preservatives, artificial colours or pesticide residue.

Food regulations prohibit the use of the word 'health' in the brand name of any food, because there is no single food that on its own will make you healthier. Just because foods are sold from a health-food shop doesn't guarantee they are better for you. Nor is there any guarantee that health foods are free of the additives and pesticides that many health-conscious shoppers wish to avoid. Because there is no code governing what a health-food store sells, each individual proprietor stocks whatever will attract people into the store.

DID YOU KNOW?

Even 'natural' foods have their own harmful toxins:

- Green and sprouted potatoes contain the toxin solanine.
- Rhubarb leaves (not the stalks), sorrel and spinach are high in oxalic acid, which is poisonous if consumed in large quantities; it's far more dangerous than any food additive—sheep and cattle have died grazing on pasture that contains oxalate weeds.
- Brussels sprouts, broccoli, swedes and turnips can antagonise the working of the thyroid gland—none of these harm us because the amounts consumed are small and can be handled by our bodies.
- Apricot kernels contain the poison cyanide.
- Comfrey, although used as a healing herb for more than 2000 years, contains toxic alkaloids, which have caused liver failure and even death.
- Cycad seeds, from one of Australia's most ancient plants, contain a powerful toxin the Aboriginal peoples used to remove by leaching the sliced seeds in a creek for many days.
- Kelp (seaweed) can accumulate toxic heavy metals and has been removed from sale from time to time because it contained dangerously high levels of arsenic.

HOW HEALTH FOOD IS SOLD TO YOU

In an era of high-tech, mass-produced goods, many people have turned nostalgically to reminders of days past, symbolised by the wholesome image of health food. Health-conscious consumers often reject the factory-made products of big business in their search for natural and pure foods. Some of the health movement's underlying messages include:

- Soils are depleted.
- Vitamins and food supplements are necessary because our food supply is deficient in nutrients.
- Our food supply is laden with 'chemicals' that are poisonous and toxic.

The marketing of health foods is based on:

- Testimonials from satisfied customers
- Endorsements from sporting personalities or celebrities
- Books by health-food gurus.

The power of suggestion (known as the placebo effect) is still as strong today as it was in the days of the snake-oil doctor and potion hucksters. If you deeply believe that a pill or food supplement will make you more vital (or cure an ailment), then there is a very good chance that it will.

Heartburn

Poor eating usually causes heartburn—either too much rich or greasy food, too much caffeine, too much alcohol, or stress and smoking are to blame. The most common scenario is when someone dines out on a rich meal, and then wakes up with heartburn during the night.

It starts when a small valve—the lower oesophageal sphincter that connects the stomach with the oesophagus (or food pipe)—is not working properly or is weakened. This causes acid to flow backwards, up into the oesophagus. Known as reflux, it causes heartburn, a burning pain behind the breastbone, which is the most common symptom.

Heartburn and reflux are not life-threatening conditions, but if it becomes chronic you need to have it checked out. It can be a warning sign of hernia or ulcer-causing bacteria. Left untreated, reflux can cause changes to your oesophagus that may lead to cancer.

MY TAKE

Various foods may cause heartburn in different individuals. For example, some people may have trouble with citrus or acidic things like pickled onions, while others may not. It's trial and error to pinpoint which foods are a problem for you.

SIMPLE WAYS TO PREVENT HEARTBURN

- ✔ Avoid big meals.
- ✔ Steer clear of greasy, high-fat foods like chips, anything deep-fried and fatty bacon.
- ✔ Avoid dishes with lots of chilli such as Thai takeaway.
- ✔ Elevate the head of your bed by at least 15 centimetres (use wooden blocks under the top legs of the mattress) to prevent the stomach contents washing back up into the oesophagus.
- ✔ Avoid too much coffee or caffeine.
- ✔ Eat slowly and chew your food properly.
- ✔ Lose weight if you need to as obesity (especially abdominal obesity) places increased pressure around your stomach; wearing tight or restrictive clothing can also make it worse.
- ✔ Avoid peppermint oil; it relaxes the sphincter at the top of your stomach—if you need to take it, buy peppermint oil in enteric-coated capsules designed to bypass the stomach and dissolve in the small intestine.

Check with your doctor if you're taking low-dose aspirin to prevent heart attacks—it can cause stomach pain, heartburn and intestinal bleeding.

DID YOU KNOW?

Milk and milky foods like custard have often been suggested for relieving heartburn. They do work like a mild antacid, but will only give temporary relief, and the calcium and protein found in milk stimulate acid production—so half an hour later, you could find yourself suffering even more.

Heart Disease and Diet

Heart and blood vessel disease is Australia and New Zealand's leading killer—almost twice as many people die from heart disease as from breast and lung cancer combined—yet it's preventable.

ARE YOU AT RISK?

Your risk of developing heart problems depends on a number of 'risk factors' such as:

- Smoking
- High blood pressure
- High blood cholesterol (both the total and the bad LDL)
- Diabetes
- Advancing years (over 50)
- Heart problems in the family
- Being overweight (especially around the middle)

- Being sedentary
- High blood triglycerides.

TEN EVERYDAY FOODS THAT KEEP YOUR HEART HEALTHY

FRUIT AND VEGETABLES

Hundreds of studies have shown that people who eat a lot of vegetables and fruit have a lower risk of heart attack and stroke. Researchers originally believed this was due to the high content of antioxidant vitamins—beta-carotene and vitamins C and E—but it's now attributed to other interesting compounds with even more powerful antioxidant capacity including carotenoids, anthocyanins and flavonoids. Fruit and vegetables also boost your folate levels, which keep homocysteine low.

RED WINE

In modest amounts, red wine is good for your heart. It could be the reason for the so-called 'French paradox'—the French have one of the lowest rates of heart disease in the world, despite their love of rich fare such as paté, croissants and high-fat cheeses. Wine's secret is its grape compounds known as polyphenols. These act as antioxidants, reduce thickening of the arteries and keep the blood flow smooth. Red wine, made with the skins and seeds of grapes, has nine to ten times more of these than white. But don't forget that the alcohol in any drink raises the 'good' HDL cholesterol, which is one of the mechanisms by which moderate drinking lowers heart disease.

GARLIC

Both fresh and dried garlic have been shown to lower the 'bad' LDL cholesterol and help dissolve clots, although the dose required is quite large for most of us—you'd need to eat three or four cloves each day, or 600–900 milligrams of powdered garlic. So add as much as you can to your cooking and you'll be helping your heart.

NUTS

Munching on a handful of nuts (30–50 grams) every day is now one of the strategies nutritionists recommend for a healthy heart. Surprised? Most of us are when for years we've been told nuts are too high in fat and will put on weight. A wave of studies over the past few years has changed thinking on nuts—they're now considered a healthy energy-packed snack that will out-perform potato crisps any way you look at it! The best way to consume nuts is lightly roasted but not salted. Toss them through salads and stir-fries, or use them in baking or as a crunchy topping.

> Each year, almost twice as many people die from heart disease as from breast and lung cancer combined—yet it's preventable.

All nuts are high in vitamin E, a heart-helpful antioxidant, as well as fibre and arginine, an amino acid, which is converted to nitric oxide in the body. Nitric oxide is a chemical 'messenger' in blood vessel cells, which causes the smooth muscle cells to relax, keeping the vessels dilated.

FISH AND SEAFOOD

Fish and seafood, eaten two or three times a week, are a powerful omega-3 boost, which helps steady the heartbeat, lower blood pressure and keep the blood free of clots (like aspirin does). Best of all, fish is low in kilojoules and cooks in minutes. Omega-3s are found in all fish and seafood but particularly in oily fish such as salmon, sardines, trout, mackerel, gemfish, mullet, herring and tuna (both fresh and canned).

TEA

People who regularly drink tea (green or black) are reported to have significantly lower risks of heart troubles. Tea's protective effects are believed to be due to its flavonoid antioxidants. They seem to maintain heart health by decreasing inflammation, lowering the tendency for clotting (an early factor in heart attacks) and by keeping the arteries more 'elastic'. These effects are obtained regardless of whether you add milk or sugar. Best of all, if you take it black with no milk or sugar, tea has no kilojoules and has the ability to both relax and revive you.

SOY

Soy is held responsible for the low rates of heart disease (and breast cancer) in Japanese and Chinese populations, where soy foods have been a staple for centuries. Soy protein lowers harmful LDL cholesterol and prevents artery 'clogging', according to more than 38 soy trials spanning 20 years. To achieve these heart benefits, you need to eat 25 grams of soy protein a day.

OATS

Oats, along with oat bran, psyllium, barley and rice bran, is high in soluble fibre, which sweeps breakdown products of cholesterol out of the body. This also means they are slowly absorbed into the bloodstream, which lessens the glucose load. But you need to eat a sizeable quantity to see your cholesterol drop. For oat bran, around one cup (around 100 grams) is required a day, which is a lot. Take it in as cereal, oat bran muffins and an oat bran smoothie. You can also substitute oat bran for half of the normal flour when baking muffins or breads.

SHOPPER'S GUIDE
PICK THE TICK

The Heart Foundation Tick has been helping Australians make healthier food choices for over 20 years. As a trusted, independent not-for-profit program, Tick continuously works with food companies to improve the nutrition of the foods we eat most often.

Tick's nutrition standards are tough and stringent so food companies work hard to earn the Tick. And once the Tick is on the pack foods are regularly random tested to ensure they continue to meet our strict nutrition standards. They must meet strict nutrition criteria and be low in saturated fat and salt, high in fibre and usually not too high in kilojoules. Companies pay the Heart Foundation a licence fee (a percentage of sales) to carry the Tick, and the income is channelled back into education, research, independent supermarket sampling and product testing. To achieve the Tick, manufacturers often reformulate and retest to meet the criteria.

By looking out for the Tick, shoppers can easily choose healthier products at a glance. They're healthier because Tick foods are lower in saturated fat, sodium (salt), and kilojoules (energy) but they also contain plenty of the good stuff like fibre, calcium, wholegrains and vegetables.

With more than 1300 products now approved to use the Tick, you are bound to find a healthier alternative to the foods you usually buy.

STEROL SPREADS

If you already use margarine, it's worth swapping to a sterol-enriched spread (brand names include Logicol and Pro-activ). Just spreading 2 to 3 teaspoons on toast or sandwiches each day is all you need to see your cholesterol go down.

Plant sterols are natural compounds found in vegetables, nuts and legumes but in low concentrations. They have a similar chemical structure to cholesterol, yet have the ability to block its absorption into the body. They are extracted from soy beans or wood pulp, and then added as a concentrate to a spread at a much higher concentration than we normally get from food.

See also **Cholesterol and Diet.**

WHOLEGRAINS

Eating more grainy breads, brown rice and wholegrain cereal is one way to reduce the risk of heart disease and some cancers. Many wholegrain foods also have a lower glycemic index (GI) than white or refined products, and will keep your blood-glucose levels on an even keel and leave you feeling fuller for longer.

Hemp Seeds

Hemp seeds are rich in omega-6 fatty acids. In Europe and North America you can buy foods made from hemp seeds and oil, including hemp milk, snack bars, pasta, bread, dressings and sauces. It is currently illegal to produce or sell hemp seed products in Australia for human consumption.

Herbs

While the market for herbal remedies such as echinacea, gingko and herbal teas is growing rapidly, let's not forget the culinary herbs that grace our meals can make a sizable contribution to our nutrition intake—if we eat enough of them.

A LITTLE NUTRITIONAL BOOST

It's easy to see why herbs are considered insignificant in the vitamin stakes, when we consume perhaps 1–2 grams at a time, compared with 120 grams of fruit. But basil, for example, is a rich source of a number of minerals, especially potassium, magnesium, and smaller amounts of iron and calcium. It also contains vitamin C, folate, vitamin B_1 and vitamin K, and scores highly for fibre and a great many antioxidants. On a weight for weight comparison, basil and parsley have almost twice as much vitamin C as oranges while dill has six times more beta-carotene than rockmelon or pumpkin.

Herbs are also surprisingly rich in antioxidants. Rosemary, thyme and oregano have been found to be rich in polyphenols, one type of antioxidant that may cut the risk of heart disease. Mint, basil and parsley are high in monoterpenes, which are thought to have cancer-delaying properties, especially with mammary tumours. Parsley is also high in coumarins, noted for their anti-coagulant and anti-bacterial effects, while extracts of rosemary are being tested to see if they can be used as a natural food-grade preservative. If you're trying to cut back on salt, use herbs freely to boost the flavour of your meals.

EASY WAYS TO ENJOY HERBS

- ✔ Extra zing—add fresh basil or mint leaves to salad
- ✔ Healthy and tasty—slice up ripe

TRY THESE

- TABBOULI—Place a couple of bunches of chopped parsley in a bowl, with some cracked wheat, garlic and tomato, and you have a delicious and nutritious herbal boost.
- PESTO SAUCE—Blend lots of basil (or you can use Italian parsley or coriander) with toasted pine nuts, olive oil and garlic.

On a weight for weight comparison, basil and parsley have almost twice as much vitamin C as oranges, while dill has six times more beta-carotene than rockmelon or pumpkin.

Popular herb partnerships

Basil—tomato, olive oil, pasta, egg, bocconcini
Bay leaves—soup, casseroles, fish, chicken
Chives—fish, seafood, ricotta, cottage cheese, potato, cucumber, omelette, chicken
Coriander—chicken, lean beef, mint, salad, avocado, soup, curries, noodle dishes
Dill—fish, egg, potato, mushroom, prawns, scallops, smoked salmon, carrot, risotto
Lemon grass—tea, soup, curries, sauces
Oregano—chicken, beef, fish, tomato, pizza, pasta, eggplant, zucchini
Rosemary—potato, pumpkin, lamb, chicken, pork, rabbit, duck, garlic, scones, breads

tomatoes and arrange over crusty bread. Top with basil and ground black pepper
- ✔ Classic with a twist—make a healthy potato salad by combining cold boiled potatoes with chopped basil, pine nuts and olive oil
- ✔ Be plentiful—use lots of oregano in your Greek and Italian cooking
- ✔ Feature flavour—coriander leaves (and often the roots as well) are used a lot in Mexican and Asian cuisines and add lots of flavour to marinades, dressings and salsas.

Herbal Supplements

> Around half of all Australians now take complementary and alternative medicine supplements.

As the combination of orthodox and complementary or alternative medicine increases, herbs and herbal supplements are steadily growing in popularity.

Studies have found that nearly 20 per cent of GPs practise some form of complementary or alternative medicine, and at least 50 per cent have an interest in the area. These numbers are likely to have increased with the introduction of university-based GP training courses in herbal medicine, and recent endorsements by peak medical bodies such as the Australian Medical Association (2002) and the Royal College of Medical Practitioners (2004) for the provision of complementary and alternative medicine to patients. Nutrition research into phytochemicals or phytotherapeutic agents, which occur in plants, also supports this growth industry.

There has been a huge rise in the sale of complementary and alternative health products worldwide and this is reflected in the acquisition of related companies by large pharmaceutical organisations. Around half of all Australians now take complementary and alternative supplements. A study profiled users as not chronically ill, but generally younger, better educated and more likely to be employed.

MY TAKE
While there's no sound documented evidence proving the safety and efficacy of herbal supplements, consumers are voting with their feet! Many herbs show great promise and have a long history of medicinal use, but questions remain over how effective they really are, what dosage is required and whether they may produce harmful side effects.

HERBAL SAFETY NOTES

While herbs are 'natural', they are not without side effects. Some can be toxic in high doses (as many drugs are when taken in excess), or trigger adverse reactions in susceptible people. Unlike drugs, research funding for herbs is low as they cannot be patented. The main criticisms of herbal medicines are:

- ✖ Poor quality control—there's no way of telling whether it's the real herb and how much of it you're actually getting
- ✖ No dosage regulation
- ✖ No purity standards
- ✖ Contaminants such as pesticide residues may sometimes be present.

Take heed of these tips when taking herbals.

- Take herbs only for minor ailments such as colds, headaches, gastro-intestinal problems or tiredness.
- Let your doctor know if you are taking them in addition to your usual medication,
- Buy reputable brands; look for standardised herbal extracts that guarantee the concentration of active ingredients.
- Don't take herbs if you are pregnant or breastfeeding without checking with your doctor first.
- Ask advice from a qualified herbalist, especially if you take other herbs or medications on a regular basis.

See also **Garlic; Ginger; Ginseng.**

OTHER HERBS AND THEIR USES

HERB	CLAIMED BENEFITS	CONTRAINDICATIONS
Aloe vera	Helps to heal wounds, burns and skin irritations and is generally reliable for external skin treatment.	Can have a laxative effect when taken orally.
Chamomile	Believed to have a sedative and calming effect. It helps treat indigestion (like peppermint), and has an anti-spasmodic and anti-inflammatory effect on the digestive system.	
Comfrey	Used in the treatment of peptic ulcers and gastritis, psoriasis and skin ulcers (topical).	Possibly linked to liver cancer.
Feverfew	It is claimed to help alleviate headaches and reduce fever. Also minimises joint pain in arthritis and has anti-inflammatory properties.	
Ginkgo	Valued in China since 2000 BC and used in Ayurvedic (traditional Indian) medicine. It may improve memory and brain function, treat headache and improve blood flow and circulation to the brain.	One of the better-documented herbs, it shows great promise.
Goldenseal (hydrastis)	Used by Native Americans for skin and eye ailments, it contains alkaloids, which possess weak antiseptic properties.	
Hawthorn	Believed to be a vasodilator (dilates blood vessels), and to reduce blood pressure and angina, improve blood supply to the heart and lessen arrhythmia. It contains large numbers of flavonoids.	
Hops	A mild sedative and sleeping aid, hops is used in beer for the bitter taste and preservative action. Contains polyphenols.	
Hypericum (St John's wort)	Traditionally used to treat colds, syphilis, tuberculosis, dysentery and worms. It inhibits bacteria and viruses and has possible anti-depressive actions.	It is becoming accepted as a non-drug treatment for depression. Photo-sensitivity toxicity limits usage. It can interact with certain drugs.
Milk thistle	Believed to stimulate the flow of bile. Research also supports its protective action against liver toxins. Milk thistle contains antioxidant flavonoids, known collectively as silymarin.	Appears to be useful in liver complaints, although more research is needed.
Nettle (tea)	A mild diuretic used frequently in folk medicine. It is also used in hair and scalp remedies. Nettle is rich in vitamin E, chlorophyll, beta-carotene and vitamin C.	
Passionflower (tea)	A mild sedative and calming agent.	
Raspberry leaf (tea)	Believed to relax the smooth muscle of the uterus during pregnancy. It also has astringent and stimulant properties. Sometimes used as mouthwash and gargle (tannins) and as a remedy for diarrhoea and stomach ailments.	
Saw palmetto	Used to treat enlarged prostates (benign prostatic hyperplasia), it contains high concentrations of sterols and has an anti-androgenic effect. Also a mild diuretic.	
Yohimbine	Believed to be a prosexual herb (aphrodisiac). Has action similar to MAO inhibitors (a class of anti-depressant drugs).	

Herbal Teas

Herbal infusions or tisanes are free of caffeine, have a refreshing taste, possess no kilojoules and may have a therapeutic effect, although scientific proof of this is limited.

Comprising extracts of leaves, flowers, bark, seeds, fruit peels and spices, many herbal teas contain vitamins, antioxidants and natural plant compounds. Herbal teas have a long history of medicinal use. For example, peppermint tea, with its refreshing tangy aroma and flavour, has been in use medicinally since the 17th century, when it was first given as a cure for diarrhoea.

SOME POPULAR HERBAL TEAS AND THEIR REPUTED THERAPEUTIC EFFECTS.

Chamomile—Has a mild sedative effect and can promote a good night's sleep. Also valued for its soothing properties, and is said to ease headaches and relax the mind.
Dandelion—Detoxifies the liver and relieves constipation.
Elderflower—A cure for hangovers.
Feverfew—Helps eliminate toxins.
Ginger—Helps overcome nausea and morning sickness.
Lemon verbena—Induces sleep.
Nettle—Eases rheumatic pain.
Peppermint—Aids digestion, settles upset stomachs and other digestive problems.
Rosehip—Made from the ripe fruits (hips) of wild roses and extremely rich in vitamin C. Said to be a mild laxative and tonic for the kidneys and gallbladder. The tea is often blended with lemon, cinnamon or hibiscus flowers.
Rosemary—Relieves tension.
Skullcap—Cures persistent headaches.
Valerian root—Calms the nerves and helps you sleep. Also said to cure headaches.

High-fructose Corn Syrup (HFCS)

High-fructose corn syrup, or HFCS, is a type of sweetener made from maize or corn. The starch is extracted from the maize and converted into various blends of glucose and fructose, a natural sugar that's also found in fruit. The main types are:

- HFCS 55—mostly used in beverages like soft drinks, fruit drinks and cordials. It contains on average 55 per cent fructose and 45 per cent glucose.
- HFCS 42—used in many solid foods and baked goods. It contains on average 42 per cent fructose and 58 per cent glucose.

Small quantities of HFCS 90 (90 per cent fructose) and crystalline fructose (more than 99.5 per cent) are also produced for 'specialty applications' (including processed foods, baked goods and beverages), and for reblending back with lower-fructose syrups.

In the US, HFCS is popular and commonly used in soft drinks because it's less expensive than cane sugar, which is what is used in Australia and New Zealand. HFCS is not widely used in foods in Australia and New Zealand, but you may see it as an ingredient on imported products.

See also **Fructose.**

Histamine

A compound found naturally in wine, beer, chocolate and matured cheese. It is commonly reported as a cause of migraines.

Honey

A golden amber liquid made by bees from the nectar of flowers, honey has been nature's sweetener for centuries and is frequently claimed to be superior to sugar. Once described as the 'nectar of the gods', today honey has largely given way to sugar (on average, we consume more than 40 times more sugar than honey). Yet it remains a favourite flavouring in foods like breakfast cereals, sauces, cakes, biscuits, honey-coated nuts, yoghurt and hams. I love honey in my lemon myrtle tea and to sweeten plain breakfast cereal. Its flavour is superb.

Being 'natural', honey is often considered to be a healthy sweetener, but nutritionally its true advantages are minor. Like other sweet foods, honey must be counted as a form of sugar when you need to watch your weight. Like sugar, it can also cause tooth decay if left to cling to teeth.

DID YOU KNOW?

In terms of kilojoules, sugar and honey rate virtually the same. One tablespoon of honey contains 270 kj, compared to 350 kj for sugar.

NUTRITIONAL VALUE

Honey is made up of around 75 per cent sugars, of which roughly half is glucose and half is fructose (although these proportions vary depending on the flowers from which the nectar was collected). The remaining 25 per cent is water, which explains why it can appear to have less 'sugar' or kilojoules than sugar (sucrose) per 100 grams.

Being derived from the flowers of plants, honey does contain small amounts of plant acids, waxes, gums, pigments and volatile oils, which have antioxidant and antibacterial properties. Honey also contains B vitamins and minerals, but the quantities are tiny and not significant nutritionally—you would have to consume enormous amounts of honey to obtain a decent intake. Unlike bread or breakfast cereals, there are not enough B vitamins in honey to metabolise the kilojoules it supplies. Analysis of honey is limited to date, but I have no doubt its natural phytochemical properties will be an area of great interest in the future.

Most commercial, blended honeys have a moderate glycemic index (GI) of 64, around the same as sugar. But some pure floral honeys—stringybark, red gum, yellow box, ironbark and others that have been produced by allowing bees access only to some types of gum trees (eucalypts)—have low GI values. Yellow box, for example, has a low GI of 35.

Growing Bodies

Parents are advised not to give babies honey during their first year of life because of the small chance of ingesting botulism spores.

NUMBER CRUNCH

One tablespoon of honey provides a trace of protein, a trace of fat, 23 grams of sugar, no starch, a trace of fibre and 270 kilojoules.

THE BEE'S KNEES OF REMEDIES

Honey has a long history of safe use as a medicinal—it appears in so many traditional remedies that one suspects an element of therapeutic truth, despite the lack of official documentation in medical journals.

A cup of hot water with lemon and honey has long been used to soothe sore throats (researchers think honey acts as a disinfectant for the mouth and throat), while many rely on hot milk and honey before bed to help them sleep. Honey is also sometimes taken for its mild laxative effect, which researchers now believe may be due to its high content of fructose, a sugar that is often not completely absorbed in the bowel.

Honey's antibacterial properties have been well known for more than 80 years, and there are many reports of its effectiveness as a dressing for minor wounds, skin ulcers and burns.

VARIETIES OF HONEY

Creamed honey—Creamed honey (also called whipped honey or granulated honey) looks like soft white honey and is thick and easy to spread like butter. It is simply honey that's been whipped to slow the natural crystallisation process. It makes the honey thicker and changes the way it feels in your mouth. Nutritionally, it has the same profile as ordinary honey. Many people prefer it, as it's less messy in the kitchen.	**Pasteurised honey**—Most of the honey sold in supermarkets has been pasteurised (heated briefly at 70 degrees Celsius and then cooled rapidly) and filtered. This makes it look clearer and more appealing on the shelf, and easier to handle and package. Pasteurisation kills yeast cells in the honey and prevents fermentation. It also slows down the speed of crystallisation. On the downside, heating reduces the enzymes, and possibly the antioxidants.	**Raw honey**—Many people believe that raw honey with its flecks made of bee pollen, honeycomb, propolis and bee wing fragments is more nutritious. This is difficult to determine, as there are no uniform standards for who can use the term 'raw honey'. Many honeys sold as 'natural' or 'raw' have still been filtered or treated mildly with heat to slow down the process of crystallisation so they remain smooth and presentable on the shelves.	**Mead (honey wine)**—An alcoholic drink made from fermented honey, water and yeast, mead can be light or rich, sweet or dry, and may be flavoured with herbs or spices. The alcoholic content of mead can range from about 8 per cent to 18 per cent. Mead is not a beer, wine or spirit in the normal sense; it is its own class of alcohol. Many historians believe it is the oldest of all the alcoholic beverages. Mead has held a pivotal place in many cultures throughout its history, which stretches back nearly 8000 years, especially in northern Europe.

However, other claims over the years—such as it being a cure for asthma, and a tonic against colds, arthritis, anaemia and heart problems—do not stand up to scrutiny.

MEDICINAL (MANUKA) HONEY

There's quite a bank of research these days behind antibacterial honeys (or medical honeys). Certain honeys are good for wound healing, but it now seems the active honeys can also relieve sore throats, mouth ulcers, sore gums and possibly indigestion. It's all due to the high antibacterial activity in honey derived from the tea tree (*Leptospermum*), or the Manuka in New Zealand.

> **DID YOU KNOW?**
>
> You don't dissolve antibacterial honey in tea or lemon juice. For maximum effect, eat 3 to 4 tablespoons each day, straight from the spoon.

Medical honeys appear to work in at least three ways—they're high in phenols, a type of antioxidant with an anti-inflammatory effect; they contain natural hydrogen peroxide, an antiseptic; and their concentration of sugars produces a high osmolarity (concentration) which can inhibit the growth of bacteria. For this reason, the undiluted honey needs to come into direct contact with the problem area.

The numbers on the label of antibacterial honeys, for example 5+, do mean something. This is a Unique Manuka Factor (UMF) rating, which means the honey has been tested for its antibacterial activity. It's like the SPF factors on sunscreen—the higher the number, the greater the antibacterial concentration. They are rare, but you can buy honeys with UMFs of 20 to 25; however, this is generally believed to be too strong and can cause adverse reactions. A UMF of between 16 and 18 is recommended for both internal and external use.

Remember most honey is *not* active. Only those labelled active or medical with a UMF of 10+ have antibacterial abilities.

Humectants

These are additives used to keep food moist. Humectants include sorbitol, mannitol and glycerin.

See also Additives.

Hunger *See* Appetite and Hunger.

Hydration

Water has been dubbed the forgotten factor in our diets, but it's the most vital of nutrients. We can survive for days, even weeks, without food, but only 4–5 days without water. It's needed for so many functions in our body. We need water to:

- ✔ Transport nutrients around the body via the blood and lymph system
- ✔ Remove wastes via urine and faeces
- ✔ Serve as a medium for the countless biochemical reactions that take place in the body
- ✔ Moisten our food to facilitate chewing
- ✔ Maintain body temperature—when we sweat, heat is released as the sweat evaporates, which cools you down.

DID YOU KNOW?

About 60 per cent of our body is made up of water. Organs like the brain and muscles contain as much as 75 per cent water.

DEHYDRATION

A US study found that significant numbers of people go about their lives in a state of mild dehydration. Dehydration occurs with only a 1–2 per cent loss of fluid, but if left uncorrected the symptoms can be significant. Over a lifetime, insufficient fluid has been linked to kidney stones, urinary tract infections and bladder cancer. Some groups are more at risk of dehydration than others. These include small children, breastfeeding mothers and the elderly.

THE TOP SIX DEHYDRATORS

- Very hot weather
- Gastroenteritis
- Diarrhoea
- Vomiting
- Extreme high-fibre diets
- Too much alcohol.

SIGNS TO WATCH FOR

Signs of mild dehydration include headache, feeling tired and light-headed, and your skin loses its plumpness and becomes flushed. Moderate dehydration can cause general weakness, rapid heart rate and an inability to think clearly. Severe dehydration will result in muscle cramps and failing kidneys.

TIPS FOR STAYING HYDRATED

- ✔ Water is the ideal drink as it's neutral in taste, has no kilojoules and is inexpensive.
- ✔ Add lemon or lime to it to improve the taste or buy an inexpensive water filter jug to remove taints from your tap water.
- ✔ Have a drink on your desk at work; aim to drink a glass of a healthy fluid every two hours so you get through those eight glasses over the day.
- ✔ Carry a drink with you in the car or on outings.
- ✔ Make it a habit to have a drink every time you take a break or go to the toilet.
- ✔ Encourage kids to drink—they are more susceptible to dehydration.
- ✔ Choose a variety of beverages to encourage a regular drinking habit.

See also Beverages.

Hyperactivity and Diet

Is your child out of control and hard to handle after eating junk food full of colours and preservatives? Are they unusually restless or irritable after eating certain foods? Hyperactivity is one of the key symptoms of Attention Deficit Hyperactivity Disorder (ADHD), and has often been linked to sugar and additives. But is this the case?

In terms of sugar, the evidence isn't convincing enough. A number of studies of ADHD children have used artificially sweetened foods as dummy controls to assess children's behaviour with and without sugar. The most recent and thorough study was carried out in the US in Tennessee, which found that even large amounts of sugar produced no significant alteration in the behaviour or cognitive performance of children. Researchers specifically selected children whose parents described them as 'sugar sensitive', but they couldn't tell when their children were on the high-sugar diet, or one of the two diets incorporating sweeteners (saccharin or aspartame).

The Royal Prince Alfred Hospital in Sydney is a leader in this field, having developed a special elimination diet to test food-sensitive children. While this should only be done under supervision, some families have noticed improvements by reducing their child's intake of preserved, coloured and highly flavoured foods.

Because kids often become unruly after parties where sugary foods are consumed, many parents blame the high load of sugar. But there's more evidence to condemn some of the other substances commonly present with sugar such as caffeine (in cola soft drinks and chocolate), artificial colours and preservatives in frankfurts, party pies, dips and pizzas. With the exception of sugar, all of these compounds are removed in a standard elimination diet when testing if certain foods are a trigger for behaviour problems.

MY TAKE
Sugar, whether it's white or brown, does not contain problem chemicals that trigger behavioural problems so there's no need to eliminate it from the diet—but that's not a green light to overindulge!

ADDITIVES, COLOURS AND KIDS

If your child is hard to handle after attending a party, it doesn't automatically mean they have ADHD. Children suffering from this disorder must also show the classic symptoms of ADHD—hyperactivity, lack of concentration and impulsivity—most of the time both at home and in the classroom, not just after a party. Remember only a small number of ADHD children are sensitive to food. If you think this applies to your child, talk to your doctor or an accredited dietitian. They can help you take steps to identify the culprits, which is not always easy.

Food triggers can be either additives or natural chemicals such as salicylates (in many fruit juices), amines (in tasty cheese) and glutamates (in soy sauce and mushrooms). The most common culprits are colours in foods like those in bright cordials, soft drinks, seasoned snack foods like potato chips with barbecue or cheese flavour, tomato sauce, sausages and coloured lollies. Other additives that can cause reactions include preservatives, antioxidants and flavour enhancers. See the checklist on page 68.

SUSPECT COLOURS

- The red food dye erythrosine (127) has been restricted to colouring maraschino cherries since 1997.
- Tartrazine (102), a yellow colouring, is suspected of provoking asthma, urticaria (hives) and mood changes
- Sunset Yellow FC (110), amaranth (123) and Brilliant Blue FCF (133) are under a cloud for being potentially carcinogenic, and for triggering reactions ranging from bad behaviour and wakefulness at night to skin rashes.

ADDITIVES THAT MAY CAUSE REACTIONS CHECKLIST

COLOURS, ARTIFICIAL	102, 110, 122–133, 142, 151, 155
COLOURS, NATURAL	160b
PRESERVATIVES	210–213, 220–228, 280–283, 249–252
ANTIOXIDANTS	310–312, 320, 321
FLAVOUR ENHANCERS	620–625

See also **Confectionery; Food Colours; Additives.**

Hypoglycaemia

Hypoglycaemia is a low level of glucose in the blood, due to excess production (or overdose) of the glucose-controlling hormone insulin. It causes trembling, sweating, poor concentration and mental confusion and can lead to coma in diabetes sufferers. It is derived from the Greek words 'hypo' (meaning under) and 'glycemia' (meaning blood glucose). People with diabetes know all about it. If you don't have diabetes, but you have vague health problems ranging from tiredness to depression, or someone tells you that you have 'low blood glucose', see your doctor and get a proper diagnosis.

THE SUGAR 'HYPO' HYPE

Sugar has often been condemned as the cause of hypoglycaemia, but this is not true. You can eliminate sugar from your diet, but this is not the entire solution to the problem.

Sugar, it's claimed, overloads the pancreas, forcing it to overproduce insulin. The insulin clears the blood of glucose and, despite having just eaten, the body tissues become starved of energy. In an attempt to correct the lack of glucose, the body instinctively puts out signals for sweet foods, which only starts the sugar-craving cycle again.

TRUE HYPOGLYCAEMIA

'True' hypoglycaemia caused by a serious medical problem is rare. A valid diagnosis requires blood-glucose levels to drop below normal, and be accompanied by shakiness, an inability to think clearly, fainting attacks and sweating. It is especially important is that symptoms are immediately relieved by eating something sweet (or by injecting glucose into the bloodstream).

Glucose tolerance tests, used to monitor blood-glucose levels after swallowing a measured dose of glucose, vary enormously from person to person. Even though they may drop low in response to the glucose-controlling hormone insulin, this does not mean you have the 'true' medical condition called hypoglycaemia.

REACTIVE HYPOGLYCAEMIA

Rebound or reactive hypoglycaemia is the common type of hypoglycaemia. It can occur in perfectly healthy people and produces a variety of unpleasant symptoms from sweating, tremor, anxiety and weakness to restlessness, irritability, poor concentration, lethargy and drowsiness.

If you have reactive hypoglycaemia, it means your blood-glucose level rises too quickly after you have eaten, causing the release of too much insulin.

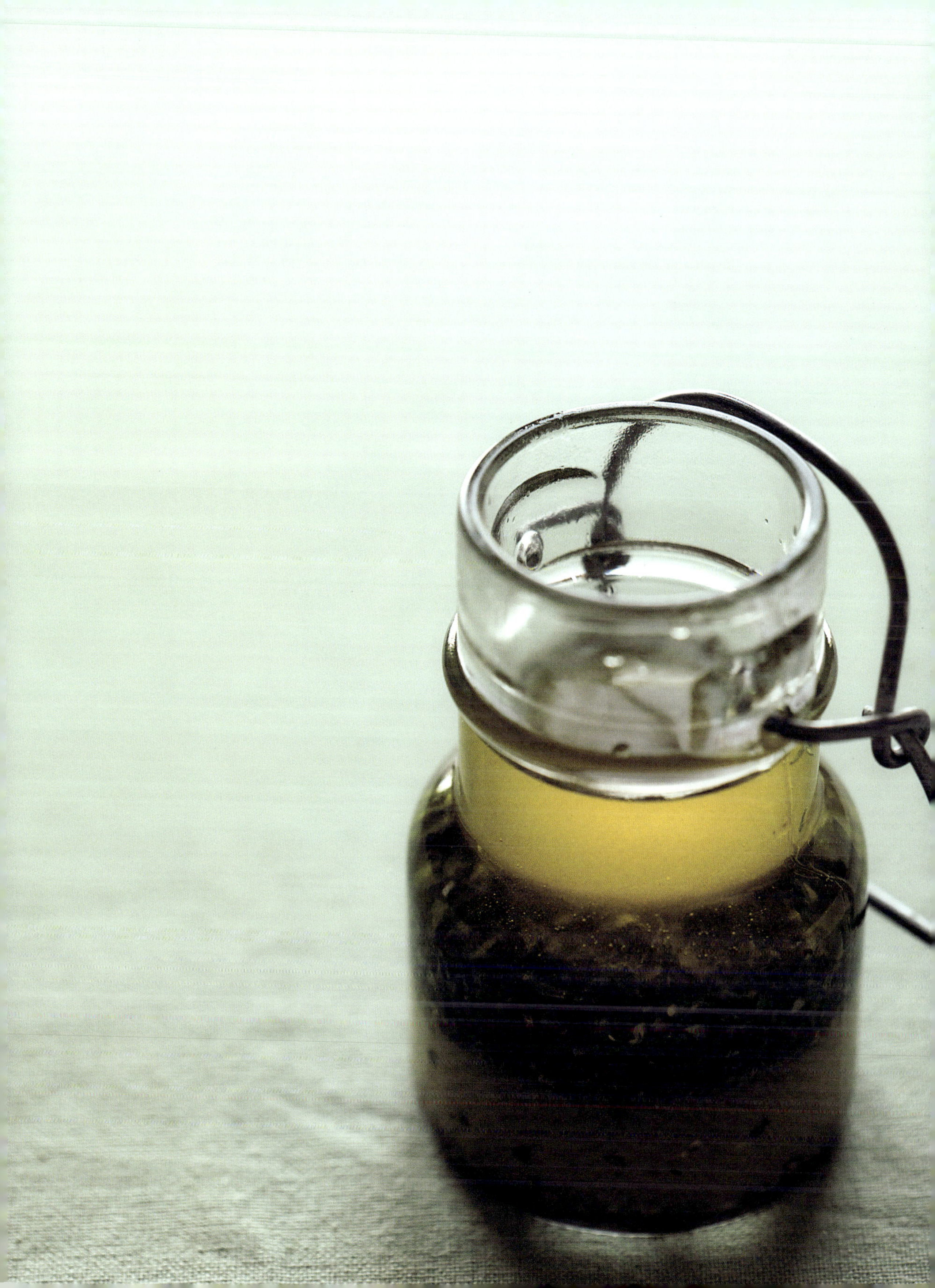

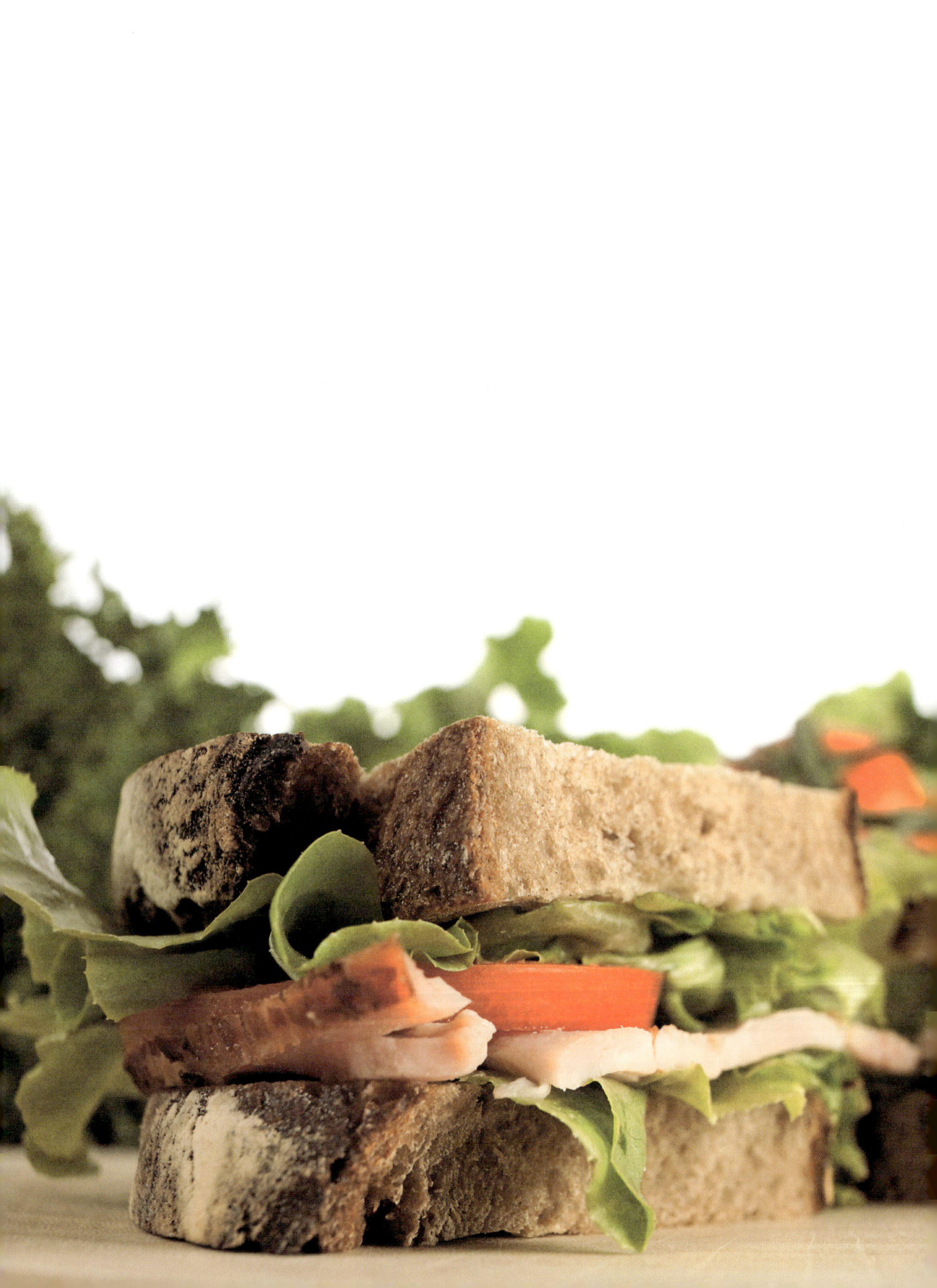

DIAGNOSIS

Diagnosis is difficult because there are no clear diagnostic criteria. Your doctor may:

- Ask you about signs and symptoms.
- Test your blood glucose while you are having symptoms.
- Check to see whether your symptoms ease after your blood glucose returns to normal after eating or drinking.

If your doctor uses an oral glucose tolerance test (OGTT) to diagnose hypoglycaemia, you have to continue it for at least 3–4 hours (the normal time is 2 hours). Your insulin levels would be measured at the same time.

TREATMENT

The aim when treating reactive hypoglycemia is to prevent large, sudden increases in your blood-glucose levels, so you won't produce excessive and unnecessary amounts of insulin and your blood-glucose levels won't plunge to abnormally low levels.

You can achieve smooth, steady blood-glucose levels by changing from high-GI foods to low-GI foods. This is particularly important when eating carbohydrate foods on their own, such as a piece of toast or a muffin. You don't have to avoid sugar but it's best to keep it low and have it with a low-GI food like sweetened low-fat yoghurt, wholegrain bread with a spread of jam or a slice of cake with milky coffee. If you can stop the big swings in blood glucose, then you will stop the symptoms of reactive hypoglycemia and chances are you will feel a lot better.

IJ

Infants and Diet

It's best for babies to be breast (or bottle) fed until 6 months of age, with the introduction of solid foods at around 6 months, together with continued breast or bottle feeding until the age of 12 months and beyond, if both mother and baby wish.

Breastfeeding is the recommended approach of the two options as it provides significant health benefits. Breastfed babies are less likely to suffer from conditions such as gastroenteritis, respiratory illness and ear infections (otitis media). Breastfeeding also benefits the mother's health by promoting faster recovery from childbirth and reducing the risks of breast and ovarian cancers in later life. Bottle feeding babies, using today's complete balanced formulas, is an acceptable option for mothers who, for a variety of reasons, can't or don't want to breastfeed.

When it's time for solid foods, introduce a new food every 2–3 days, according to their readiness and what the family eats. Introduce one new food at a time so that any reactions can be readily identified. Talk to your early childhood nurse about what solids to introduce and when.

Infertility and Diet

Infertility affects one in six couples, according to recent studies in Europe and the US. There are many reasons for infertility – for women, there may be structural problems like blocked fallopian tubes, a disease of the uterus like fibroids or endometriosis or an ovulation failure where the eggs don't ripen and release when they're supposed to. Diabetes, polycystic ovaries, age and thyroid disorders also affect ovulation. For men, low sperm count may be the cause, or the sperm's motility may be slow or their tails damaged so they have trouble navigating up through the uterus to the eggs.

EATING FOR FERTILITY

Before heading down the in vitro fertilisation (IVF) road, consider trying a high-fertility diet. This diet aims to boost the intake of certain micronutrients and improve insulin sensitivity through diet, weight control and increased physical activity.

Tackling insulin is important for women as it helps correct polycystic ovarian syndrome (PCOS), the leading cause of female infertility.

Research has also found that eating a balanced, nutritious diet contributes to higher fertility rates. A recent study by the Harvard School of Public Health and Harvard Medical School followed a group of 17,544 married women for eight years as they tried to become pregnant or became pregnant. It found that the women with the lowest rate of infertility (and most likely to fall pregnant) were those who ate fewer trans fats, less sugar, more low-GI foods such as pasta and grainy bread, and more protein from vegetables than from animals, had a good intake of iron, took multivitamins, exercised daily, kept their BMI between 20 and 25, and (surprisingly) consumed more full-fat dairy products.

WHAT WOMEN CAN DO

Eat a diet rich in fruits, vegetables, wholegrains, nuts, low-fat dairy and proteins to increase your energy and ensure you are getting all the nutrients your body needs.

Cut back on all refined carbohydrates and swap these foods for low-GI foods and wholegrains, which don't trigger such big rises in insulin and helps to manage PCOS and create regular ovulation. They will also boost your folate and other B vitamins, fibre and antioxidants intake.

If you need to, now is a good time to lose excess weight before you start trying to conceive. Couples often find that they become pregnant once one or both partners lose weight. Being overweight can hinder the function of your reproductive system and alter hormone levels. But don't be silly and try fad diets that can jeopardise your health.

Exercise at least three times a week for a minimum of 30 minutes to help maintain your weight and keep hormone levels normal.

Keep your alcohol intake light—fewer than five standard drinks a week. While research into the effect of alcohol on fertility is inconclusive, some studies have shown a slight link between drinking and infertility.

Quit smoking, even if you have just a few cigarettes a day.

WHAT MEN CAN DO

Make sure you're taking in sufficient zinc, selenium and other minerals, which aid in healthy sperm development. Studies show that short-term zinc deficiencies can reduce sperm volume and testosterone levels. Zinc also plays an important role in producing sperm, protecting its genetic material and helping it live as long as possible after ejaculation.

Eat foods rich in vitamin C and other antioxidants. These help prevent sperm defects and boost motility. Vitamin E works with selenium to prevent sperm damage.

Limit alcohol. Less is best with alcohol, especially during the 3 months prior to trying to conceive. Studies show that drinking alcohol daily can reduce testosterone levels and sperm counts and raise the number of abnormal sperm. There is a link between men who drink more than two drinks a day and lower birth weights.

Quit smoking. Smoking cigarettes and marijuana can decrease the number, motility and development of sperm.

Inflammatory Bowel Disease (IBD)

See **Crohn's Disease.**

Insomnia and Diet

Getting enough solid, quality sleep is essential for your health and wellbeing. Sleep gives the body a chance to rest, recuperate and repair. It gives the brain a chance to process the activities of the day and it plays an important role in memory formation. But research shows about one-third of us toss and turn every night, waiting for that peaceful slumber to descend, or we fall asleep only to be wide-eyed at 3 am. With longer working hours and increasingly stressful lifestyles, more and more of us are running into sleep-deprivation problems.

Lack of sleep leads to many health problems. Apart from leaving you tired and irritable, it can lower your immunity, make your memory poorer, reduce productivity and worsen insulin resistance. Lack of sleep has been linked to an increase in weight and type 2 diabetes.

While 7–8 hours sleep each night is usually recommended, there are many people who only need 6–7 hours and feel fine. Whatever your sleep needs, you should have enough quality sleep to wake up feeling refreshed and alert with energy the next morning. If you are having trouble meeting your sleep needs, try adjusting your diet and relaxing by following some of the techniques I suggest below, before going to your doctor for a prescription for sleeping tablets.

WHAT YOU CAN DO TO GET YOUR FULL 40 WINKS

AVOID ALCOHOL OR KEEP IT MODERATE

While it is common to think a bedtime nightcap helps you to relax, feel drowsy and nod off to sleep, in fact, it actually reduces the quality of sleep you get by giving you a fragmented, fitful sleep. Alcohol is a diuretic so too much alcohol may wake you up in the middle of the night and send you off to the toilet. So enjoy one or two drinks a night—but no more.

NO BIG MEALS AT NIGHT

Don't overindulge late in the evening with a heavy meal. A full stomach needs a couple of hours to digest and interferes with a relaxing sleep. On the other hand, a light snack before bed helps some people doze off. This could be a glass of warm milk, cheese and crackers, stewed fruit with yoghurt, a piece of toast with honey or jam or a small bowl of cereal with milk.

SKIP CAFFEINE AFTER 4 PM

Caffeine is a stimulant well known for its ability to keep the mind alert and switched on. This is great in the morning, but not conducive to a peaceful sleep. It's best to skip coffee, tea, cocoa or energy drinks with guarana (a source of caffeine) in the late afternoon or evening—especially just before bed!

THE MILK MYTH

A warm glass of milk before bed is an age-old tonic many people swear by. The theory is milk acts as a mild sedative, possibly due to its tryptophan (a component of protein), which is converted into serotonin, a 'calming' chemical. No-one knows for sure if this is the full explanation or if it's merely psychological, but if it works for you, it's worth doing. And it will boost your calcium at the perfect time—calcium uptake by bones peaks during the night.

EXERCISE

Be active throughout your day so you are physically tired at night. Walking in the fresh air is particularly beneficial, but any form of activity including swimming, dancing, cycling, tennis or yoga is fine. Avoid strenuous activity in the two hours before going to bed.

UNWIND WITH LAVENDER

Light a burner with lavender oil, slip into a warm bath with lavender or sprinkle a few drops onto a tissue under your pillow

ESTABLISH A REGULAR BEDTIME

A regular time for sleep works with your body's internal 'clock' and gets you into a natural pattern. Your body knows when to wind down and when to wind up in the morning. Travelling across time zones or varied work shifts interferes with this natural sleep pattern and can leave you out of kilter with your sleep.

Apart from leaving you tired and irritable, lack of sleep can lower your immunity, make your memory poorer, reduce productivity and worsen insulin resistance.

RELAX AND UNWIND

In the hour before bed, don't do any work. Instead, take a bath with aromatherapy oils, listen to soft music or read a good book. You could also try relaxation exercises like Tai

Chi or yoga, or practise some deep breathing with long stretches. Take time out and meditate on a peaceful place you have been to or a happy time in your life. Perhaps write a to-do list for tomorrow so you don't worry about it over the night. Avoid watching the late-night news or listening to loud music.

KEEP IT COOL AND DARK

Make sure your bedroom is dark, quiet and at the right temperature. It's better to sleep in a cooler room than to be too hot and have fitful sleep.

Insulin Resistance *See* Diabetes; Metabolic Syndrome.

Inulin

This is a substance found in chicory root and in lesser amounts in onion, artichoke, garlic, rye and banana. It activates the growth of 'friendly' bacteria in the large bowel. It can also act as a fat substitute, creating a rich creamy taste without the fat.

Iodine Deficiency

Iodine is a mineral that's a component of the thyroid hormones. It's essential for normal growth, physical health, metabolism and brain function.

Iodine can't be stored in the body so tiny amounts must be consumed regularly. If you don't get enough iodine, you may not be able to make enough thyroid hormone. This can lead to hypothyroidism—a condition where a person's metabolism slows and they put on weight, become tired easily and feel the cold. Severe iodine deficiency can seriously impair mental and physical growth, causing a condition known as cretinism. Largely eliminated from the developed world, cretinism is still observed in some areas, such as regions of Bangladesh, Chad, China, Indonesia, Nepal, Peru and Zaire. A milder form can still be found in developed countries though (where it's given the name of iodine deficiency disorder or IDD).

43 per cent of Australians are iodine deficient.

RECOMMENDED DAILY INTAKE

Children 0–8 years—90 micrograms
Children 9–13 years—120 micrograms
Adults and children over 14—150 micrograms
Pregnant women—220 micrograms
Lactating women—270 micrograms.

FOOD SOURCES

Iodine is scarce in our food supply. The main source comes from saltwater fish and seafood (prawns, crab, mussels and

DID YOU KNOW?

Since 2009, most bread in Australia and New Zealand now contains iodised salt to assist the 43 per cent of people who are iodine deficient. Only bread was chosen for fortification to ensure that we don't take in too much iodine (excess can be just as much as problem as deficiency). This is particularly important for children, who have a lower body weight and so are more sensitive to iodine excess, and for people with thyroid conditions. Organic breads are exempt, as are bread mixes for home baking.

oysters), as well as seaweeds such as nori and kelp, which are common ingredients in Japanese cuisine, though at low levels. Moderate sources of iodine are found in dairy foods like milk, yoghurt (although contents have reduced in recent years) and eggs. Smaller quantities are found in vegetables and meat, but the exact quantity depends on the concentration of iodine in the soils in which they were produced. For example, Tasmanian soils are low in iodine—the reason for the many iodine fortification programs there since the 1950s.

IODINE AND PREGNANCY

When the demand for iodine is high, such as during pregnancy and breastfeeding, an iodine supplement may be a good idea. It's feared that many women don't eat that much bread, so will not be benefiting from the supplementation of bread with iodine. Most multivitamin supplements, available from chemists and health-food stores, contain between 50 and 150 mcg of iodine. Discuss your needs with your doctor.

IODISED SALT

Iodised salt is a common source of iodine in many countries, but it is not used by the food industry. This means foods such as ham, cheese, crackers, potato crisps, fries and olives do not contain iodine, even though they pack in a lot of salt.

Though one of the main sources, less than 5 per cent of table salt is sold as iodised salt in Australia. Iodised table salt contains 25–45 micrograms of iodine per gram of salt, and was once a good source. But over the past 10 years or so, for good health reasons, we've cut back on table salt. Despite being extracted from seawater, sea salt and salt flakes are not a good source of iodine.

FOODS HIGH IN IODINE	MCG
200 g carton yoghurt	127
10 king prawns	45
1 cup milk	50
1 large egg	37
Thick slice of fortified bread	35
120g fillet of white fish	45
100g can salmon	30
4 sardines, canned in oil	14

CHILDREN WITH IODINE DEFICIENCY

Insufficient iodine inhibits thyroid hormones and can interfere with normal brain development in babies and young children, resulting in low IQs. Slowed thyroid function can ultimately produce goitre. Children with iodine deficiency suffer poor control of body movements and hearing problems, have an IQ 10 to 15 points below normal and are more likely to have attention deficit hyperactivity disorder (ADHD).

Iron

Iron is an essential part of haemoglobin, the red colouring of blood, which helps carry oxygen to every part of the body. Iron is also part of the muscle protein myoglobin, which explains why athletes need to check their iron for peak performance. It also plays a role in many enzymes and co-enzymes, especially those involved with the immune response.

RECOMMENDED DAILY INTAKE

Children 1–3 years—9 milligrams
Children 4–8 years—10 milligrams
Children 9–13 years—8 milligrams
Boys 14–18 years—11 milligrams
Girls 14–18 years—15 milligrams
Women 18–50 years—18 milligrams
Women over 50 years—8 milligrams
Pregnant women—27 milligrams
Lactating women—9 milligrams
Men of all ages—8 milligrams

Iron deficiency is the most common nutrition problem in the world.

Growing bodies
Young children under 2 years are at risk of iron deficiency—they are growing fast, can be fussy eaters and are sometimes over-dependent on milk. The signs of iron deficiency in children are delayed psychomotor development and poor capacity for exercise. In babies, those with a low birth weight or that are pre-term are the ones to watch.

IRON AND WOMEN

Iron is especially critical for women for two reasons. First, women need more than double the amount of iron men do because of the monthly blood loss through menstruation and the demands of pregnancy. Second, most women do not eat enough iron to meet their body's needs. Most research shows that around 40 per cent of women have inadequate iron intakes. Skipping meals, constant dieting and not eating enough meat are three of the most common reasons.

SOURCES OF IRON

RED MEAT

This is the best source of iron and being haem iron it is well absorbed by the body. Red meat has twice as much iron as chicken and three times as much as fish. Generally, the redder the meat, the richer it is in iron. In the average Australian diet, meat, chicken and fish account for 20–30 per cent of the total iron intake.

CEREAL GRAINS, VEGETABLES, LEGUMES, NUTS AND EGGS

All these contain iron, but it is non-haem iron and therefore not absorbed as well. Of these foods, grains make the greatest iron contribution to our diet, with around 30 per cent coming from fortified breakfast cereals and bread.

IRON DEFICIENCY

Iron deficiency is the most common nutrition problem in the world. It affects around 35 per cent of people in developing countries, and about 8 per cent of people in affluent countries like Australia and New Zealand. Because it's not life threatening and affects mainly women and young children, the issue of iron deficiency has never received enough attention, until now.

Look out for early warning signs that you may be iron deficient—tiredness, lack of energy, poor stamina with little ability to do physical work or exercise, frequent infections due to lowered immune response and feeling the cold more than usual.

ABSORBING IRON

Popeye was wrong! There is plenty of iron in spinach, but it's not well absorbed. In spinach and other vegetables, the natural fibre and oxalates bind to much of the iron so it cannot pass into the body.

COMPARE

RED MEAT One small serve of red meat (100 g cooked)	VEGETABLES One serve of cooked vegetables (200 g cooked)
Iron present—4.1 mg	Iron present—6.4 mg
Absorption into the body —approx. 20%	Absorption into the body—approx. 5%
True iron contribution—0.8 mg	True iron contribution—0.06 mg

The bottom line: we absorb about 1000 per cent more iron from red meat than from spinach.

WHO'S LIKELY TO RUN LOW?

- ✔ Women with heavy periods
- ✔ Pregnant women
- ✔ Teenage girls experiencing rapid growth and the onset of menstruation
- ✔ Vegetarians
- ✔ Athletes with intense training programs
- ✔ Young children under the age of 2
- ✔ People with coeliac or Crohn's disease.

MY TAKE

To enhance iron absorption, consume non-haem iron food sources with other foods high in vitamin C. For example, have a glass of orange juice with your spinach pie.

ANAEMIA AND SUPPLEMENTS

The body's iron is in delicate balance—too little leads to problems, but so does too much. It's best to obtain iron as nature intended from food, rather than rely on supplements. Nevertheless, when your iron levels are low, a supplement can help, but it pays to choose one well. The most common form of iron in supplements is slow-release ferrous sulphate, but this can cause constipation or an upset tummy. Ferrous gluconate, ferrous fumarate and chelated forms of iron are more readily absorbed and may cause fewer problems. All are non-haem forms of iron. Take them on an empty stomach as food can inhibit their absorption by up to 50 per cent. Taking them every second day is also less likely to trigger unpleasant side effects.

IRON EXCESS

Iron excess is usually caused by the accidental high intake of iron tablets. It can cause gastrointestinal upset or constipation and may interfere with the absorption of zinc. In toddlers, accidental swallowing of iron supplements can be fatal. A maximum of 45 mg a day is the limit for adults.

HAEMOCHROMATOSIS

Chronic iron overload is one of the most common, yet least-often diagnosed disorders affecting the population. It is more common than cystic fibrosis but much less well known. It is the abnormal and excessive absorption of iron from food. The excess iron is retained and deposited in various joints and organs throughout the body, particularly the liver, which becomes enlarged and can lead to cirrhosis, cancer of the liver and premature death if it goes untreated.

Other serious conditions caused by an excess of iron are diabetes, arthritis and heart disease. One in 100 Caucasians will experience the condition, and it will be as high as one in 80 in people of Celtic ancestry. There are often few obvious symptoms, just the presence of ongoing complaints such as chronic fatigue, joint pains, or bronze colouring of the skin. Treatment involves blood donations on a regular basis to reduce the iron level in the body.

Irradiation

Irradiation is the process of using ionising energy to kill pests and bacteria and slow down the ageing process, to help preserve fruit and vegetables. Food is exposed to gamma rays from a radioactive source such as Cobalt-60, inside a protected chamber. The rays pass straight through food (just like X-rays), destroying some or all of the organisms that cause it to spoil. Sometimes called cold pasteurisation, food irradiation has been studied for more than 50 years. NASA first started using irradiation to sterilise meat for astronauts to take with them in space back in the 1970s, and the process is still used by NASA today.

Use of irradiation is today gaining wider acceptance. It can be used to replace the practice of spraying food with harmful chemicals such as ethylene oxide (a possible carcinogen), now banned in many of the countries that receive exports from Australia and New Zealand.

DID YOU KNOW?

The number of irradiated foods on our shelves is extremely low, as is the case overseas. To date, the only approved foods are dried herbs and spices (which often carry high levels of harmful bacteria), herbal infusions (teas) and tropical fruits like mango, papaya, lychee and rambutan (to control fruit fly).

SHOPPER'S GUIDE

All irradiated foods or those containing irradiated ingredients must be labelled as 'Irradiated' or 'Treated with ionising radiation'. Some countries feature a circular radura symbol on the label.

IS IT SAFE?

Experts from the US, UK, Australia and the United Nations have determined that irradiation to a maximum dose of 10 kilogray (unit of absorbed ionising radiation), is acceptable. At this level, it's believed to present no toxicological hazard and introduces no special nutritional or microbiological problems. Irradiation was approved in Australia and New Zealand in 1999 for specific foods on a case-by-case basis, and is subject to ongoing public consultation and a demonstration of the technological need for it.

Nutritionally, irradiation can affect the levels of vitamins B_1, B_6, C, E, folate and fatty acids in food, but other vitamins, proteins, carbohydrates and minerals suffer little damage. Remember, however, that all cooking and processing will reduce these sensitive vitamins to some degree—drying fruit causes a drop in vitamin C, while pasteurisation of milk reduces a fraction of its B vitamins.

Irritable Bowel Syndrome (IBS)

Irritable bowel syndrome (IBS) can be a distressing and sometimes embarrassing problem. Doctors are not sure of the exact cause of IBS, but they do know that the nerves of the bowel become overly sensitive and the muscles of the bowel fail to work in unison like they should.

IBS comes and goes. Many times, there are no obvious reasons for an IBS attack. Often stress, diet or infection can trigger symptoms or make them worse. For many people, food will often make symptoms worse due to either stimulation or intolerance.

WHAT YOU CAN DO

STRESS LESS

Relaxation techniques, regular exercise and trying to reduce the amount of stress in your life can help to reduce IBS.

AVOID FIBRE—FOR SOME

A high fibre intake used to be the standard dietary modification for IBS, but not everyone finds it helpful. Some people find too much fibre upsets their system rather than improving things—personal trial and error will tell. If you're constipated you should aim to increase your intake of vegetables, wholegrain breakfast cereals, fine wholemeal bread and fruit. Make this increase gradual. It may take a week or so to notice the effect. If you're on an elimination diet that is fairly low in fibre, introduce a tablespoon of unprocessed bran and bran cereal two to three times a day, or take a fibre supplement based on psyllium (like Metamucil and Fybogel) or sterculia (Normacol).

MY TAKE

Remember, modifying your diet is only one aspect of treatment. Unless you are certain that a particular food or group of foods causes you problems, there is no need to eliminate foods entirely. A balanced diet is important for health and energy.

AVOID WINDY FOODS

Avoid wind-producing foods as the gas can upset your system. Notorious culprits are Brussels sprouts, cabbage, cauliflower, onions, legumes (lentils, chickpeas), dried fruit (raisins, prunes), spices and anything with whole seeds. Others include fizzy drinks and certain sweeteners such as sorbitol, mannitol and xylitol (used in sugar-free chewing gum). Remember to eat slowly and avoid swallowing air.

ADD ACIDOPHILUS

Friendly bacteria from probiotic yoghurts or acidophilus capsules can normalise your bowel bacteria, but you must take them regularly.

REDUCE LACTOSE LEVELS

Some individuals find it best to avoid lactose (the sugar found in milk and soft cheeses), as it can be the cause of bloating and diarrhoea.

CHECK FOR FOOD INTOLERANCES

Intolerance to the natural chemicals found in food such as amines, salicylates and glutamates is common in IBS. It's wise to follow an elimination diet such as the low-FODMAP diet under the advice of an accredited dietitian to work out what are your problem foods.

DOES THIS SOUND LIKE YOU?

- Tummy pain that is relieved once you have been to the toilet
- Gassiness or flatulence all the time
- Frequent bloating and abdominal discomfort
- Irregular bowel movements
- Frequent episodes of diarrhoea, often passing mucus as well
- Diarrhoea alternating with constipation.

If you regularly experience one of more of these symptoms, you could have IBS. Talk to your doctor for more advice.

WORK OUT YOUR TRIGGERS

Keep a food diary to help you understand what foods aggravate your system. Coffee, alcohol, tomatoes, milk, wheat and preservatives have all been reported as common offenders.

TALK TO YOUR DOCTOR

Stay in contact with your doctor or gastroenterologist who can help you with medication to help relieve cramps, bulking agents to keep regular, peppermint oil capsules for spasms and anti-diarrhoea tablets.

See also **Digestive Disorders; FODMAPs.**

Isoflavones

These are compounds found in soy beans and other legumes that have oestrogen-like qualities.

J

Juice

There's no doubt fresh fruit juices (with no added sugar) can be nutritious and healthy. They are:

- ✔ Healthy and natural
- ✔ Full of vitamins, minerals, enzymes and antioxidants
- ✔ Rich in fruit and vegetable nutrients such as vitamin C, beta-carotene (which is converted to vitamin A in the body), folate, vitamin B_1, niacin, vitamin K, potassium and magnesium
- ✔ Easy to drink—great for fussy eaters who won't usually touch fruit or vegetables, or ideal for someone who is underweight or recovering from chemotherapy and can't eat much
- ✔ Better than other less-nutritious drinks (including soft drinks and cordial).

THE NEW FAST FOOD

In recent years, juice bars have made juice the new fast food. Vitamin-packed, fresh and made while you wait, they seem so good for you! A whole new market has been created for fresh juices and smoothies—orange, carrot and peach, guava and pineapple, apple and celery or watermelon, mint and beetroot. These tasty combinations are often enhanced with a shot of wheatgrass, guarana, green tea, echinacea or ginseng. But where do they fit in a healthy eating plan?

A serving of fruit juice is a small glass—just 200 ml (about ¾ cup). While juice does provide vitamin C and other phytonutrients, it also contains about 5 teaspoons of sugar per glass, the same as soft drink.

Drinking 100 per cent fruit juice gives the appearance of ultimate health. After all, they were part of the raw food movement and have long been advocated by natural health practitioners. Juices are said to be an integral part of detox regimes, used to 'cleanse the digestive system', 'draw out toxins' and 'alkalinise the body'. Some of these claims are groundless, but are capitalised on by advertisers to highlight the virtues of juice.

THE JUICE TRAP

While there is a lot to love about juice, there are drawbacks. Juice is concentrated fruit and packs a lot of kilojoules. It is very easy to consume too much.

With the fruit's skin (and source of fibre) removed, you lose the natural brake that stops you consuming too much. When you eat whole foods with their skin on and high-fibre structure intact, there's more chewing involved so you take longer to eat them. As they fill the stomach and the intestines, working like gastric banding surgery, your eating is slowed and your stomach gets full—giving you the signal to stop eating. This doesn't happen with juice.

Juice is usually sold in large sizes by juice bars, and is equivalent in food value to four or five pieces of fresh fruit, yet it takes only a fraction of the time to drink. It's a trap for health-conscious people and can be a way to put on weight—they may be healthy kilojoules but they are still kilojoules and you can all too easily pile on the kilos if your lifestyle is sedentary (as it usually is these days) and you don't exercise enough to burn it off!

TIPS FOR HEALTHY JUICE CONSUMPTION

- ✔ Think of a juice as more like a mini-meal or a substantial snack, rather than just something extra to quench your thirst.
- ✔ Drink water if you're thirsty (no kilojoules) and eat whole fruit.
- ✔ Order the smallest-size juice you can, share with a friend or drink half now, half later.
- ✔ Add vegetable juice, which dilutes the sugars and kilojoules so it's not so concentrated. Try adding carrot, spinach, tomatoes or other green leafy veggies like celery.
- ✔ Dilute juice with water or sparkling mineral water.
- ✔ If you have a juice extractor and make your own, you know exactly how much fruit you have used. Throw in some pulp for fibre and dream up new concoctions with herbs or spices for extra zing.
- ✔ Remember to eat two serves of whole fruit each day as well.

SHOPPER'S GUIDE

One medium 200 g apple provides 3 g fibre and 300 kJ and takes a relaxing 5 minutes to eat. One 600 ml apple juice provides zero fibre and 1300 kJ, and you can gulp it down in a couple of minutes.

READ THE LABEL

FRUIT JUICE

This is 100 per cent juice and no added water. It may contain up to 4 per cent added sugar, depending on the seasonal sweetness of the fruit, but the sugar added would appear on the ingredient list.

FRUIT JUICE DRINK

This is 25–50 per cent fruit juice and is sweetened with sugar. Blackcurrant, guava or lemon juice usually contain only 25 per cent juice because of their tartness; apple, pear and pineapple contain 50 per cent; orange, grapefruit and others are 35 per cent.

WHEATGRASS JUICE

Promoters of wheatgrass claim a single 30 ml shot gives you the vitamins and minerals found in 2 kg of green vegetables. They will tell you it does everything from purifying the liver to washing drug residues out of the body. But while wheatgrass is nutritious, so is any other leafy green vegetable such as spinach, basil or parsley. If you liquefied these vegetables, you would get similar nutrient-rich liquid—it's just easier to swallow in liquid form than chomping your way through a large salad. If the juice is squeezed from fresh growing shoots, it will offer the maximum vitamins, as they won't be destroyed by storage or heat. High in vitamin C, folate, minerals and plant antioxidants, wheatgrass is nutrient-packed. Just don't expect it to do everything it's hyped to do. And yes, it does taste just like cut grass!

FRUIT JUICE CORDIAL

This must contain a minimum of 25 per cent fruit juice, but only 4–5 per cent juice when made up with water. It may also contain sugar, flavours and colours.

See also Berries; Beverages, Citrus Fruit; Fruit.

Junk Food

Most of us can instantly recognise junk food when we see it. It's usually applied to things like ready-to-eat and convenience foods—things eaten on the run or without a knife and fork. This includes potato chips and fries, cheese snacks, movie popcorn and other salty packet snacks as well as lollies, chocolate, confectionery, biscuits, doughnuts, cakes, soft drinks, sugary breakfast cereals, ice-creams and most fast food including hamburgers, nuggets, pizza, hot dogs, meat pies, sausage rolls and wedges.

But the term is hard to define. In my opinion, it's any foods that are over-processed and high in fat, salt, sugar, refined starches or kilojoules with little nutritional value. They're often dubbed 'empty kilojoules' as they contribute little to nutrition and lots to your kilojoule intake and waistline. Junk food advertising is banned or restricted during children's television viewing hours for these reasons.

MY TAKE

Think of junk food as an 'extra' in a healthy balanced diet. Don't eat it every day and eat only small serves when you do. If you're overweight—limit these 'extra' foods to no more than once a week, and only have them if you are eating a balanced diet and being physically active. If you're not overweight—you can probably fit in one or two 'extra foods' a day as long as you are active and have had your daily serves of vegetables, fruit, meat, dairy and wholegrains.

WHY IT'S BAD FOR YOU

There's nothing wrong with having the occasional burger now and then, but consuming a diet based primarily on junk food (as many younger people do today) is a worry. Here's why:

- It's soft, easy to chew and swallow, cheap and served in large portions or meal deals. Designed to be tasty and easy to consume, it is a major contributor to the obesity epidemic.
- It often lacks important vitamins and minerals, especially vitamins B and C, fibre, potassium, magnesium and omega-3.
- It has been highly processed and its main ingredients are refined carbohydrates (white bread in buns and pizza bases, white rice with takeaways, peeled potatoes for fries and chips). There's little wholemeal or fibre.
- It's packed with additives to prolong the shelf life and enhance the colour, flavour and texture.
- It's high in salt, which is a risk factor for high blood pressure, and sets the scene for stroke, kidney disease, fluid retention and heart disease in later life. Once your tastebuds get used to its saltiness, it's hard to eat normal home-cooked meals.
- It's high in 'bad' fats such as trans fat and saturated fats, which contribute to high blood cholesterol and heart attacks.
- If you fill up with energy-dense, nutrient-poor junk food, you don't leave room for healthy, nutrient rich meals and snacks.

They're often dubbed 'empty kilojoules' as they contribute little to nutrition and lots to your intake and waistline.

KL

Kelp

Kelp is a seaweed that is rich in iodine and a range of other minerals and vitamins. It is said to perk up your whole system and help slimmers 'burn fat'. Kelp is one of four components of a popular weight-loss supplement, along with lecithin, vitamin B_6 and cider vinegar. Unfortunately, this mixture neither 'dissolves unwanted fat' nor 'stimulates the thyroid gland to raise the metabolic rate', so it is of questionable value to dieters. It is the strict low-kilojoule diet that accompanies the supplement that is responsible for the weight loss.

Ketogenic Diet

This is a very low-carbohydrate diet, with a high intake of fats and proteins that causes accumulation of unoxidised fats in the blood and urine. The ketogenic diet is not recommended for weight reduction as there are many side effects (including nausea, fatigue, constipation and bad breath), and it raises blood fat levels. Under medical supervision, a ketogenic diet is used to help control seizures in children with epilepsy.

Kilojoules

This is the unit of energy used to measure the level of energy in food and diets. In the metric system, the kilojoule replaces the kilocalorie (commonly called just calorie). One kilocalorie equals 4.186 kilojoules (4.2 or 4 is close enough for a quick conversion).

See also **Energy.**

L

Labels and Claims

All food labelling in Australia is governed by food standards legislation; you can find out more on the Food Standards Australia New Zealand (FSANZ) website. A food label carries useful information about a product, but only if you know what you're looking for.

DATE MARKING

The time of best eating quality is indicated on food by a 'Best Before', 'Use By' or 'Baked On' date. Foods with a shelf-life of more than two years do not have to carry a date, nor do ice-creams on sticks, whole fresh fruit and vegetables, sandwiches or filled rolls made and sold on the premises.

'Use By' dates are generally found on perishables and short shelf-life foods such as fresh meat packed at the supermarket, milk and yoghurt. Products should be eaten or thrown away after this date, as the food is not safe to eat, even if there are no signs of spoilage.

'Best Before' dates apply to most cereals, biscuits, snack foods, flour, eggs, and canned and frozen foods. The food is not spoiled immediately after the date and can

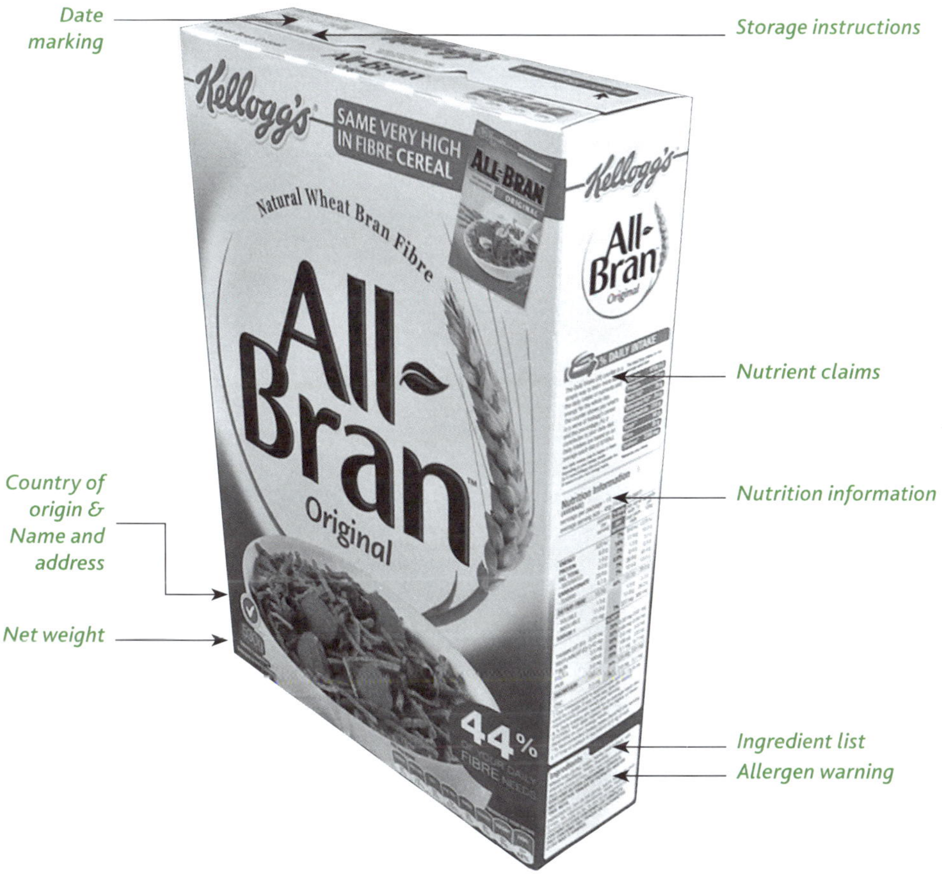

be sold if stored properly and in good condition, but its quality has begun to decline.

'Baked On' dates are usually on bread and other bakery goods made on the premises.

INGREDIENT LIST

All ingredients must be stated in descending order of weight, from most to least. The ingredient with the largest proportion is listed first, followed by the second, third and so on. Additives are included by their functional name, for example PRESERVATIVE, followed by either their chemical name (SODIUM METABISULPHITE) or their code number (223).

ALLERGEN WARNINGS

For allergy sufferers, the presence of fish, shellfish, eggs, milk, nuts, sesame, gluten, soy bean, added sulphite in high concentrations, royal jelly, bee pollen or propolis must be declared. It is usually in or near the list of ingredients.

NUTRITION INFORMATION PANEL (NIP)

This shows the energy in kilojoules (calories), protein, fat (total and saturated), carbohydrate (total and sugars) and sodium in an average serve and in 100 grams of the food. Some foods also show fibre, potassium, mono-unsaturated fat, polyunsaturated fat and trans fat, depending on whether they make a claim about these.

COUNTRY OF ORIGIN

This identifies the country or countries in which the food was grown, made or processed. In Australia, if the food is made from imported ingredients or from local and imported ingredients, this must be listed. New Zealand does not require country of origin labelling. If you like to buy Australian products, here's what you need to know.

PRODUCT OF AUSTRALIA means each significant ingredient has been produced in Australia and virtually all the production processes occurred here as well.

MADE IN AUSTRALIA means more than 51 per cent of production costs have been in Australia or the product has been substantially transformed in Australia. This labelling statement is under review.

STORAGE INSTRUCTIONS

For best quality (and safe) eating, follow the manufacturer's instructions.

NET WEIGHT

This is the actual weight of food, without the extra weight of any packaging. In canned foods it includes any liquid—it is not the drained weight.

NAME AND ADDRESS

The name and address of the manufacturer, packer, distributor or importer must be clearly identified for consumers.

WHAT NUTRITION CLAIMS REALLY MEAN

Many products make bold nutrition claims on their packaging to grab your attention. Some can be confusing, while others are misleading.

97 PER CENT FAT-FREE

This really means that the food contains 3 per cent fat, but saying it the other way around makes it sound better for you! Only low-fat foods with 3 per cent fat or less can make this claim. It is also the same with 98 per cent fat-free and 99 per cent fat-free labels.

BAKED NOT FRIED

This often appears on snack foods and implies that the food is low in fat. For some snacks, like pretzels, this is true (i.e. they have less than 3 per cent fat) but for others, like biscuit snacks, it means they are lower in fat (around 25 per cent less) but not necessarily low in fat. Check the nutrition panel if in doubt.

CHOLESTEROL-FREE OR NO CHOLESTEROL

These are confusing terms. They do not mean no fat. Many foods such as oil, margarine, nuts, avocadoes and snack foods can be free of cholesterol, but remain high in fat. All plant-derived products are free of cholesterol anyway. Stop worrying about dietary cholesterol—it is saturated fat and trans fat that matters most.

COOKED IN VEGETABLE OIL

Palm oil, a tropical oil with 50 per cent saturated fat, is commonly used to fry snacks and fast foods. While it qualifies as a vegetable oil (with no cholesterol), it differs greatly from the unsaturated vegetable oils consumers are familiar with such as canola, soy bean, sunflower and cottonseed oil. If one of these oils is used in the food, it will generally tell you on the pack. If not, you can assume it is palm oil or a hydrogenated (hardened and therefore saturated) vegetable oil.

GLUTEN-FREE

This means there is no wheat, rye, triticale, barley, oats or malt present, and there must be no detectable gluten.

HIGH IN FIBRE

The food must contain at least 3 grams of fibre per serve to qualify for this claim, and this can be verified from the nutrition panel on the back of the package. Wholegrain breakfast cereals and mixed grain breads would meet this type of claim.

VERY HIGH IN FIBRE

Products that contain 6 grams of fibre or higher per serve can be classified as very high fibre. Bran breakfast cereal, baked beans and lentils would qualify as some of these. You can verify this from the nutrition panel on the back of the package.

HIGH IN PROTEIN

Only foods containing at least 5 grams of protein, or those with 12 per cent of its kilojoules deriving from protein, can carry this label. Most lean cuts of meat and chicken, eggs, milk and cheese would meet this claim.

LITE OR LIGHT

This can mean a number of things and not necessarily that the product is low in kilojoules or fat. Be sure to check what part of the food has been 'lightened'. Here are some examples:

- Light beer is low in alcohol, not fat
- Light cheese contains less fat and salt
- Light ice-cream has less fat but more sugar and thickeners
- Light olive oil has a blander flavour, but the same amount of fat as regular oil
- Light potato crisps are thinly sliced and lightly salted, but may still have the same amount of fat as regular chips.

NO ADDED SUGAR

This applies to food that does not contain added cane sugar, honey, glucose, fructose, malt, malt extract or maltose. But they may be just as high in natural sugars and provide similar kilojoules. The label must tell you how many kilojoules of sugar there are in 100 grams or 100 millilitres of the product. Be aware there are many names for sugar. They can appear as:

- Sucrose (the chemical name for sugar), the sugar in cane sugar
- Fructose (fruit sugar), occurring naturally in fruit and honey
- Glucose
- Dextrose (another name for glucose)
- Golden syrup
- Treacle
- Concentrated pear juice or syrup.

If some form of sugar appears as one of the first three ingredients, the food is generally high in added sugar.

Growing bodies

We began implementing a traffic light classification system in school canteens in 2006. Green, amber and red indicate the differing nutritional value of foods. **Green** foods are everyday foods such as fruit, vegetables, lean meats and grains. **Amber** foods are moderate in added fat and/or sugar and/or salt. They provide some nutritional value but can contribute to excess kilojoules if consumed in large serve sizes. Examples include full-fat dairy foods, processed meats, commercially prepared hot foods, snack-food bars, 100 per cent fruit juices, reduced-fat ice-creams. **Red** foods vary but generally include those high in fat, sugar and sodium (salt), as well as soft drinks. Red foods are allowed in some schools occasionally, while others ban them outright.

Understanding the nutrition information panel

Each bar supplies 650 kilojoules (or 155 calories) of energy. It also contains 2 grams of protein, 4 grams of fat (of which 2 grams are saturated fat), 29 grams of total carbohydrate (of which 15 grams are sugars). Deducting 15 from 29 means that there is 14 grams of starch coming from the flour, oats and nuts. The sugars from honey, dates, apple puree and sugar make up the 15 grams of sugars.

There are four bars (four serves) in the pack, each weighing 40 grams. The nutrition table relates to one bar (defined as a 'serve') and also to 100 grams, so you can compare an equal weight of this food with others in a fair way.

The figures in the 'per 100g' column are equivalent to percentages. Thus 10 grams of fat per 100 grams means that the bar contains 10 per cent fat, which is moderate (bread contains 2 per cent, sweet biscuits around 30 per cent).

Muesli bars with apple and honey

160 g net weight

NUTRITION INFORMATION

Servings per pack: 4 **Serving size: 1 bar (40 g)**	**Per bar**	**Per 100 g**
Energy	650 kJ 155 Cal	1625 kJ 385 Cal
Protein	2 g	5 g
Fat, total	4 g	10 g
Saturated	2 g	5 g
Carbohydrate	29 g	73 g
total sugars	15 g	38 g
Dietary fibre	2 g	5 g
Sodium	5 mg	12 mg

INGREDIENTS: WHOLEMEAL FLOUR, HONEY (18%), DATES, ROLLED OATS, VEGETABLE OIL, APPLE PUREE (6.3 %), SUGAR, DESICCATED COCONUT, EMULSIFIER (LECITHIN), WALNUTS, HUMECTANT (SORBITOL), SPICES.

Each bar contains 2 grams of dietary fibre. Per 100 grams, the dietary fibre content is 5 per cent, which is a significant amount, around three-quarters of that of wholemeal bread.

Each bar contains 5 mg of sodium.

Wholemeal flour is the major ingredient, being listed first, followed by honey, dates, rolled oats and so on.

The percentage of honey and apple are quoted because these two ingredients are mentioned specifically in the product name.

Sorbitol is used here as a humectant to stop the bar drying out and to maintain the chewy texture. It can also function as a sweetening agent in sugar-free foods.

The spices would be similar to household spices and in this product there is a commercial mix of stable cinnamon, nutmeg and lemon oil.

Lecithin is used here as an emulsifier.

REDUCED FAT

These foods contain less fat than regular products, but may not necessarily be low in fat—there is usually 25 per cent less fat than there is in its regular counterpart. The most common examples of these are reduced-fat milk, cheese, ice-cream, mayonnaise, sour cream and dairy desserts. The product must show a comparison with the reference food. Fat can also be listed as:

- Vegetable oil (in snack foods and sauces)
- Vegetable shortening (in muffins and cakes)
- Ghee
- Lard
- Suet, dripping
- Coconut cream
- Copha
- Triglycerides.

MY TAKE

You will often see claims like 'fresh' or 'natural' on labels. 'Fresh' applies to foods that have not been preserved in any way, while natural should be reserved for foods containing no additives (other than natural additives and flavours). Be sure to check the ingredient list.

HOW LOW DO YOU GO?

If you're trying to cut back on fat, salt and sugar and eat plenty of fibre, here's an easy guide to what figures you should check out on the nutrition information panel.

NUTRIENT	PER 100 g COLUMN	PER SERVE COLUMN
Fat	3 grams (3 per cent) or less	-
Sugars	15 grams (15 per cent) or less	-
Sodium	120 milligrams or less	-
Fibre	-	3 grams per serve or more

REDUCED SALT

Foods containing at least 25 per cent less salt than their regular counterparts can carry this label.

%DI LABELS

You may have spotted the %DI on packaging. It stands for 'Percentage of Daily Intake'. The label looks like a series of thumbnails and is a graphic representation of how much a serve of a food will contribute to your daily intake. It's a voluntary front-of-pack label scheme adopted after broad industry consultation including the Dietitians Association of Australia. It is used by more than 2000 products on supermarket shelves.

The label is based on the recommended amounts of energy and nutrients an average adult needs each day—energy (kJ), protein, fat, saturated fat, total carbohydrate, sugars, fibre and sodium.

While it seems like a great idea, the problem is the figures are based on an average adult diet, and you may need more or less, based on your age, height, weight, sex and how much activity or exercise you do. To find out what you should be eating, visit their website at www.mydailyintake.net and use the calculator to work out what your BMI and your actual daily energy requirements are.

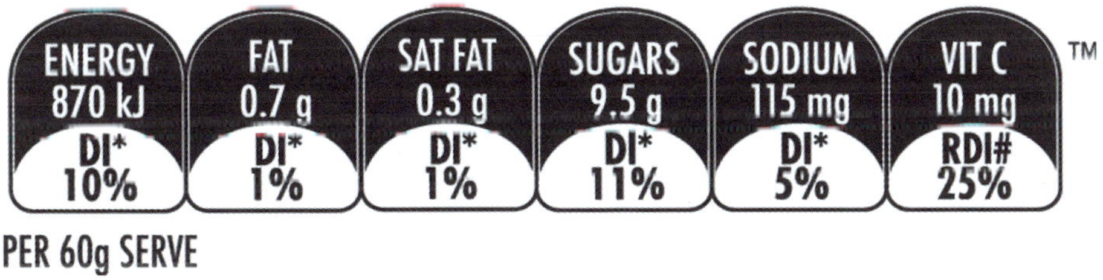
ENERGY 870 kJ DI* 10%
FAT 0.7 g DI* 1%
SAT FAT 0.3 g DI* 1%
SUGARS 9.5 g DI* 11%
SODIUM 115 mg DI* 5%
VIT C 10 mg RDI# 25%
TM
PER 60g SERVE

See also **Additives; Organic Food; Wholegrains.**

Lactase

This is an enzyme that splits milk sugar, lactose, into its components glucose and galactose. All babies are born with lactase to digest breast milk but in many it disappears after infancy. About three-quarters of the world's adults do not possess lactase and are unable to digest lactose from milk.

See also **Lactose Intolerance.**

Lactic Acid

Lactic acid is acid produced by fermentation of lactose, found in yoghurt, buttermilk and most cheese. It is also formed in muscles from glucose when oxygen supply is inadequate, as it may be during intense exercise.

Lactose Intolerance

Can't drink milk? Get tummy pains and bloating when you drink milk? One in 10 adults suffer from lactose intolerance, a condition where they are unable to digest dairy foods, mainly milk. Drinking too much causes pain, bloating, wind and even diarrhoea.

Lactose is a sugar naturally occurring in milk. It is made up of two simple sugars, glucose and galactose, and is a natural component (about 4–5 per cent) of the milk of all mammals including cows, goats, sheep and humans. Lactose intolerance occurs when there is not enough of an enzyme called lactase in the small intestine to break down the sugar allowing it to be absorbed. Around 90 per cent of adults from Asia, Africa, the Middle East, some Mediterranean countries, Australian Aborigines, Maori and Pacific Islanders are lactose intolerant. After infancy, they are unable to digest lactose in large quantities, and their traditional diets reflect this. Any 'milk' products they consume are 'cultured' (such as yoghurt, buttermilks and soft cheeses), with the live bacteria converting much of the lactose into a safer lactic acid.

MY TAKE
Don't confuse lactose intolerance with milk allergy, which occurs via a different biological mechanism involving the body's immune system.

Lactose intolerance is much less common in anyone of northern European descent, whose ancestors herded dairy cows and drank a lot of milk, consequently retaining the enzyme needed to split the lactose molecule. It can, however, occur short term, whenever the digestive tract is affected, for example after a bout of gastroenteritis or in certain illnesses like coeliac disease or HIV infections.

GOOD NEWS ON MILK

One of the most common misconceptions about intolerance to lactose is that it means no more dairy. The good news is that milk and other dairy foods—important sources of protein, calcium and B vitamins—don't need to be completely eliminated. Research shows most people with low enzyme levels can have up to one glass of milk with meals every day, without symptoms of lactose intolerance.

MANAGING LACTOSE INTOLERANCE

- ✔ Eat foods containing lactose as part of a meal rather than on an empty stomach—milk with your cereal and fruit may pose no problems, but a strawberry milkshake on its own can give you bloating and an upset tummy.
- ✔ Reduce the amount of foods containing lactose you eat at any one time. Eating a small amount often is likely to be better tolerated that a large quantity from time to time.
- ✔ If you are really sensitive, stick to low- to moderate-lactose foods like cheeses and ice-cream. Avoid milk.
- ✔ Look for milks labelled 'No lactose' or 'Lactose-reduced'.

- ✔ Talk to your pharmacist about liquid enzyme drops. These are added to regular milk and left for 24 hours in the refrigerator, breaking down the lactose.
- ✔ Try regular milk instead of skim—it has a slightly lower lactose level.
- ✔ Yoghurt is better tolerated than milk as around 30 per cent of its lactose has been broken down to lactic acid by the friendly bacteria present.

GETTING YOUR CALCIUM

If you eliminate all milk, yoghurt and cheese from your diet, you're eliminating the major sources of calcium. If you replace milk with soy milk, make sure you choose one that has calcium added. A calcium supplement is also a good idea, too, particularly for children or pregnant women.

FOOD SOURCES OF LACTOSE

FOOD	LACTOSE (g)
HIGH	
½ cup milk, evaporated	13.4
1 cup skim milk, skim	12.5
200 g tub natural, low-fat yoghurt	12.2
1 cup milk, full cream	11.5
MODERATE	
2 scoops ice-cream	4.7–5.9
1 tablespoon cream	0.4–1.0
1 tablespoon creamed cottage cheese	0.3–0.9
1 tablespoon cream cheese	0.4–0.5
LOW	
1 teaspoon butter	0.2
1 slice cheddar cheese	0.1
1 slice edam, Swiss or gouda cheese	negligible
Soy drink or rice drink	0

Growing bodies

Regular cow's and goat's milk contain about 4 per cent lactose, so neither is suitable for lactose intolerant children. Choose low-lactose and lactose-free cow's milk in fresh or long-life form. Look for brand names such as Zymil. Or, if your child doesn't like milk, hard yellow cheeses (cheddar, parmesan) have very little lactose, but still contain the other nutrients of milk.

Laxatives *See* Constipation and Laxatives.

Lecithin

Lecithin is made by the body as a component of bile and acids by the liver, and aids in the digestion and transport of fats. It is a major constituent of brain and nerve tissues and is used in the structure of cell membranes.

Commercial lecithin is a fatty substance containing phospholipids sold as granules or capsules. It is also commonly used as an emulsifier in food products (code number 322), allowing oils and water to mix in a range of foods from bread, mayonnaise, margarine, oil sprays and chocolate.

Unlike vitamins or minerals, lecithin is not an essential nutrient, but does contain choline and inositol, two compounds often associated with the B vitamins. Lecithin is generally extracted from soy bean, but egg yolks, legumes and grains such as maize are alternative sources. It is high in polyunsaturated fats, which accounts for early reports that it could lower cholesterol. It is expensive, however, and you could get these fats much more cheaply from polyunsaturated oils or nuts.

Although analysis is limited, it is probably rich in vitamin E, which means it is able to protect polyunsaturated fats from oxygen attack. Two tablespoons of lecithin granules supply 10 grams of fat and 335 kilojoules.

MY TAKE

For most people, lecithin is of limited value.

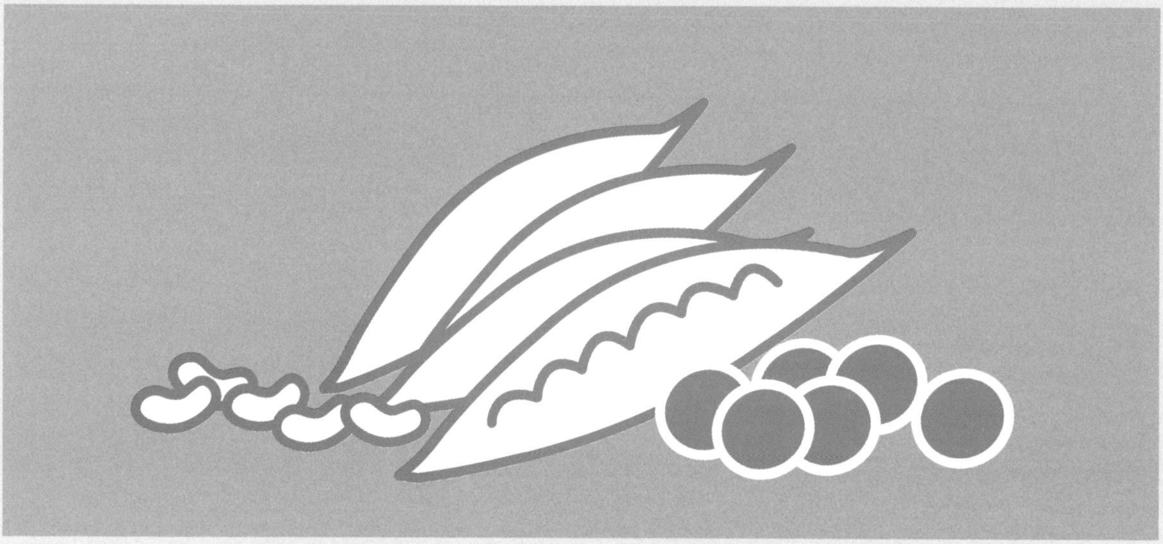

Legumes

Legumes are one of our best food friends. Also known as pulses or beans, they are nutritious, versatile and budget-friendly. It's definitely worth getting to know how to cook them if you're vegetarian—they should be a staple protein source—and for the meat eater, they extend the protein of meat or chicken (add a can of kidney beans to a mince recipe or casserole and you save on cost and still have a nutritious high-protein dinner).

Legumes are the dried edible seeds of plants from the *Leguminosae* family. The green beans and peas we enjoy as vegetables with our meals belong to the same family but they are nutritionally different because their water content is so much higher and that changes their nutrient levels.

SHOPPER'S GUIDE

Aim for two serves or more per week as a starchy vegetable alternative—more if you are vegetarian. One serve is half a cup of canned beans or cooked lentils or split peas, or a small 100 g serve of canned baked beans.

NUTRITIONAL VALUE

Beans, lentils and split peas have almost no fat (apart from soy beans) and are packed with fibre, protein, B vitamins and minerals, and heart-friendly phytonutrients. All have a similar composition except for soy beans, which contain a higher amount of quality protein and oil.

All legumes boast one of the lowest levels of GI of any starchy food, meaning they fill you up and keep hunger away. If you can swap some of your potatoes or rice for beans (or mix in half and half), you'll reduce the overall GI of your diet because your body digests them slowly. This is primarily because their starch breaks down relatively slowly (or incompletely) during cooking and they contain tannins and enzyme inhibitors that also slow digestion.

A few years ago, researchers were hopeful that legumes, particularly soy beans, could alleviate menopausal symptoms (because of the phytoestrogens or plant hormones they contain), but later research has shown their benefits are mild, if they occur at all. More certain is the fact that a healthy diet containing a wide variety of foods (including soy and legumes) is ideal at this stage of life.

NUMBER CRUNCH

Half a cup of canned chickpeas (drained) weighing 75 grams supplies 5 grams of protein, 0 grams of fat, 12 grams of carbohydrate, 1 gram of sugar, 4 grams of dietary fibre and 415 kilojoules.

DID YOU KNOW?

Cooking legumes in fresh water (not the water you soaked them in) reduces the chances of wind, as does eating small amounts regularly—your body becomes used to them. Canned beans don't seem to be as powerful as dried and cooked ones either. You can also try adding a tiny amount of powdered asafoetida spice to the pot during cooking—no more than a quarter of a teaspoon per cup of dried beans or lentils.

CANNED VS HOME-COOKED

Don't feel guilty about using canned beans! The process of soaking and cooking beans often deters consumers, but canned beans make a convenient and nutritious alternative. Mostly equivalent to home-cooked beans, there is some loss of B vitamins during canning but it is not significant. The protein, fibre and minerals remain unchanged. The only disadvantage with canned beans is that they tend to be softer in texture. If you like a firmer texture, you'll probably need to cook your own. Baked beans are the most popular of canned beans, either as a snack or as a light meal, and are generally made from haricot beans cooked in a tomato sauce.

MY TAKE

Lentils are so quick and easy to use, it makes them my pick from among the legumes. Learn to love them, especially if you have diabetes or need to shed weight. No matter how much you eat, they have only a small affect on your blood-glucose levels.

LEGUMES AND WIND (FLATULENCE)

Legumes of all sorts, including baked beans, are renowned for producing flatulence, and many jokes. This is due to their high fibre content—at around 6 grams of fibre, a small 100 gram can of beans has as much fibre as three slices of grainy bread or a bowl of bran flakes. They also contain indigestible sugars called raffinose, stachyose and verbascose that reach the large bowel intact, where they are fermented by resident flora. Believe it or not, this is good for colonic health, increasing the proportion of good bifidobacteria and reducing potential pathogens. However, not all legumes will make you windy, and not everyone has the problem to the same extent.

EASY WAYS TO GET MORE BEANS

- ✔ Served with grainy toast, baked beans make a quick, nutritious, high-fibre meal.
- ✔ Add a drained and rinsed can of beans to soups, one-pot meals and pasta sauces.
- ✔ Mix half a cup of cooked or canned beans through macaroni, couscous or rice dishes.
- ✔ Add half a cup of red lentils to the meat sauce when making spaghetti Bolognese.
- ✔ Serve a bean salad at barbecues and buffets with green beans and celery for extra colour and crunch.
- ✔ Make a chilli sauce with kidney beans and serve with tacos or tortillas.
- ✔ Enjoy a lentil or split-pea soup as a winter warmer.
- ✔ Sprout your own and sprinkle over a salad or stir-fry.
- ✔ When you feel like a curry, try a chickpea one or serve your favourite curry with dhal.

BEANS

Beans are a good source of protein, low-GI carbs, soluble fibre and B vitamins. Their minerals like iron, zinc and

Types of beans

Adzuki beans
Black beans
Black-eyed beans
Borlotti beans
Butter beans
Broad beans
Cannellini beans
Chickpeas (garbanzo beans)
Haricot beans
Kidney beans
Lima beans
Mung beans
Pinto beans
Romano beans
Soy beans

calcium are not as well absorbed as the iron and zinc from meat or the calcium from dairy foods. Adding a food that's rich in vitamin C improves the absorption of iron. Soy beans have almost twice as much protein as other beans and lentils and their protein is of higher quality. They also have a high oil content, which is polyunsaturated with some omega-3s. All beans are great for chilli dishes, soups and casseroles or as a side dish, salad or salsa. They are also gluten free.

LENTILS

Types of lentils
Green/brown lentils
Puy or French lentils
Red lentils

Lentils are the perfect slow-acting food, and since they cook quickly (no pre-soaking needed) there's no excuse not to add them to soups, salads and dishes such as pilaf. One of the oldest legumes and integral to the cuisines of the Middle East, India and eastern Europe, lentils are important for their protein, iron, zinc, potassium and fibre. All colours and types of dried lentils have a similar nutritional value including B vitamins and minerals like potassium, magnesium and zinc.

PEAS

Types of peas
Blue peas (or whole dried peas)
Green or yellow split peas

Peas are another little gem from the legume family containing lots of cholesterol-lowering fibre that is not only good for heart health, but also great for preventing blood glucose 'spikes'. Most of us when we think of split peas think of soups or dhal. But you can also use them in salads and other side dishes. Dried peas are a good source of vegetable protein and slow-digesting carbs like other legumes, and also contain vitamin C, iron and B group vitamins.

LUPINS

Lupin or sweet lupin is high in protein and fibre, low in fat and contains natural antioxidants such as carotenoids (which account for its golden-yellow colour) and tocopherols. Lupin has been earmarked as a major competitor to soy beans as an ingredient in vegan sausages, noodles, breads, muffins and breakfast cereals.

Eating foods containing lupin flour can help cut your food intake without going hungry, thanks to the fibre and protein content. It is an excellent alternative to both wheat flour and soy products. It is higher in lysine than cereals, and is rich in the amino acid arginine, which is a precursor of nitric oxide, a vasodilator in blood vessels. Like other legumes, it is gluten-free and its starch is slowly digested, so as an ingredient it could help lower the GI of breads and breakfast cereals.

> A few years ago, researchers were hopeful that legumes, particularly soy beans, could alleviate menopausal symptoms, but later research has shown their benefits are mild, if they occur at all.

The downside is lupin allergy. Major food manufacturers are currently holding back from using lupin flour due to the likelihood of it provoking a severe allergic reaction like peanuts (botanically a legume). It appears that people with peanut sensitivity may have cross-reactivity with lupin or the allergy may arise for no known reason.

Currently, food producers are not required to label lupin as a potential allergen, unlike gluten or soy. Immunologists suggest that anyone allergic to peanuts be tested for lupin sensitivity before eating foods made with it.

See also Soy.

Light (Lite) Foods

They seem to be the answer to our diet prayers—you eat, and enjoy, the same food, but consume less fat and fewer kilojoules (calories). To a dieter, it sounds just perfect! Light foods generally refer to those that have lowered the fat, sugar or alcohol content to reduce kilojoules. This is usually by around 25–30 per cent, but in some cases it may be as little as 10 per cent or even zero, having been lightened in colour or texture. Whatever part of the food is lightened must be stated on the label.

CLASSIFYING LIGHT PRODUCTS BY FAT AND KILOJOULES

You can divide light foods into three groups based on the amount of fat and kilojoules they save you. We reckon that if you aren't getting a 30 per cent saving in fat and kilojoules, it isn't worth the trade down! Here are the ones that are worth the swap.

GROUP ONE—SUPER SAVERS

These save you more than 30 per cent fat (or sugar or alcohol) and save kilojoules. These will really make a difference to your diet efforts.

LIGHT MILK

On the label, full-fat milk doesn't look that high in fat at only 3.5 per cent or 3.5 grams per 100 millilitres. However, if you drink 2 cups or 500 millilitres each day, that fat intake quickly rises to a hefty 17 grams (almost a quarter of your recommended daily intake). By buying light, you'll save on fat and also saturated fat, the 'bad' fat that's implicated in heart disease.

LIGHT CREAM

You'll drop around half the fat and kilojoules by making the switch to light cream. It's fine to make a sauce or 'finish off' a soup with, but remember it doesn't whip up well.

LIGHT CREAM CHEESE

This is another way to cut the fat by half and save yourself about 40 per cent in kilojoules. The spreadable texture is maintained with cottage cheese and skim milk.

LIGHT COCONUT CREAM

Coconut cream is usually high in fat and saturated fat, but by buying light you can reduce this by about half. There is great variation between brands though, so it pays to check the label and look for a brand with 11 per cent or less.

GROUP TWO—SOME SAVINGS

These light foods are not worth giving up the taste of the real thing for. Even if they save you fat, they don't save you many kilojoules as the fat is replaced with extra sugar or starch to maintain a smooth creamy texture or an attractive taste for baking. They are useful for reduced saturated fat or sodium though—so compare the label.

LIGHT PEANUT BUTTER

Regular peanut butter is half fat, thanks to the natural oil of peanuts. Switch to the light version and you get a huge drop in fat content from 53 to 38 per cent. But you will make only a 12 per cent saving in overall kilojoules because starch thickener and sugar have been added to keep it spreadable.

SHOPPER'S GUIDE

- ✔ Buy the light version but keep to the same portion you normally eat. Even if a light food has 50 per cent less fat, the kilojoules only drop by 40 per cent at the most.
- ✔ Fat adds flavour. If you take the fat out, you have to put something else in to give a light food enough flavour and texture. This is often sugar, fruit puree or starch and these add kilojoules.
- ✔ Read the label and check what is being lightened—is it the fat, salt, alcohol or just the texture or colour?
- ✔ Watch how small the serve size is. Many light products are packaged in smaller sizes so it looks like you're saving lots simply because you're eating less food.
- ✔ Sometimes it's more enjoyable to eat a small amount of the 'real thing' than lots of a light substitute. Sit down, savour a small serve slowly and you'll feel satisfied.

LIGHT ICE-CREAM

Again you save on fat, but not much in kilojoules as extra sugar and additives like maltodextrin have to be added to maintain a creamy texture.

LIGHT MICROWAVE POPCORN

You'd think that less fat would translate into a lot less kilojoules, but sadly it doesn't! You drop the fat by 43 per cent but only save 16 per cent of the kilojoules.

LIGHT CHOCOLATE

Everyone loves chocolate so a light bar offers pleasure without guilt—until you look closer. Often the saving is simply due to a smaller bar size. For example, a regular fun-size bar weighs 22 grams while the light alternative weights only 16 grams. You save because you're eating 6 grams less chocolate overall.

GROUP THREE—NO SAVINGS

These light foods give you no saving in fat or kilojoules.

LIGHT OLIVE OIL

Light olive oil has exactly the same fat and kilojoule count as regular oil, but without the strong flavour. Don't be fooled by this one!

LIGHT INSTANT GRAVY POWDER

Light gravy powder has the same fat and kilojoules but 40 per cent less salt.

See also **Weight Loss.**

Lignans

This is a group of phytoestrogens widely distributed in oilseeds (of which linseed has the greatest concentration), cereal brans, seaweed, legumes, vegetables and fruits.

Linoleic Acid (LA)

This is an essential omega-6 fatty acid that is a precursor to the longer-chain fatty acid arachidonic acid (AA). Food sources include most vegetable oils including sunflower, safflower, corn, peanut and grape seed oils, wholegrains, nuts, seeds and wheat germ.

Listeria

Listeria (technically *Listeria monocytogenes*) is a microorganism that may cause an infection that can be picked up by eating contaminated food. It causes few symptoms in healthy people, but can lead to serious illness or miscarriage in the unborn or illness in newborns.

During pregnancy, it's crucial to avoid eating any suspect food. This also applies to people whose immune systems cannot fight off infections and to people over 70.

Listeria bacteria are found widely in nature but they can be higher in things such as pre-prepared foods, raw foods or cooked foods that have been kept for some time after they have cooled down.

HOW TO AVOID IT

Risk of infection can be greatly reduced by good hygiene practices at home and taking care with ready-to-eat foods when out. You can take precautions to avoid listeria by:

- ✔ Eating only freshly prepared and well-washed food
- ✔ Following good food hygiene such as washing and drying hands
- ✔ Reheating foods to 'steaming' hot
- ✔ Refrigerating leftovers immediately and not keeping them any more than one day
- ✔ Buying from places that look clean, have a busy turnover and/or make foods to order (i.e. not selling sandwiches that have been made up hours before).

HIGH-RISK FOODS

- Soft cheeses (brie, camembert, ricotta and feta)—hard cheese, cream cheese and cottage cheese are safe if eaten when very fresh
- Paté and cold deli meats such as ham and salami
- Takeaway cooked chicken, particularly cold chicken used in sandwiches
- Raw seafood such as oysters and sashimi
- Smoked seafood (canned is safe)
- Pre-prepared sandwiches
- Ready-prepared salads
- Soft-serve ice-cream and unpasteurised dairy products
- Fruits and vegetables that are prepared, pre-packaged or served from smorgasbords or salad bars.

Liver Cleansing

Diet regimes to 'cleanse the liver', such as *The Liver Cleansing Diet* made famous by Dr Sandra Cabot's bestselling book, are based on the notion that our liver is the 'supreme organ of metabolism' in the body. If the liver is cleansed and detoxified, the theory goes, it can get on with its job of regulating metabolism and burning fat and weight loss becomes effortless. Such diets claim that a cleansed liver will also fix a long list of other ailments such as liver disease (cirrhosis or hepatitis), gallbladder problems, irritable bowel syndrome, chronic fatigue syndrome, arthritis, allergies and migraines. It's even supposed to delay ageing and increase longevity. The diet is usually supported by a number of natural liver remedies such as psyllium, taurine (an amino acid), dandelion, milk thistle, globe artichoke and slippery elm bark.

While the diets may be healthy in themselves, there's no research to support the theory they 'cleanse the liver' or provide a cure for liver disease. All evidence is anecdotal; there have been no independent clinical trials published in peer-reviewed journals. In fact, these diets may even result in compromising the nutritional status of those with liver disease. No-one knows for certain whether it's necessary to cleanse the liver. Certainly it can do no harm to avoid alcohol and rich or fatty food, as many people do after the excesses of Christmas. But whether this stops the liver ageing or fatty deposits is uncertain.

See also **Detox Diets.**

Locavore

This is a term used to describe people who are interested in eating food that is locally produced and has not been transported long distances to market. Some groups consider food grown within a '100 mile' radius (that's around 160 kilometres) of their location to qualify. Others seek food grown in home gardens or grown by local communities who are interested in sustainability. Foods such as tea, coffee, chocolate and spices pose a challenge for locavores.

See also **Sustainable Eating.**

Low-carb Diets, Foods and Beverages

Diets low in carbohydrates are usually based on meat, chicken, fish, eggs and non-starchy vegetables, with little or no bread, potato, rice, cereal, sugar or fruit. They are often touted as the sure-fire way to shed fat, making enticing claims about rapid weight loss without hunger or food restriction.

Low-carb diets are not new. As often happens in nutrition, things get recycled and this particular weight-loss regime tends to surface every so often under a new guise. In the 1970s, protein was big and the *Dr Atkins' Diet Revolution* was top of the bestseller list (*The Dukan Diet* has now taken over). At other times, a high-protein diet has been sold as *The Demis Roussos Diet* (devised by an overweight opera singer in a long caftan), *Sugar Busters Diet*, *Scarsdale Medical Diet*, *Boston Police Diet*, *Woman Doctor's Diet* and *Dr Stillman's Quick Weight Loss Diet*.

Most low-carb diets start off with an initial period of virtually no carbohydrates at all, for example the Atkins starts with a 14-day 'induction period' where you eat 'only fish, fowl or flesh'. No bread, potato, rice, cereal, pasta or sugars are permitted, and the carb intake is as low as 20 grams per day (one slice of bread is 15 grams). Once the dieter moves to the Atkins Ongoing Weight Loss (OWL) phase, carbohydrates are gradually re-introduced while testing

WHAT ARE LOW-CARB FOODS?

There's no official definition of low-carbohydrate products in Australian food standards, as there is for low-salt, low-fat, high-fibre or diet foods. Low-carb generally means there is less than 10 g per serve (a slice of bread has around 15 g so it's not much). There are three things to be mindful of when considering a low-carb diet:

- Lowering or removing the carb content does not necessarily mean the food is lower in kilojoules. Some products are even higher in fat than their regular counterpart—items like chocolate brownie bars or chunky peanut butter are essentially refined and overly sweet and not the ideal fare for dieters to eat.
- Genuine low-carb foods have both a lower carb and a lower kilojoule count (many are low-fat as well). These products will make a useful addition to a weight-loss diet as they have fewer kilojoules per serve. For example, pasta, bread and cereals can be modified to offer a 30 per cent reduction in carbohydrate per serve by substituting a protein-rich grain or high-fibre flour for part of the wheat.
- Many diets simply remove the carbohydrate component, e.g. the bread, potato or rice from a meal. Burger King introduced a bun-less burger in 2004, while many dieters replace bread with crispbread or eat a dinner consisting of meat or fish with non-starchy vegetables or a salad. This was typical of the dinner meals in the *CSIRO Total Wellbeing Diet*.

DID YOU KNOW?

Gram for gram, pure protein has around the same kilojoules as carbohydrates, so whether you opt for a small steak or more pasta you won't blow your day's kilojoule budget.

There's no need to cut out all carbohydrates—the right types are an important nutrient in a healthy balanced diet.

the urine for ketones which supposedly indicate that the body is in a 'fat-burning' mode (which has no proof behind it—it merely shows that there is insufficient glucose and that the body is trying to break down fat for energy). Carbohydrate intakes in this phase range from 20 grams to 100 grams, which is still below the recommended minimum safe intake.

MY TAKE

From a health viewpoint, irrespective of whether you are trying to lose weight or not, it's better to drink less alcohol than take in fewer carbohydrates. Therefore, my choice would be a light beer. You cut back on alcohol AND save on kilojoules.

See also **Beer; Carbohydrates; Weight Loss.**

CUTTING CARBS FOR WEIGHT LOSS

There's no need to cut out all carbohydrates (both sugar and starchy foods)—the right type of carbohydrates are an important nutrient in a healthy balanced diet. However, studies from both Australia and overseas show that a diet containing higher protein and moderate carbohydrate (with low-GI carbs) is beneficial for dieters. A diet with a ratio of higher protein and a lower carb rate is satiating and keeps you fuller for longer; requires less insulin, a hormone which encourages fat to be stored and slows fat burning; may help preserve muscle mass, which is more metabolically active; and can help reduce triglycerides (a type of blood fat like cholesterol).

A 375 ml bottle or can of beer contains about 11 g of carbs, compared with 40 g for a can of fizzy drink.

LSA

LSA is an acronym for linseed (flaxseed), sunflower seeds and almonds that have been ground into a coarse meal. Most LSA mixes are half linseed, with the remainder sunflower and almonds. It's useful to provide unsaturated fats, omega-3 oils for vegans, B vitamins, protein and natural fibre. It helps digestion and regularity and is a nutritious boost to skin and hair.

With its pleasant nutty flavour, you can add a daily tablespoon of LSA to muesli or cereal, or mix it into smoothies or yoghurt. Replace a couple of spoons of flour with LSA in home-baked bread and muffins.

Ideally it should be ground fresh each day. If you can't, make up enough for three or four days, and store in an airtight container in the refrigerator.

Lunch

Lunch is important in helping to maintain momentum during the day and avoid that mid-afternoon slump known as the '3 pm low'. This low is so common that I suspect there must be an underlying biological reason behind it. Maybe our bodies weren't meant to work for eight hours straight. The clever Spanish and Italians have formalised this low point with the siesta, which makes great body-sense to me—after lunch, they nod off with a short nap that keeps them out of the hot midday sun and rejuvenates them for the second half of the day. Of course, most of us don't have this luxury, but if you've skipped lunch or eaten an inadequate meal, you'll feel even more drained of energy and unable to concentrate, and be much less efficient.

This battle against our body's in-built circadian rhythm is also the precise point where most diet intentions come unstuck. It's a difficult point in time when office workers need something to keep themselves going. How many times have you snuck out for a coffee (and usually a muffin)?

MY TAKE
This is the best lunch-break advice I've read over the years (and practised myself) to ward off the slump:
***1.** Get outdoors and go for a walk to take in fresh air and recharge the brain. This works best when it's a little cold and fresh outside. On a hot summer day, go for an invigorating swim, or a lunchtime session in an air-conditioned gym.*
***2.** Eat a high-protein lunch based on tuna, salmon, chicken, hard-boiled eggs or cold meat with salad, rather than a sandwich, roll or pasta meal.*

THE IDEAL OFFICE LUNCH BOX

It pays to select a slower-digested, low-GI meal that will stick with you longer and prevent your energy levels from flagging through the afternoon:

- ✔ Swap white bread for grainy bread.
- ✔ Avoid white rice if you order takeaway—ask for thin hokkien noodles instead.
- ✔ Go for legumes like baked beans on grain toast or chickpeas in a salad with tuna or lentil curry.
- ✔ For a healthy and budget-friendly option, bring in leftovers from dinner for lunch the next day or a frozen soup, which can thaw and be reheated.

Lutein *See also* **Eyesight.**

This is a carotenoid and antioxidant, which appears to protect against loss of vision in the elderly.

Lycopene

An important carotenoid found almost exclusively in tomatoes and tomato products.

Lysine

An amino acid (component of protein) classified as essential because it cannot be made in the body. Although present in animal proteins, it is of special importance, as it is not found in a number of grain proteins—including those of corn, rice and wheat—and therefore needs to be obtained via the consumption of complementary protein from legumes.

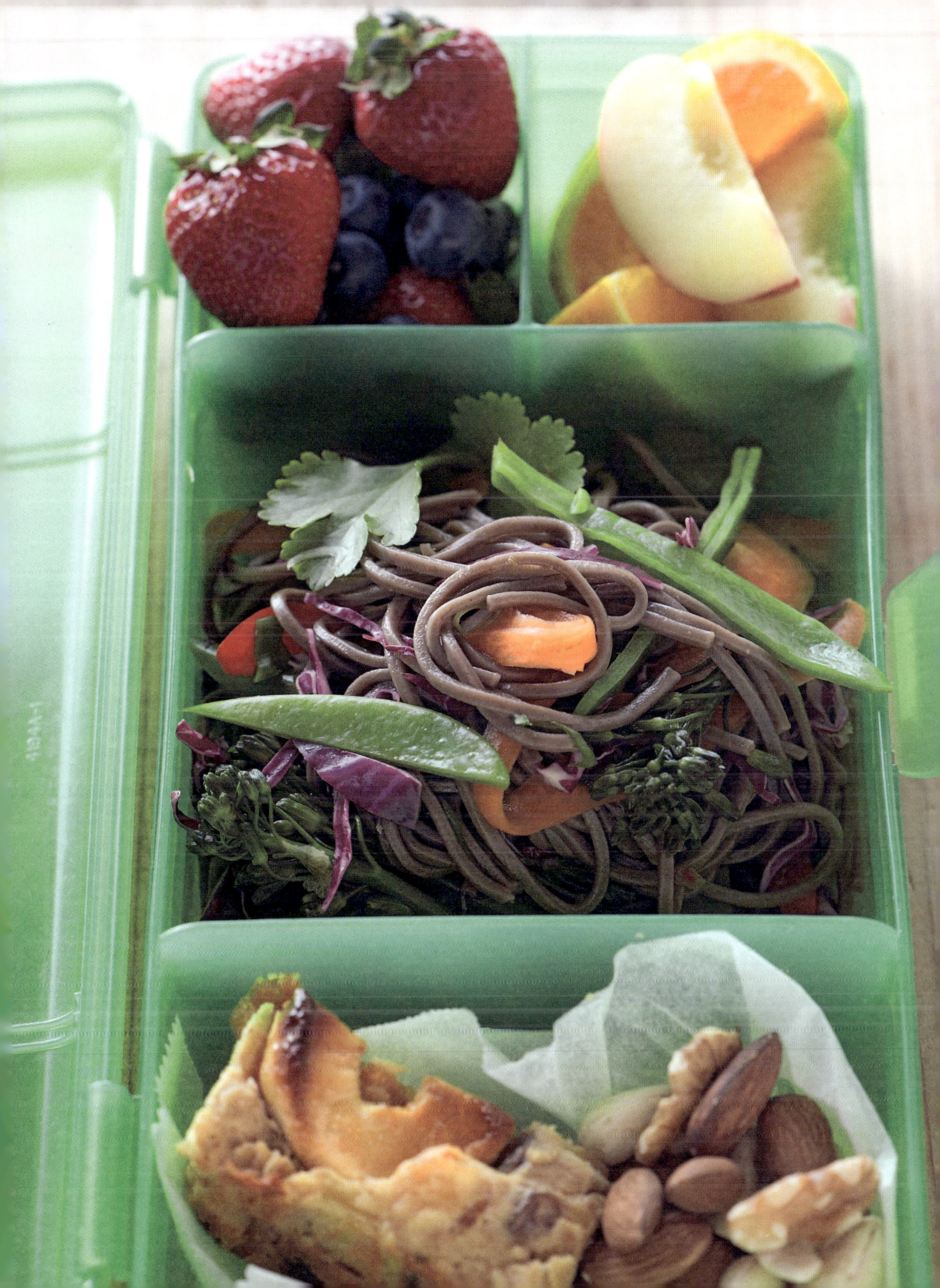

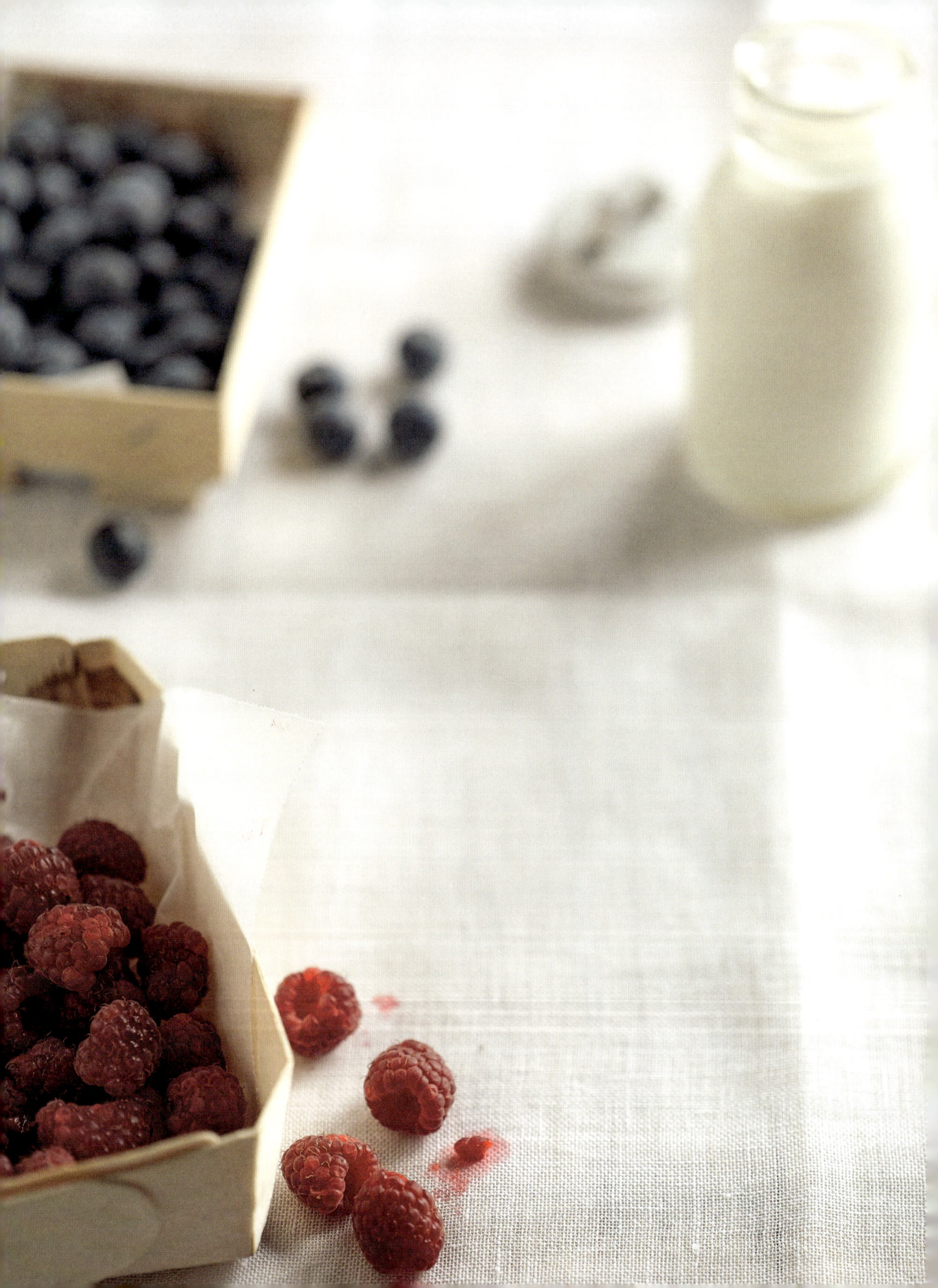

M

Macrobiotic Diets

MY TAKE
Overall it's a low-fat, high-fibre, mainly vegetarian diet. Although it counteracts the excesses of modern refined foods (a plus in my view), it can be marginal in important nutrients such as iron, zinc and calcium as well as vitamin B_{12} and omega-3s. For this reason, I would not recommend this diet.

Macrobiotic ('macro' meaning 'large' and 'bio' meaning 'life') diets are centred on the consumption of unprocessed, unrefined and seasonal food as much as possible, and are based mainly on wholegrains, vegetables, legumes and sea vegetables. There is no single macrobiotic diet; they vary depending on cultural background, seasons and circumstances.

Wholegrains, vegetables and beans are thought to create balance (yin), while meat, poultry, eggs and salt are considered to be concentrated and heavy and create stagnation (yang). Macrobiotic diet food portions are generally broken down like this:

- 40–60 per cent—well-chewed wholegrains, especially brown rice
- 25–30 per cent—vegetables
- 5–10 per cent—legumes
- 5 per cent—miso soup
- 5 per cent—sea vegetables
- 5–10 per cent—traditionally or naturally processed foods.

You can eat fish and seafood, seeds and nuts, seed and nut butters, seasonings, sweeteners, fruits and beverages occasionally—maybe a couple of times a week. Organic meat can be eaten from time to time.

Magnesium *See* **Minerals.**

Maltodextrin

This is a predigested starch that may be used as a carrier as well as a thickener or texture-modifying agent in many foodstuffs. It may be produced from wheat, corn or potato starches.

Manganese *See* **Minerals.**

Margarine *See* **Spreads.**

Maltose

Maltose or malt sugar is produced when starch is broken down, or in the malting of barley or wheat grains.

Meat (Red)

As hunters and gatherers, we obtained a substantial portion of our kilojoules eating meat. When we became farmers around 10,000 years ago, meat continued to play a key role in our diet, prized for its flavour and nutritional value, as well as its social significance.

Today, what we serve with our meat meal is important too, as we need plenty of vegetables and salad. Many of us love to tuck into steak and three veg, steak and salad, or a roast with the works. These combinations are good for our overall nutrition.

NUTRITIONAL VALUE

Meat gives us valuable, high-quality protein with all the essential amino acids required by the human body. It is also very filling and satisfying for the kilojoules it provides, which is a big help to anyone on a weight-loss diet.

Eating red meat is a great way to get a boost in nutrients often in short supply in modern diets. It is rich in minerals like iron and zinc (in a readily absorbed form), B vitamins (particularly B_{12}) and omega-3 fatty acids. The most valued of these is the iron content, which occurs as haem iron—the type most easily absorbed by the body. We need iron for healthy blood, the development of our brain, the functioning of our immune system and work performance. It is somewhat ironic that women, who have the greatest nutritional requirement for iron, are the smallest consumers of meat, depriving themselves of the best form of iron from food.

RED MEAT

Meat that falls into this category includes beef, veal, lamb, mutton, pork, horse, goat, venison and kangaroo.

A small piece of grilled rump steak (weighing around 125 grams) provides an adult with two-thirds of their daily protein needs, half of their iron, zinc and niacin and all of their vitamin B_{12}, as well as lesser amounts of other vitamins. It also has 6 grams of fat (including 2 grams of saturated fat and 70 milligrams of cholesterol), which is not high compared with fast food.

SHOPPER'S GUIDE

Trim lamb is a healthy alternative. Try lean cuts such as easy-carve boneless leg roasts, lamb strips, fillets, steaks, cubes and cutlets—a frenched lamb cutlet with no visible fat is 65 per cent lower in fat than the traditional rib loin cutlet.

THE FAT

These days, thanks to the breeding of leaner beasts and trimming of fat by butchers, the arbitrary classification of trimmed meat is fairly similar in fat and kilojoules to skinless poultry.

Three factors influence the amount of fat cover on a meat carcass: the breed of cattle (crossbreds with Charolais, Simmental or Limousin lines have less fat than the more common Herefords), feeding (grass-fed animals have less fat than grain-fed) and stocking rates.

Always choose lean cuts, trim away visible fat and use cooking methods such as grilling or roasting on a rack (which allow fat to drain away), to reduce the amount of fat and saturated fat in your diet.

One serve is 125 grams of cooked meat (150 grams raw weight becomes around 125 grams when cooked). For example:

- 2 slices roast meat
- 2 medium chops
- 1 small steak
- ¾ cup mince.

MINCE MATTERS

Mince is the most popular cut of meat. It is versatile and liked by children. It can be fattier than

It is somewhat ironic that women, who have the greatest nutritional requirement for iron, are the smallest consumers of meat, depriving themselves of the best form of iron from food.

Q

I've heard meat causes bowel cancer. Is this true?

A

There's been a suspicion that meat is linked to colorectal cancer for some years now, but the link is only there if the meat is charred, processed or preserved. This is an important distinction. Colorectal cancer is the most common cancer in Australia, with more than 12,000 new cases each year. So, don't bring home the bacon! Avoid processed meats such as bacon, ham, salami, corned beef and some sausages. Why? Processed meat is preserved by smoking, curing or salting or by the addition of preservatives. These methods of preserving meat can produce cancer-causing substances. Take care cooking meat too (especially when barbecuing); don't burn or char it.

DID YOU KNOW?

Kangaroo and venison are the leanest of the red meats. Kangaroo is 98 per cent fat free and its very modest fat content consists mainly of polyunsaturated and monounsaturated fats. It is also very low in cholesterol.

straight cuts of meat though, so it pays to buy the lean or extra-lean mince, which must have less than 10 per cent fat.

Good-quality regular mince has around 20 per cent fat and a good amount of protein, iron and B vitamins. If you do use this mince, be sure to use low-fat cooking methods—grill burgers, instead of frying them, skim excess fat from the top of your mince casserole before serving, or shallow-fry or bake meatballs and koftas rather than deep-frying them, and then drain well on kitchen paper to get rid of excess oil.

GROWTH HORMONES

The issue of hormones in beef has surfaced recently thanks to a large supermarket's marketing claim that they sell 'hormone-free' beef.

Extra hormone has been used in beef since 1979, and now about 40 per cent of Australian cattle are raised using Hormone Growth Promotant (HGP), a supplement of naturally occurring hormones (oestrogen, testosterone and progesterone) that are found in most animals. HGPs are present at much lower levels than the natural hormone levels found in many common foods including soy beans and eggs. The hormone comes in the form of small implants that are placed under the skin on the back of the ear, slowly releasing a low dosage over a period of time—usually 100–200 days. It causes no harm to the animal and it's been tested and approved by the Australian government and the World Health Organization.

HGPs improve the growth rate of cattle (by 15–30 per cent), and help them convert feed to meat more efficiently (by 5–15 per cent). This means that the beef producers are more competitive and their impact on the environment is reduced. The biggest difference for the consumer is to the tenderness of certain cuts, particularly sirloin and scotch fillet. However, you'd be hard-pressed to notice much variation, and any difference can be negated by the use of simple techniques like ageing beef a little longer and different methods of hanging the carcase.

Personally, I think there are bigger problems to worry about with meat such as buying grass-fed (not grain-fed) beef, as most are in Australia, trimming away the fat and getting the size of your portion right. And eating larger serves of vegetables with your steak or chops. But if it bothers you, shop at the supermarket or butcher shop that claims to sell hormone-free or buy organic meat. Remember that the supermarket advertising this claim is only talking about its fresh meat. Other beef products such as meat pies, packaged beef soups and stocks, or smallgoods like corned beef and beef sausages may or may not be reared with hormones.

See also
Barbecuing; Iron; Protein.

Mediterranean Diet

Switch to a Mediterranean diet and live a longer, healthier life. It's perfectly suited to our warm sunny climate with its salads, easy vegetable dishes, seafood and fresh fruit.

Widely regarded as one of the healthiest ways to eat, those on a Mediterranean diet are less likely to suffer from heart disease, high blood pressure and certain types of cancer. Research supports this. The rate of heart disease among Greek people when they first migrate to Australia is low compared with that of Australians. But once the first generation of Greek Australians grows up, their heart disease rates rise to approach that of the locals. This is because they have replaced the traditional plant-based dishes of the Mediterranean diet with food more dense in kilojoules, including larger serves of meat, chicken, sweets and fast foods.

MEDITERRANEAN DIET STAPLES

The Mediterranean diet is the traditional eating pattern of the countries around the Mediterranean Sea including Spain, southern France, southern Italy, Greece, Turkey, Lebanon and Morocco. There is no single Mediterranean diet—it can be generally described as a variety of fresh, colourful, delicious dishes that feature in a hospitable lifestyle. The emphasis is always on fresh seasonal vegetables, fruit, legumes, fish and seafood, garlic, herbs and spices and olive oil, with only small quantities of meat and dairy products and few processed foods. Desserts, when served, will generally be based on fruit—not cream or chocolate!

The health benefits associated with the diet cannot be attributed to a single food. But there are some factors we know are particularly helpful. The generous use of olive oil means the diet is high in mono-unsaturated fats and low in both saturated and polyunsaturated fats. Tomatoes, garlic, red wine (in some countries) and vegetables all add antioxidants, while seafood contributes plenty of omega-3s, a heart-friendly factor.

GARLIC AND ONION

Renowned for its wonderful taste, garlic has been shown to keep the blood flowing freely, help reduce cholesterol and improve the flexibility of the blood vessels. In its raw form, it has mild antibacterial properties, stopping the growth of harmful bacteria and yeasts. Onion is a close cousin of garlic and delivers the same health benefits, along with plenty of vitamin C.

TOMATOES

Tomatoes are a big feature. Besides being a good source of vitamin C, they contain lycopene (which gives the red colouring), an antioxidant that fights against oxygen's damaging effect on body cells. Cooking tomatoes and adding oil increases the absorption of lycopene.

SEAFOOD

An Italian restaurant that doesn't dish up calamari, mussels or lemon sole is unimaginable. Fish and seafood dominate the Mediterranean diet and provide powerful omega-3 fats as well as protein and the minerals iodine and potassium. Omega-3s are known to reduce the risk of heart disease, by lowering the amount of triglycerides (blood fats), thinning the blood and preventing irregular heartbeats (arrhythmia).

PASTA

Of all the starchy carbohydrates, pasta is the one nutritionists love. It's low in fat, has little salt and is low GI. It's also blessed with protein and B vitamins, plus a little iron and calcium. For a filling, non-fattening meal, top your pasta the Mediterranean way—with tomatoes or a tomato sauce, capsicum, zucchini or other vegetables, chickpeas, seafood and fresh herbs like basil or oregano. Enjoy versatile couscous too, a pasta that's usually made from durum wheat semolina but can also be made from barley or corn. Use wholemeal pasta for added health benefits and try spelt or Kamut pasta for variety.

SHOPPER'S GUIDE

Food shopping in Mediterranean countries is a real treat. Bustling marketplaces are bursting with an abundance of fresh produce—onions and garlic, artichokes, eggplants, tomatoes, sweet peppers, mushrooms, cucumbers, okra, zucchini and a multitude of leafy greens and lettuces, fresh herbs such as rosemary, flat-leaf parsley, coriander and oregano, as well as seasonal fruits like figs, lemons, limes and oranges create sensational colour and aromas.

OLIVE OIL

Olive oil contains over 70 per cent monounsaturated fat, among the highest of all the oils. If you buy extra-virgin cold-pressed oil, it will also give you natural antioxidants such as polyphenols and carotenoids as well as some vitamin E. Extra-virgin olive oil is from the first pressing of olives and is low in acidity. It is usually reserved for salads and dressing cooked zucchini or other vegetables. Pure (regular) olive oil is usually a mix of extra-virgin and refined olive oil, sold in large tins. Save this one for cooking.

LEGUMES

Harvard researchers persuaded 26,000 Greek people to record their food intake for eight years, and they found that eating less red meat and more legumes like peas, beans and lentils cut the risk of cancer by 12 per cent. It is recommended you eat legumes as a meal at least once a week—they are easy on the budget, nutritious, filling, low in kilojoules and low GI.

LEAFY VEGETABLES

Dark-green leafy vegetables are a big feature in the Mediterranean diet. Excellent sources of magnesium and plant omega-3 fats, they can be steamed, boiled or served raw. They come in a wide variety including spinach, rocket, endive, chicory, amaranth and mustard greens (sold in Australian supermarkets as choy sum, bok choy and Chinese spinach). Greeks like to dress them by adding oil, lemon and vinegar and serving with vegetables and starchy foods, which boosts the flavour, and creates a nutritious, low-GI meal.

LEMONS

What a great way to add flavour—squeeze them on fish, put a slice in your tea or drizzle over salad leaves. They are a feature of one of my favourite main meals—slow-cooked Greek leg of lamb with lemon, garlic and rosemary. Always on my shopping list, I wonder why on earth didn't I plant a lemon tree years ago. Like other citrus fruits, they are nutritional all-rounders, but packed especially with vitamin C, which enhances iron absorption, speeds up wound healing and reduces the risk of heart attack. They also provide small amounts of minerals and some B vitamins. Don't just juice them—bring out the zester and enjoy the nutritional goodies in the skin.

NUTS AND SEEDS

Traditional snacks in the Mediterranean diet include pumpkin seeds, roasted chickpeas, almonds and walnuts, which add fibre, good fats, vitamins and minerals to your intake.

YOGHURT

A daily staple in the Mediterranean, yoghurt is used in drinks, salads, dips and desserts, and on its own with a drizzle of honey and a sprinkle of chopped nuts. Packed with calcium, protein and B vitamins (especially riboflavin), it offers the nutrients of milk but in a more concentrated form.

RED WINE

Red wine contains antioxidants known as polyphenols and resveratrol and can increase 'good' cholesterol. It is enjoyed with meals in many Mediterranean countries but in moderation.

THE MEDITERRANEAN LIFESTYLE

Research shows that exercise, stress reduction and strong social support all contribute to a reduced risk of heart disease.

The traditional Mediterranean diet and lifestyle is conducive to this. People buy fresh produce from local markets and prepare meals from scratch, rather than eating pre-prepared, highly processed and takeaway foods. There's also more physical labour incorporated in the everyday living, i.e. walking or riding to the shops for provisions, mixing dishes by hand rather than with a processor and picking vegetables daily from the garden. Community ties are strong, and families come together for an unhurried midday or evening meal providing opportunities to share, relax and unwind.

See also Citrus Fruit; Fish; Garlic; Legumes; Oils; Seafood; Vegetables; Yoghurt.

Medium-chain Triglycerides

These are smaller-sized fats—ordinary fats and oils are long-chain triglycerides. They are broken down faster and more completely in the digestive tract and go directly to the liver, where they are used as a source of energy and not stored as body fat, as ordinary fats are. They were developed in the 1950s to help people with trouble absorbing regular fats and are usually derived from coconut oil.

Men and Healthy Eating

Real men don't eat quiche, or so that urban myth goes. When compared with women, men are generally not well informed on nutrition. They don't take as much interest in their health or in healthy eating and they don't consult doctors and health professionals as often. Perhaps because of this, men tend to be less healthy than women and are more overweight, usually in the form of that really life-threatening potbelly.

The bad news is that this weight is the visceral fat linked to the trio of unhealthy 'highs'—high blood pressure, high blood glucose and high blood fats, as well as type 2 diabetes and heart disease. The good news is that it is much easier to shrink tummy fat cells than hip and thigh ones through healthy eating and being more active.

Taking an interest in nutrition is the first step in turning around what is generally a less than healthy diet. Men typically don't eat enough wholegrains, vegetables and fruit, yet they eat plenty of processed food including fatty meats and salty snacks, drink too much alcohol, salt their food more and eat larger portions. Research shows men usually only change these habits when they get a 'scare' such as a heart attack or diabetes. Here are some tips for helping blokes improve their diet before it comes to that.

MAKE A CHANGE

- ✔ Take an interest in what you eat.
- ✔ Cook a meal for your partner or family at least once a week.
- ✔ Do the grocery shopping occasionally.
- ✔ Let your kids see the man cooking up a storm.
- ✔ Eat more variety, not the same thing out of habit or whatever you grew up with.

HEALTHY SWAPS FOR BLOKES

✖ Potato crisps	✔ Pretzels, rice crackers or salted beer nuts
✖ Burger with the lot	✔ Regular burger with tomato and lettuce
✖ Meat pies	✔ Steak sandwich
✖ Meat lover's pizza or cheesy-crust pizza	✔ Thin and crispy marinara pizza
✖ Fried chicken	✔ Barbecue, wood-fired or rotisserie chicken
✖ Nachos with all the trimmings	✔ Soft tortillas with lean beef, beans, tomato and guacamole
✖ Beer (full strength)	✔ Low-carb or light beers (the kilojoules are around the same) ✔ A nip of spirits with soda water or diet ginger ale
✖ Soft drink	✔ Diet soft drink, sparkling mineral water or tomato juice
✖ Chocolate milk (full fat)	✔ Low-fat chocolate milk or the smallest-size milk carton you can buy

- ✔ Give the bacon cheeseburger stack a miss—order something lighter and healthier next time.
- ✔ Switch to wholemeal bread and cereals for fibre.
- ✔ Salad and veggies aren't just 'rabbit food'—they should be a staple in your diet.
- ✔ Don't salt food before tasting it.
- ✔ Help with the kitchen clean-up (this one will earn you serious brownie points).

Menopause and Diet

Menopause—those years when a woman's hormones begin to decline—can be a blessing or a curse. Around 80 per cent of women experience unpleasant symptoms like hot flushes, night sweats, vaginal dryness, weight gain, moodiness and irritability. A small number will sail through those years between 45 and 60 with nothing more than irregular periods.

However it affects you, this is a time to pay attention to your daily diet. Good food and a healthy lifestyle can help avoid menopause-related problems like weight gain, heart disease and osteoporosis. There are also various remedies and supplements on the market, touted to relieve menopausal troubles, but in general, the research into these has been inconclusive.

MY TAKE

Twenty years down the track, clinical trials have not proven the benefits of soy's phytoestrogens. They have found little or no effect, even when given in concentrated form as supplements. In fact, some research found supplements can increase the risk of breast cancer. Similarly the trials of menopause supplements such as dong quai or wild yam have not produced significant results. It's wise to talk to your gynaecologist about these and whether they can harm or help your medication.

THREE WAYS TO CHANGE YOUR LIFE DURING THE CHANGE OF LIFE

1. MINIMISE THE MID-LIFE SPREAD

As we age, our metabolic rate gradually slows so it becomes easier to put on kilos, especially around the stomach. This abdominal fat deposition is also due in part to the drop in hormones at the time. However, weight gain does not have to be automatic; it can be prevented with healthy eating and exercise. Menopause is often associated with fewer family commitments, increased socialising and a decrease in sport and other physical activity. So fight mid-life spread by keeping up moderate daily exercise like walking, yoga or aerobics, and maintain lean muscle with light weight training to keep your metabolism up.

2. KEEP YOUR BONES STRONG

Menopause accelerates the loss of calcium, magnesium, potassium and other minerals from bones, setting the scene for osteoporosis as we age. Rate of loss is high—as much as 20 per cent a year following menopause. Fractures affect around 50 per cent of elderly post-menopausal women.

It is much easier to prevent osteoporosis than to treat it, and you need to consider calcium long before menopause begins. The peak bone density you achieve in your early twenties is critical to warding off osteoporosis in later years. However, you can still save your bones by reducing the rate of calcium loss or by increasing calcium (and vitamin D) intake in later years. The recommended intake for women over 55 is 1300 milligrams a day, which is higher than that of younger women, and usually requires a combination of dairy foods and a calcium supplement.

Calcium-rich foods or supplements are important but need to be combined with hormone replacement therapy to enable the calcium to 'move into the bones'. Calcium alone is of little use. Aim for:

- Eat at least four serves of calcium-rich dairy foods each day such as yoghurt, enriched milks, reduced-fat cheese and fortified soy milks.
- Consider a supplement of calcium with vitamin D.

- Start a weight-bearing exercise program such as regular walking, dance, exercise classes, tennis or golf.
- Check with your doctor about hormone replacement therapy or other bone-maintaining medications. Eat mineral-rich foods like vegetables, fruit, herbs, wholegrains and nuts.
- Avoid too much phosphorus from fizzy drinks (phosphoric acid is used as a preservative).

DID YOU KNOW?

The research into soy and hormones was initiated in the 1990s after doctors noticed that Japanese women were only one-third as likely to report menopausal problems as women in the US or Australia. In fact, there is no word in the Japanese language for 'hot flush'! This was attributed to soy, which is a staple food eaten daily in large amounts.

3. KEEP YOUR HEART HEALTHY

Heart disease looms during menopause as the protective effect of female hormones wanes. In fact, figures in the US estimate that menopause triples the risk of heart disease for women, putting them on a par with men. Maximise heart health by watching your fat intake and incorporating moderate aerobic exercise along with regular blood testing to monitor cholesterol and blood pressure.

EAT FOODS RICH IN PHYTOESTROGENS (PLANT HORMONES)

Today's common advice is to consume soy as soy foods. Soy contains a group of natural compounds known as isoflavones, a group of phytoestrogens that are similar in structure to our own oestrogens. As such, it was originally believed they have the potential to 'top up' oestrogen levels during the years when women's ovaries wind down their production of oestrogen. The mechanism seems logical; isoflavones have been shown to bind to the body's receptors for oestrogen, and it's possible they participate in the body's hormone interplay. This is backed up by studies, which found that soy can extend the length of a woman's menstrual cycle.

Other sources of these plant hormones are lentils, chickpeas and other beans, salad sprouts and linseed (flaxseed), but the concentrations in these are not as high as in soy foods.

See also **Weight Loss; Heart Disease and Diet; Osteoporosis and Diet.**

Metabolic Rate

Metabolism is the collective word for all the processes by which your body converts food into energy. Think of metabolism as your body's engine, burning fuel (kilojoules or energy) and regulating your energy needs. How fast your engine runs is called your metabolic rate.

Many factors determine this rate. Some of these you can control, like the level of activity, the ratio of muscle to body fat and the number of meals you eat throughout the day, but there are three key contributing factors which you can't do anything about.

Genes—some people are lucky to be born with a high metabolism, while others spend most of their time in the slow lane.

Gender—men typically have faster metabolisms than women, because they have less body fat and more muscle.

Age—the reality is that metabolism slows down as we age because we tend to lose muscle and become

SHOPPER'S GUIDE

Don't bother throwing supplements that claim to increase your metabolism in your shopping basket. Sales of these pills that 'enhance fat oxidation' or are 'metabolism boosters' are booming, but there is little evidence they have any real weight-loss effect. They usually contain things like chromium picolinate (supposedly to help insulin work better), guarana (a herbal form of caffeine), iodine (to boost the thyroid), chilli extract, vitamins and various herbs. If there is any effect, it's quite small—much less than what you can achieve by a heart-pumping workout or a session doing weights—and not long term. Without changing your diet and exercise routine to build your muscle mass, you'll be wasting your money.

more sedentary. An average 45 year old burns 400 fewer kilojoules a day than a 25 year old. You can delay this by staying physically active over the years, and building muscle mass through strength training or weights.

See also **Weight Loss.**

DID YOU KNOW?

Many people complain they can't lose weight because they have a 'slow metabolism'. It's actually rare to find someone with a genuinely sluggish metabolic rate. Often, it's simply a matter of regular exercise and a healthy diet.

Metabolic Syndrome (Syndrome X or Insulin Resistance)

Made popular recently by many diet books, this syndrome may sound to you like something from outer space. In reality, it's a real problem that has been around for some years and is increasingly recognised by doctors and dietitians. It's a term you'll be hearing more about as it relates to our obesogenic lifestyle.

Metabolic syndrome refers to a cluster of risk factors that can lead to type 2 diabetes, heart disease, polycystic ovarian syndrome (PCOS), gallstones, cataracts and a number of different types of cancer. Researchers originally coined the term Syndrome X, but later renamed it after they'd worked out how it centred on one's metabolism and insulin resistance.

RISK FACTORS

- Are you obese?
- Is your excess weight mostly around your middle?
- Do you have high blood pressure?
- Is your day mostly sedentary, with little moving around (be honest!)?
- Do you have high blood-glucose levels, diabetes or impaired glucose tolerance?
- Do you have high blood fats (LDL cholesterol or triglycerides)?
- Are you a smoker?

If you answer yes to two or more of these questions, you should see your doctor for a check up and detailed advice.

MANAGEMENT

The cornerstone of treatment is your lifestyle. You need to be active and eat a healthy diet that will help you lose weight. Of course, the first thing to do is have a chat to your doctor or to an accredited practising dietitian, but here are some tips.

FEWER REFINED CARBOHYDRATES

Pop diet books proclaim that if you just cut out carbohydrates, all your problems will disappear. Unfortunately it's not that simple. Rather than eliminating all carbohydrates, be more selective. Choose less of refined high-GI types such as those in white bread, white rice, pastries, biscuits, muffins and some breakfast cereals, and more of the low-GI varieties such as grainy breads, rye crackers, wholegrain breakfast cereals, pasta, fruit and legumes.

MORE FIBRE

People who eat more foods rich in fibre such as fruit, vegetables, legumes, wholegrain breads and bran cereals have lower risk factors associated with this syndrome.

MORE LEAN PROTEIN

There's no need to follow a Dr Atkins high-protein, high-fat diet but boosting your protein intake is helpful. A serve of lean protein such as canned tuna, lean red meat or chicken without the skin at meal times will give you greater satisfaction for longer and demand less insulin. This means you will be less hungry and likely to snack between meals, and have fewer swings in your blood-glucose levels.

GOOD FATS

High blood fats and heart disease that go along with metabolic syndrome need special attention. Keep your total fat intake down to help with weight control and make sure that any fats you do use are healthy. Choose vegetable fats such as sunflower, safflower, canola or olive oil and spreads made from these. Omega-3 fats from fish are also important, so make sure you try to eat some at least twice a week. I'd recommend also trying the new omega-enriched milks, breads and spreads.

REV UP THE EXERCISE

Exercise can prevent or reverse many of the unhealthy metabolic changes that contribute to metabolic syndrome. Increase your general day-to-day activity levels by using the stairs, walking to the shops and getting up to turn the TV off. Invest in a pedometer and start counting your steps—your goal could simply be to walk 1000 more steps a day, or aim higher and go for 7000 or 10,000 steps!

See also **Carbohydrates; Glycemic Index; Weight Loss.**

Microwave Cooking

This is high-energy radiation that heats water particles within food. Its main advantage is rapid cooking and thawing. Microwaving is similar to steaming and there is no browning of food.

Like pressure-cooking, microwaving food retains a high proportion of vitamins and minerals—more than boiling, as it uses little or no water so you don't leach out the nutrients into the surrounding water. Because the cooking process is fast, heat-sensitive vitamins like B and C are not broken down. Most other nutrients are not affected adversely by any cooking method. In fact, cooking improves the digestibility of most proteins and increases the availability of lycopene and other fat-soluble vitamins. The mineral and fibre content does not change.

MY TAKE

The notion that microwaving 'nukes' food and destroys nutrients is not true. With a microwave now in about 80 per cent of homes, one would think any harmful effects over the past 40 years would have been evident by now. I regard microwave cooking as safe and one of the healthier ways to cook vegetables, along with steaming and pressure-cooking.

Milk and Milk Alternatives

One of our basic foods, cow's milk is the basis of all dairy products and is a major ingredient in foods like yoghurt, cheese, custard, white sauces and many soups. Milk is considered essential during childhood to supply protein, vitamins and bone-building calcium. For the first two years of life, milk is the largest single item of food consumed.

Milk is a complete food, containing all vitamins and minerals. It consists of 88 per cent water with around 4 per cent protein, 4 per cent milk fat and 4 per cent lactose or milk sugar. The protein in milk is high quality, supplying all of the eight essential amino acids required by humans. Milk fat or butterfat is high in saturates with over 60 per cent saturated fat, 33 per cent mono-unsaturated fat and less than 5 per cent polyunsaturated, so low-fat milks are recommended for those on cholesterol-lowering programs.

Milk is rich in calcium and its calcium is better absorbed than from other foods. A 300 ml carton of milk (whole or skim) contains some 350 mg of calcium, which is one-third of the recommended day's intake of 1000 mg for adults. Without milk (or its calcium-rich products yoghurt and cheese), it is quite difficult to reach this total of 1000 mg, and obtaining sufficient calcium in the teenage and early adult years is critical to the prevention of osteoporosis or brittle bones.

As well as calcium, milk is a good source of the minerals phosphorus and potassium. Milk carries B group vitamins, particularly riboflavin (vitamin B_2). Full-cream milk also carries vitamins A and D, which are fat-soluble. Milk's riboflavin is susceptible to sunlight and milk in plastic bottles exposed to direct sunlight may lose up to 50 per cent of this vitamin in two hours. Paperboard cartons significantly reduce the penetration of light but do not block it completely. So don't leave your milk out in full sun.

Milk, whether full fat or skim, has a low GI.

FINDING THE ONE RIGHT FOR YOU

There are a lot of different varieties of milk in our supermarkets, and they all vary in cost. In my opinion, nothing beats standard reduced-fat milk in terms of value for money. It provides your family with bone-building calcium and phosphorus, protein, carbohydrate and riboflavin, and it's low in saturated fat. However, if you have a particular condition such as osteoporosis or heart disease, the specialised milks that are more concentrated in calcium and/or vitamin D, or carry sterols or omega-3s, may be beneficial.

Growing bodies

With our overweight sedentary population, nutritionists now recommend anyone over the age of 2 consume reduced-fat or low-fat milks. But full cream still has a place, particularly for hungry teens and growing children who burn up a lot of energy, or for anyone who is underweight.

FULL-CREAM MILK

The original milk, with around 3.8 per cent milk fat, this still remains the biggest seller in the milk market. Like all milks, it offers quality protein, calcium and B vitamins as well as the fat-soluble vitamins A and D (along with oily fish and margarine, it's one of the few food sources of vitamin D which we usually get from sunlight on our skin). The downside is if you tend to drink it by the glass, it ends up contributing a fair amount of saturated fat.

REDUCED-FAT MILK (OFTEN LABELLED 'LOW-FAT')

Reduced-fat milks (Lite White, Lite Start, Physical, Rev, Trim) contain 1 to 1½ per cent fat, which is around one-third of what's found in full cream milk. Children over the age of 2 can drink reduced-fat milk. Vitamin A and D levels are lower than in full-cream milk as the natural vitamins are removed when the fat is removed. Some milks may have added vitamin A and D to replace those removed; others have extra protein or calcium added. These are a good choice for families with older children.

LOW-FAT MILK

Low-fat milks (Hi-Lo, Physical No Fat) have less than one per cent milk fat, with some as low as 0.15 per cent. They are made by combining skim with non-fat milk powder or by ultra filtration. They are usually richer in calcium, protein and lactose and have a 'fuller' flavour, which most people find more acceptable than skim milk. Some of these milks can fall into the no-fat category—it's just how the manufacturer has chosen to label them.

SKIM MILK, NO-FAT

Skim or no-fat milks (Shape, Pura Tone, Skimmer, Skinny Milk) contain less than 0.15 per cent fat, so are virtually fat-free. This means they have half the kilojoules and virtually none of the fat or cholesterol of full-cream milk. With the fat, however, go the fat-soluble vitamins A and D, which is why skim milks are not suitable for infants (you'll see this listed on the label). However, they still carry all the protein and calcium of regular milk.

In days gone by, skim milk had a 'watery' taste with less flavour than reduced-fat milks. These days, low-fat milks have a better taste thanks to extra milk solids added or the presence of gums to thicken it. This is the milk to drink if you have to be absolutely strict about a fat-free diet (e.g. gallbladder problems, liver troubles).

HIGH CALCIUM

Calcium-boosted milks (Pura Boost, Hi-Lo, Calcium Plus, Anlene) are the highest in calcium per 100 millilitres or per glass so are an easy way to maximise your intake without having to drink a lot. Most are low-fat and contain added vitamin D and sometimes phosphorus, both of which are needed to build bones. These milks are more expensive than regular milks, so if you're getting enough calcium in your day, there isn't any need to spend the extra money. Still they're worth buying if you can't eat a big volume of food and you've been diagnosed with osteoporosis or bone fractures (or come from a family with a history of it).

LACTOSE FREE

Lactose-free milk starts out as regular milk that is first pasteurised and homogenised. A natural enzyme is then added and the milk is packaged and stored for 1–5 days while the enzyme goes to work breaking down the milk sugar. By the time you buy it, the lactose has been converted into two simple sugars that are more easily digested. Lactose-free milk can be used in exactly the same way as regular milk for cooking. Zymil is the only lactose-free fresh milk available in Australia. It has the same level of protein, fat, calcium and vitamins as regular milk, but without the lactose (milk sugar). It is also available in reduced-fat and long-life versions.

NUTRITION COMPARISON OF DIFFERENT MILKS

Per 100 ml (just under half a glass)

TYPE	KILOJOULES	FAT (g)	CALCIUM (mg)
Full-cream milk (regular)	265	3.5–4.0	118
Reduced-fat milk	212	1.4	134
Skim milk	148	0.1	120
High-calcium milk	241	1.4	200
Goat's milk (full cream)	253	3.5	180
Sheep milk (full cream)	396	6.0	170
Lactose-free milk	196	1.5	125
Plant sterol milk	174	1.0	123

PLANT STEROL MILKS

Milks containing added plant sterols (Pura Heart Active, Logicol) are designed for people with high cholesterol. Like the sterol spreads, the plant sterols block the absorption of cholesterol and so reduce your cholesterol levels. A serve (250 millilitres) contains 0.8 grams of plant sterols. To get the cholesterol-lowering benefits of plant sterols, research shows you need to consume 2–3 grams of plant sterols each day, which is equal to three glasses or 750 millilitres (you could also eat a combination of plant sterol milk, spread and yoghurt). These milks do cost more. If money is not a problem, then go for the plant sterol milks. Remember you need to drink the milk every day (or consume enough of the milk, spread or yoghurt to total three serves). They won't work if you don't!

A2 MILK

Growing bodies

Omega-3 milks are an easy alternative for children who won't eat fish.

Cow's milk contains six (four casein and two whey) proteins. The most common are beta-casein A1 and beta-casein A2. Most milk on the market is high in beta-casein A1, while milk high in beta-casein A2 (from herds bred to produce it) is marketed and trademarked as A2 milk. The difference is that during digestion these two proteins break down into different chemical compounds. A1 breaks down into the casomorphin BCM7, which A2 supporters claim causes a diverse range of disorders from heart disease and diabetes to autism. There have been a number of animal (rat) and epidemiological studies—both the New Zealand Food Authority and the European Food Safety Authority (in 2009) reviewed all the A2 and BCM7 research, and found there is 'insufficient evidence' to prove that A1 milk BCM7 has a negative effect on health.

OMEGA-3 MILKS

Omega-3 can now be found in some specialty milks like Farmers Best or Logicol, in a bid to improve heart health and reduce inflammation-related problems like arthritis. The inclusion of omega-3 from fish oil or DHA extract in milk does incur an extra cost, with these milks costing more than regular milks.

GOAT'S MILK

Except for a significantly lower level of folic acid, goat's milk is very similar to cow's milk in nutritional value and apart from a slightly higher fat content, provides approximately the same amounts of protein, calcium, most other B vitamins and lactose. Its proteins also have the same immune cross-reactivity as those in cow's milk, so drinking it will trigger a reaction in susceptible people. So, if you are genuinely allergic to cow's milk, you will most likely react just as badly to goat's milk. Be aware that most goat's milk is sold raw (unpasteurised) and may carry potentially dangerous bacteria, even though strict hygiene measures are followed during milking. It should not be fed to infants under the age of one.

UHT (LONGLIFE) MILK

UHT stands for ultra heat-treated. It means the milk is subjected to a much higher temperature during pasteurisation, which inactivates all bacteria and enzymes but does not harm the protein or vitamins. It is then packed aseptically and, if unopened, keeps for about five months unrefrigerated. Once opened, however, it must be refrigerated. It is available as regular, reduced-fat, low-fat and skim milk.

FARMERS BEST

This milk is made by removing almost all the saturated fat from regular milk and replacing it with a little mono-unsaturated fat, so it's healthier for the heart. It was one of the earliest 'modified' milks. At 1.4 per cent, Farmers Best has a similar fat content to light milks, but a lot less saturated fat. Only one-third of the total fat is saturated compared with two-thirds in other milks. It tastes better than skim milk and you get more calcium.

ORGANIC MILK

Organic milk is produced from cows that are reared in a humane way without antibiotics or hormones administered. They graze on pasture that is free from synthetic fertilisers and pesticides. The milk ideally should be packed in recyclable paper containers and is usually not homogenised (so the cream rises to the surface instead of being dispersed throughout). To ensure you're buying the genuine thing, look for a milk that carries a certification logo from one of the organic bodies such as National Association of Sustainable Agriculture Australia (NASAA), Biological Farmers of Australia (BFA) or Biodynamic Research Institute (Demeter).

RAW MILK

Raw unpasteurised milk is sometimes sold at health-food shops 'for cosmetic use' and is sought after by alternative health groups for its 'friendly bacteria' and enzymes. The benefits of raw milk need to be weighed up against the risk of disease. In Australia, all milk sold for consumption must be pasteurised by law. Pasteurisation involves a brief heat treatment, which inactivates disease-producing bacteria that could cause TB or brucellosis. However, the process may also inactivate some of the bioactive substances in fresh milk that have health benefits, and it may also slightly reduce levels of vitamins.

SOY AND OTHER MILK ALTERNATIVES

If you have a special dietary need such as lactose intolerance or milk allergy, or you follow a vegan diet and wish to avoid dairy products altogether, you can substitute with the following 'milks' made from soy beans, almonds, oats and rice. Outside of city areas, you'll mostly find them sold in UHT tetra-packs (not chilled). Choose calcium-enriched products if you drink them regularly or give them to children.

NUTRITION COMPARISON OF ALTERNATIVE MILKS

Per 100 ml

TYPE	KILOJOULES	FAT (g)	CALCIUM (mg)	PROTEIN (mg)	CARBS (mg)
Soy milk (regular) *	270	3.4	120	3.6	4.9
Soy light *	170	0.9	120	2.6	3.9
Almond milk	175	0.4	3.0	0.3	9.1
Oat milk	260	1.9	120	1.0	10.0
Rice milk	210	1.2	120	0.3	9.5

*Check the label—many of these milks are fortified with added calcium, but it's not absorbed as well as the calcium from cow's milk.

SOY MILK

Available in full-fat and low-fat versions, soy milk is similar to cow's milk in nutrients and kilojoules, but it can vary a great deal in its calcium content. Soy milk can be made in two different ways, which may influence your choice at the supermarket:

- It can be made from whole beans that are soaked, heated and then crushed to extract the milky juice, which is blended with water, sweeteners like malted barley and sugar, vegetable oil and salt. It is generally lower in calcium (20–80 milligrams per glass) but rich in protein and B vitamins. It is regarded as more 'natural'.
- It can contain soy protein isolate powder, which is processed from defatted soy flour and contains around 90 per cent pure protein. This is blended together with water, oil, sweeteners like sugar or maltodextrin, gums, emulsifier, vitamins, mineral salts and calcium. This is generally fortified with vitamins A, B_1, B_2, B_{12} and calcium to a level similar to milk (250–290 milligrams per glass). It generally has a better flavour and less 'beany' taste.

ALMOND MILK

Made from ground almonds, almond milk is low in carbohydrate, protein and kilojoules. It comes into its own if you're allergic to both dairy and soy. Plain, unsweetened almond milk can be used as a substitute for regular milk in most recipes. It has a pleasant nutty

DID YOU KNOW?

There's little scientific evidence for the theory that milk makes mucus. Milk and dairy products do not cause asthma, runny noses or ear infections—they can leave a thick whitish coating on your tongue or phlegm at the back of the throat, but this is not mucus. In fact, a study by Adelaide researchers found no association between milk and mucus in healthy adults who were inoculated with the common cold virus. Those adults who initially said they felt milk affected them recorded more congestion and coughs, but not more nasal secretions. So don't eliminate milk from your diet or that of your child; you will only remove the major source of calcium that can lead to the risk of brittle bones later in life.

flavour that makes a nice milky coffee and teams well in desserts and Middle Eastern recipes. Vanilla flavour and sugar, or a sweetener (such as agave), are often added to commercial almond milks. You can make your own almond milk at home by swirling ground whole almonds with water in a blender then squeezing the liquid out through a fine sieve or mesh. It has a low GI of 25.

OAT MILK

Popular in Sweden, oat milk is made from a solution of ground oats and water. It has a light semi-sweet taste, so substitutes well for low-fat or skim milk. Commercial versions are often fortified with calcium so that nutritionally it will come close to cow's milk. Oat milk has some fibre and contains vitamin E, folic acid, minerals and natural phytochemicals. In addition to the oats and water, it may also contain some type of oil and barley malt or flour. It has a moderate GI of 69.

RICE MILK

Rice milk is typically processed from brown rice and is essentially a source of carbohydrate (24 grams per 250 millilitre glass). The milks that have been tested to date have very high GI values (92 and 79) like their parent rice.

Mindless Eating

Mindless eating is commonplace in the modern world. In my opinion this is often overlooked as a cause of obesity. Distracted by watching TV or a movie, we mindlessly fill our mouths, short-circuiting our fullness signals; we keep on eating, unaware of the huge amounts we're putting away. The modern food supply encourages a grazing mentality via fast-food drive-ins, vending machines full of junk food and confectionery counters at every retail outlet. What's more, it actually encourages us to eat while doing other tasks. Whether it's popcorn at the cinema, desktop dining while you work, dashboard dining as you drive or dinner in front of the TV—it all leads us to eat more than we need.

Dr Brian Wansink, director of Cornell's Food and Brand Lab, has carried out some fascinating studies on the hidden forces behind our food choices, and how easy it is to eat without thinking. He says most of us overeat because we are distracted or are surrounded by junk food served in large portion sizes. We eat as if it's our mission to finish everything! His book, *Mindless Eating*, was a real eye-opener for me—and I suspect for most of us. It shows why you may not realise how much you're eating, what you're eating, or why you're even eating at all! You'll certainly never look at movie popcorn the same way again.

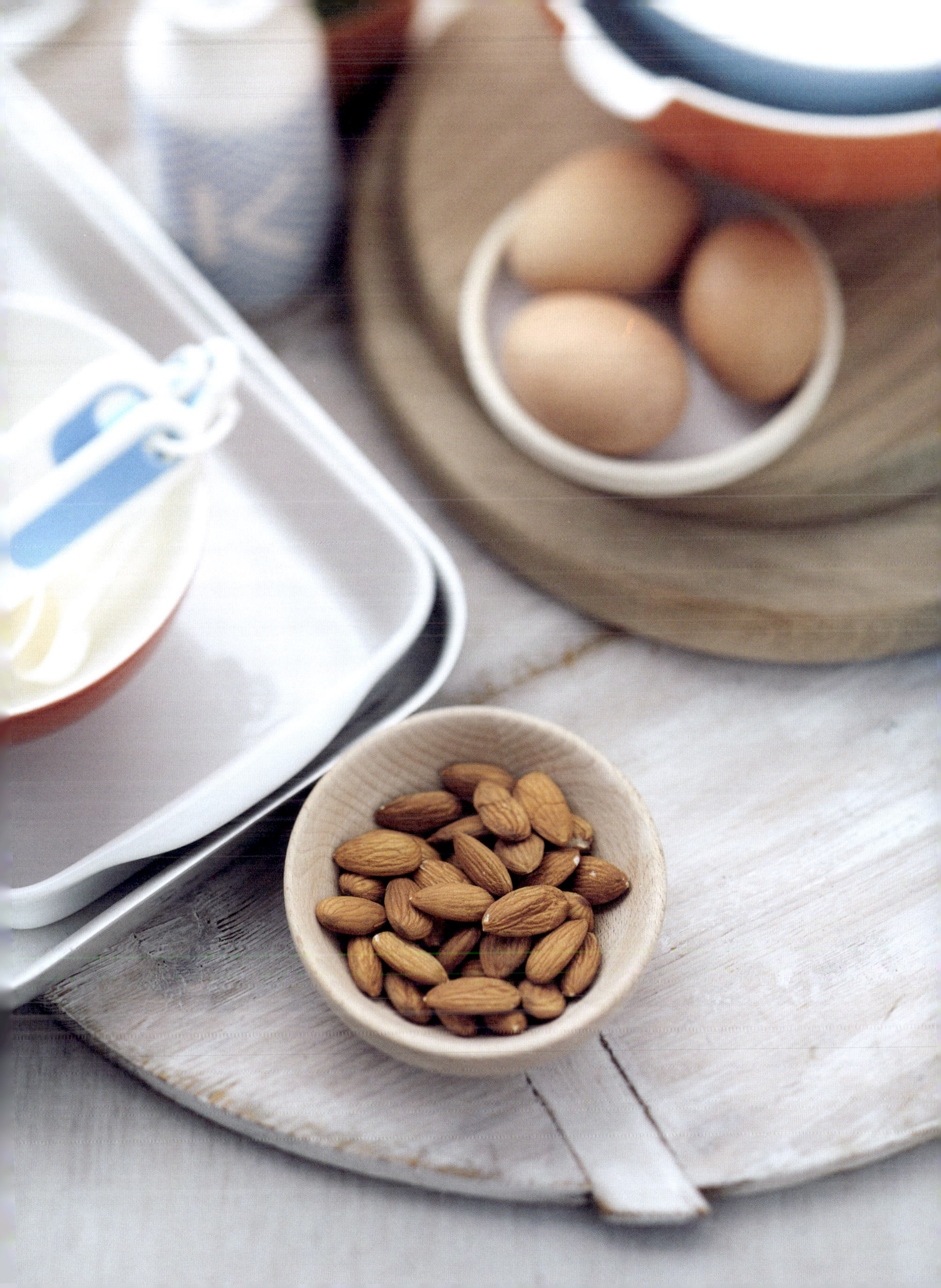

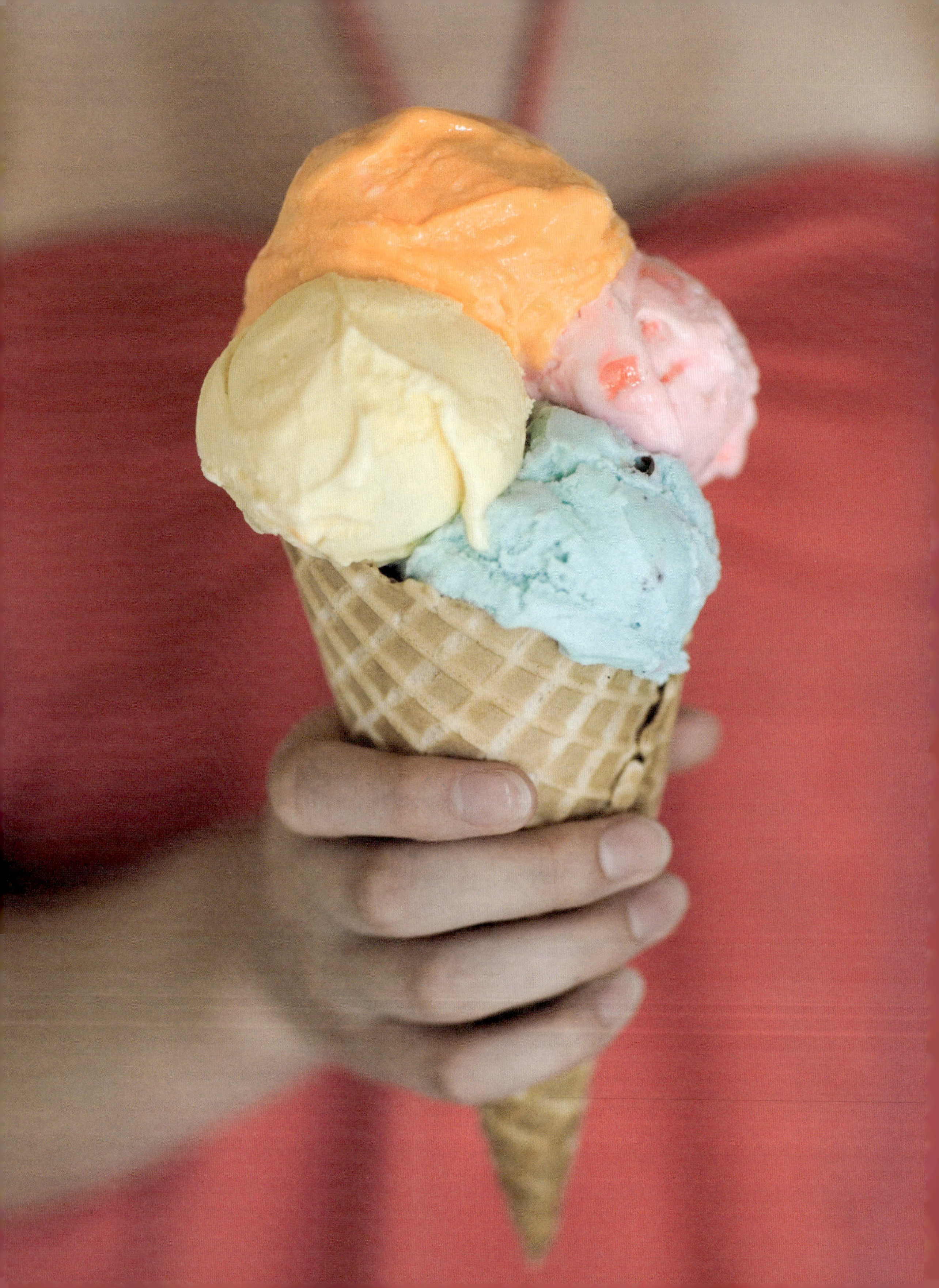

Wansink's approach encourages small, almost effortless environmental changes to save 100 calories (420 kilojoules) each day for slow and steady weight control. Called the 'mindless margin', this represents a painless way of under-eating. As he says, the best diet is the one you don't know you're on!

SIX STEPS TO EATING WITH AWARENESS

To help yourself learn to eat with awareness, try these simple first steps to prevent mindless consumption. Your goal is to be conscious of how you're eating and what your stomach registers. When you're in touch with what is going on inside, you'll know the exact moment you are physically satisfied rather than over-full or stuffed. It's the best technique for weight control and works regardless of what sort of diet you're on. I follow these steps every day and highly recommend this way of eating!

See also **Appetite and Hunger; Weight Loss.**

1. Sit down to eat, even if it's only for a snack. Turn off the TV, laptop and phone, and don't read. Let the food be the centre of your attention.
2. Take two deep breaths before you eat. Pause to reflect on what you're about to eat, being respectful of the dish in front of you and thankful for the food (a little like saying grace). This is an easy step to follow even when eating out or with others.
3. Chew each mouthful thoughtfully, paying attention to the flavours and textures—some health-food advocates have suggested at least 30 times per mouthful! Put your knife and fork down between bites.
4. If you know you're a fast eater, try eating with chopsticks or with your non-dominant hand to slow things down.
5. Plate up normal (not diet) portions of food.
6. Eat slowly and make the meal last at least 20 minutes.

The evidence is also piling up that Grandma was onto something when she told us to sit down to eat (elbows off the table), chew our food properly and leave the table feeling as though we still had room for a little more. She was possibly a fan of The Great Masticator, Horace Fletcher (1849–1919), who believed chewing food 32 times before swallowing would increase your strength and decrease your food intake. He certainly lost a considerable amount of weight eating this way.

THE RESEARCH
THE POPCORN EXPERIMENT

Wansink and his researchers offered a free bucket of popcorn to moviegoers in return for answering a few (dummy) questions about the movie once it was over. Half the moviegoers got a medium-size bucket weighing 120 g, while the other half were given the large-size, bigger-than-your-head bucket weighing 235 g. Weighing the leftovers in the buckets after the movie, the researchers reported that the big-bucket group ate 53 per cent more popcorn (an average of 725 more kilojoules) while mindlessly munching. That's roughly the equivalent of 21 more dips into the bucket. Wansink repeated the experiment with stale, 14-day-old popcorn and got similar results. After the movie, the researchers asked the moviegoers to describe the popcorn and they weighed how much popcorn was left in the containers. Even though they described the popcorn as 'stale' and 'terrible', moviegoers with the larger containers still ate 34 per cent more than those given the medium-sized containers.

THE BOTTOMLESS SOUP BOWL

I found myself fascinated by his ingenious bottomless soup bowl experiment where he and his colleagues invented a soup bowl that secretly refilled itself, so you never managed to eat your way to the bottom. The results were as you may have guessed—people eating out of the bottomless bowl ate and ate and ate, often eating three times more than normal without realising! The message is simple—people don't listen to their stomach. They don't know when to stop. We see this time and again at buffets, yum cha restaurants and family dinners where food is on display in unlimited amounts.

Mineral Water

Mineral water is water containing minerals or other dissolved substances that alter its taste or give it supposed therapeutic value. Salts, sulphur compounds and gases are among the substances that can be dissolved in the water. Mineral water can often be effervescent. Mineral water can be manufactured or can occur naturally from springs.

Traditionally, mineral waters would be consumed at their source, often referred to as 'taking the waters at the source' or 'taking the cure', and such sites were referred to as spas, baths or wells. Well-known brands include Perrier, Vichy and Evian. In modern times, it is far more common for mineral waters to be bottled at their source and then distributed for consumption. In many places, the term mineral water is often colloquially used to mean any sort of carbonated drink.

HOW IT COMPARES WITH SODA WATER

Also known as carbonated water, sparkling water or seltzer water, soda water is plain water into which carbon dioxide gas has been dissolved. It usually contains low levels of a number of salts (ranging from added table salt and sodium citrate to sodium bicarbonate, potassium bicarbonate, potassium sulphate or disodium phosphate). These additives are included to emulate the slightly salty taste of homemade soda water, which in the past was made by 'charging' a refillable seltzer bottle by filling it with water and then adding carbon dioxide.

Contrary to popular opinion, today neither soda nor mineral water are high in sodium. The vast majority of mineral waters have less than 10 milligrams per 100 millilitres of water and are suitable for a low-salt diet. A few mineral waters may have a higher concentration due to the natural salts in the particular spring where they are bottled, but these are the minority. Always check the label for one with less than 120 milligrams per 100 millilitres (equal to 1.2 grams per litre) if you need to watch your sodium intake.

Minerals *See tables on following pages.*

Minerals form the hard bony structure of the body, but they are also vitally important in chemical reactions and in regulating water balance, nerve response and muscle contraction. They are usually classified as major or trace minerals.

We need major minerals like calcium, phosphorus, magnesium, potassium, sodium, chlorine, iron and sulphur in larger amounts. We know of at least 17 trace minerals including zinc, copper, iodine, fluorine, manganese, chromium, selenium, molybdenum and cobalt as being necessary for good health, but because of the difficulties of measuring such tiny amounts, we may need more. It's important to remember that an overdose of any mineral has toxic effects. Overdoses can happen by consuming too many supplements (such as when toddlers swallow iron tablets), and by contamination from pollution (mercury accumulation in long-living fish).

Molybdenum *See* **Minerals.**

MINERAL	WHAT IT DOES	BEST FOOD SOURCES	RECOMMENDED DAILY INTAKE	SAFE UPPER LIMIT
CALCIUM	Forms the hard structure of the bones and teeth Prevents rickets and osteoporosis Aids muscle contraction and nerve functioning Aids in clotting of the blood and enzyme activity May prevent high blood pressure, premenstrual syndrome (PMS) and kidney stones.	Milk, cheese and yoghurt (both full-cream and low-fat), canned salmon and sardines (including the small edible bones), wholegrains, cereals, breads, tofu, soy drinks (fortified), sesame seeds, prawns, broccoli, ice-cream, milk chocolate, nuts (particularly almonds, Brazil nuts, hazelnuts), dried figs.	1000 milligrams	2500 milligrams
CHROMIUM	Facilitates normal growth Forms part of an organic complex called the Glucose Tolerance Factor, which enhances the action of the hormone insulin to regulate blood glucose.	Brewer's yeast, yeast extract, egg yolk, liver, kidney, lean meat, wholegrains, wholemeal bread, bran, cheese, wine, oysters.	25 micrograms (women), 35 micrograms (men)	It is not possible to set an upper limit, but no adverse effects have been reported with doses ranging from 200 to 1000 micrograms daily, mostly in the form of chromium picolinate for diabetes.
COPPER	Forms a component of enzymes Partners iron in formation of red blood cells Aids formation of melanin pigment in skin and hair Aids functioning of the nervous system.	Oysters, crab, lobster, mussels, liver, kidney, nuts, yeast, cocoa powder and wholegrains.	1.2 milligrams (women), 1.7 milligrams (men)	10 milligrams
FLUORIDE	Facilitates structure of healthy bones and teeth Increases resistance of teeth to dental caries Possibly prevents osteoporosis.	Fluoridated drinking water; small amounts are found in fish (especially if eaten with the bones) and tea.	3 milligrams (women), 4 milligrams (men)	10 milligrams

See also Calcium; Osteoporosis.

See also Fluoride.

MINERAL	WHAT IT DOES	BEST FOOD SOURCES	RECOMMENDED DAILY INTAKE	SAFE UPPER LIMIT
IODINE	Prevents goitre and promotes normal functioning of the thyroid gland Aids brain function.	Fish, shellfish, seaweed, iodised salt. It is also found in iodophores, compounds sometimes used to sterilise food-processing equipment.	150 micrograms	1100 micrograms
IRON	Prevents anaemia Acts as a key component of haemoglobin (the red colouring of blood cells) and myoglobin (muscle protein) Acts as a component of many enzymes.	Lean red meat, liver, kidney, heart, chicken, fish, dark-green leafy vegetables, iron-fortified breakfast cereals, wholemeal bread, legumes, eggs, cocoa powder and dried fruit.	18 milligrams (women), 8 milligrams (men)	45 milligrams
MAGNESIUM	Provides structure for the bones Functions in many enzyme systems Controls muscle contraction and nerve function (together with calcium, sodium and potassium).	Widely distributed in foods, but the richest sources are milk, wholegrain cereals, wholemeal bread, green leafy vegetables (spinach, parsley, cabbage, sorrel), lean meat, nuts, bananas and peas.	320 milligrams (women), 420 milligrams (men)	350 milligrams
MANGANESE	Acts as an activator of many enzymes.	Widely distributed in many foods, but the richest sources are nuts, wholegrains, cereals, vegetables and oils.	5 milligrams (women), 5.5 milligrams (men)	No upper limit has been set, but up to 11 milligrams a day is considered safe
MOLYBDENUM	It is vital in iron utilisation, alcohol detoxification and the metabolism of wastes.	Widely distributed in many foods—vegetables, legumes and grains provide the most, but this depends on the molybdenum content of the soil in which they were grown.	45 micrograms	2000 micrograms
PHOSPHORUS	Occurs as a partner with calcium in the mineral structure of bones and teeth Combines with many B vitamins to form energy-release factors A component of proteins and nucleic acids.	Widely distributed in foods—meat, milk, cheese, eggs, yeast extract, bran and wheatgerm are excellent sources.	1000 milligrams	4000 milligrams

See also Iodine.

See also Anaemia; Iron.

MINERAL	WHAT IT DOES	BEST FOOD SOURCES	RECOMMENDED DAILY INTAKE	SAFE UPPER LIMIT
POTASSIUM	Controls the transmission of nerve impulses and maintains cell membrane differential in conjunction with sodium Part of many enzyme systems Counteracts the adverse effects of excess sodium on blood pressure.	Widely distributed in nuts, yeast extract, dried fruit, instant coffee, bran, wheatgerm, raw vegetables, lean meat, fish and fruit (fruit juice in particular).	2800 milligrams or 72 millimoles (women), 3800 milligrams or 97 millimoles (men)	No firm data but more than 10,000 milligrams (10 grams) in a single dose may cause cardiac arrest
SELENIUM	Inactivates free radicals as part of the antioxidant enzyme glutathione peroxidase Maintains resistance to disease Treatment for Keshan disease, a selenium deficiency disease in China Can protect against heavy metal poisoning from mercury, cadmium and silver Acts against cancer and heart disease.	Nuts (particularly Brazil nuts), fish, seafood, liver, kidney, lean meat, chicken, eggs, mushrooms, garlic and grains, although their content depends on the selenium content of the soil.	60 micrograms (women), 70 micrograms (men)	400 micrograms
SODIUM	Controls the transmission of nerve impulses, in conjunction with potassium Helps maintain water balance Assists the transport of amino acids and glucose.	Foods high in sodium are largely commercial or processed foods. Natural unprocessed foods all contain sodium but in very low amounts. Very high sources are table, sea and vegetable salts, anchovies, monosodium glutamate (MSG), soy sauce, bottled sauces, gravy powder, stock cubes, yeast extract, salami, ham, deli meats, cheese, olives, canned vegetables, packet soups, salted nuts, cornflakes and potato crisps.	460–920 milligrams or 20–40 millimoles, equivalent to 1.2–2.4 grams salt or ¼ to ½ teaspoon per day	2300 milligrams (100 millimoles) or less a day due to the adverse effects of salt on blood pressure. Most of the population already consumes more than this.

See also Potassium.

See also DASH diet; Salt.

MINERAL	WHAT IT DOES	BEST FOOD SOURCES	RECOMMENDED DAILY INTAKE	SAFE UPPER LIMIT
ZINC	Aids the healing of wounds and cuts Facilitates normal taste, smell and sight Makes up many enzymes Provides hard structure of the bones Assists sexual maturation and reproduction—concentrated in sperm and prostate Said to prevent or shorten the duration of the common cold, but results are inconclusive.	Lean meat, liver, kidney, chicken, seafood (especially oysters), milk, wholegrains, wholemeal bread, legumes and nuts.	8 milligrams (women), 14 milligrams (men)	40 milligrams

See also **Calcium; Iron; Potassium; Zinc.**

Mood and Food

There's no denying the food we eat affects our mood and how well we think. Almost every vitamin or mineral deficiency can cause some sort of psychiatric symptom such as fuzziness, irritability, poor tolerance to stress, tension, anxiety, nervousness and depression.

The big contributors that affect our mood are caffeine, alcohol and blood-glucose levels, but everything we eat will make a difference in some way. Here's how you can keep your brain in top working order and boost your mood.

MY TAKE

Avoid low-carb diets such as Atkins. They've been found to have detrimental effects on mood. Many dieters find they feel sluggish and depressed, and experience a greater food preoccupation.

DON'T GET DEHYDRATED

Your brain as a whole contains as much as 75 per cent water and needs to be well hydrated to perform at its best. Disorientation is one of the early warning signs of dehydration. Nutritionists recommend you drink around eight glasses of fluid a day, more if it is humid or if you've been sweating. Water is the ideal fluid as it's inexpensive and has no kilojoules, but other fluids including weak black or herbal tea, broth, diluted juice and sugar-free drinks also count towards your eight glasses.

KEEP ALCOHOL SOCIAL

Alcohol is a central nervous system depressant. When consumed in excess, alcohol has the potential to be mood altering or disturbing. Limit your intake to one or two glasses a day, with some alcohol-free days each week.

SWITCH TO LOW-GI CARBS

Glucose is the brain's primary fuel. While fat and protein can be converted into glucose, the process takes time and is not as efficient as eating carbohydrates. But you want your carbohydrates to release their energy slowly over time, and keep your blood-glucose levels even, so go for the low-GI types. These also provide B vitamins (thiamin, niacin, folate) that help release energy from food.

MAXIMISE YOUR OMEGA-3s

It's thought omega-3s can help improve your mood, keep you mentally sharp and reduce the risk of depression and dementia. Fish oil supplements have been found to be an effective mood stabiliser in studies of people suffering bipolar disorder (manic depression). Researchers believe that fish oil works via a similar mechanism of action to that of current mood stabilisers lithium and valproate. Countries where intakes of omega-3 are low, such as New Zealand, Canada and Germany, all have a high (around 5 per cent) prevalence of major depression. Countries like Japan and Taiwan have some of the highest fish intakes in the world, and have less than 1 per cent depression rates. Each cell of the myelin sheath, which 'insulates' communicating neurons, is about two-thirds fat. The omega-3 fatty acids are incorporated into the phospholipids of the membranes surrounding each cell, which are crucial for cell-to-cell signalling. Once incorporated, they enable the cell membranes to be flexible which ensures the signals can move swiftly.

> **CALMING CARBS**
>
> Changes in brain serotonin levels are now believed to set the scene for sleep by inducing feelings of calmness and serenity. Serotonin is a neurotransmitter made in the body from the amino acid tryptophan. Foods such as milk, malted products and others rich in carbohydrates lead to an increase in brain levels of tryptophan and therefore serotonin, and are thought to help in getting to sleep.

GET YOUR B VITAMINS

B vitamins such as B_1 (thiamin), B_6, B_{12} and folate in supplement form have been shown in some studies to improve mood and mental function. You don't have to take pills though; everyday grain foods such as oats, wholegrain cereals, wholemeal breads, lentils and other legumes can do the trick. Go for low-GI, high-fibre or wholegrain foods.

> **Growing bodies**
>
> It's believed the 30 per cent drop in a new mother's DHA levels immediately after giving birth may be a key factor in postnatal depression. The developing baby draws heavily on the mother's supply of omega-3 during pregnancy. This may be alleviated by eating more fish.

AVOID JUNK FOOD

Recent studies show eating foods rich in kilojoules and poor in nutrients may change the way the brain works. Studies on rats have shown junk food can trigger the same addiction-like response in the brain as heroin, with similar changes in the brain's reward circuits in both obese and drug-addicted rats. Eating food is associated with the release of dopamine, and the more that is released, the greater the degree of pleasure.

EAT REGULARLY THROUGH THE DAY

You will recognise that empty feeling when you're running low and need to eat to boost your thinking. Always keep a food stash in your desk drawer; canned fish, beans, fruit and rice pudding store well, as do crackers, nuts and low-fat muesli bars.

CUT DOWN ON CAFFEINE

Caffeine is useful for boosting your concentration, alertness and good mood, but drink it in moderation as it can also increase anxiety and mood swings. One or two coffees or energy drinks a day poses no problem for most people but don't get into the caffeine habit.

GET OUTSIDE

Just five minutes of outdoor exercise in a green space can boost mental health, according to UK researchers. Being out in nature, whether it's a park or garden or by the sea, can rapidly improve mood and self-esteem. If you work in a stressful workplace, taking a short walk at lunchtime in the fresh air is highly recommended.

MSG

Does the number 621 mean anything to you? If you're wary of additives or you read the labels as you shop, you'll recognise 621 as the code number for MSG, or monosodium glutamate. There was a time when the three letters 'MSG' created widespread fear. Today, scientists have cleared MSG of being a harmful ingredient, but it remains on the 'avoid' list for many health-conscious consumers.

Suspicions about MSG first began back in 1968, when Dr Robert Kwok penned a letter to the prestigious *New England Journal of Medicine* describing a cluster of symptoms he called the 'Chinese Restaurant Syndrome'. He noticed that within half an hour of eating a meal at his favourite Chinese restaurant, he often felt a burning sensation at the back of his neck, followed by headache, weakness and sometimes heart palpitations. The symptoms were only temporary, lasting about 45 minutes, causing discomfort rather than long-term harm. He wondered if other doctors had noticed it. Although his was not a formal study, from that time on MSG has been under a cloud.

WHAT IT IS

Monosodium glutamate is the sodium salt of glutamic acid, one of the most abundant amino acids in nature. Glutamate can exist in a 'free' form or be 'bound' to protein. It is found in virtually all protein foods such as meat, chicken and fish, but it is the free form of glutamate that has the flavour-enhancing properties. MSG in this free form provides a similar flavouring function as the glutamate that occurs naturally in food. It is believed to stimulate the tastebuds on the tongue and increase the flow of saliva.

MSG in its free form was originally extracted from natural protein-rich foods such as seaweed. For more than 1200 years, Japanese cooks improved the taste of their meals with a soup stock made from seaweed, high in glutamates. The Japanese have long appreciated this meaty flavour, having a specific name for it—*umami*—and regard it as the fifth addition to the four basic tastes of sweet, sour, salty and bitter.

Today, MSG is made from starch, corn sugar or molasses from sugar cane, or sugar beets. You can buy crystals of MSG in large packets in Asian supermarkets, as it is a popular additive at the Asian table, much like salt and pepper.

ADVERSE REACTIONS

According to three major reviews of MSG's safety by international regulatory authorities including the Joint FAO/WHO Expert Committee of Food Additives (JECFA), MSG is safe for the general population at the levels typically used in foods and restaurant meals. No upper limits have been placed on its use.

A very small number of people may experience some reaction to large amounts of MSG when consumed in a single meal, but there is no robust evidence to suggest that MSG is a significant trigger factor in more serious reactions such as asthma attacks.

MSG is not a common trigger for food sensitivity in the way that sulphites or colours may be. If you think you have an intolerance to MSG, do not try and work it out yourself. It doesn't usually occur on its own, but with other sensitivities. Make an appointment at an allergy clinic or with an accredited practising dietitian.

WHERE YOU'LL FIND MSG

Glutamate occurs naturally in virtually all foods including meat, fish, poultry, vegetables and even breast milk. Tomatoes, mushrooms and aged cheeses tend to have high levels of free glutamate, giving them plenty of flavour.

MSG is also often included to boost flavour in savoury packet foods such as Asian noodle meals, gravies, dried soup and sauce mixes. The quantities added to commercial foods range from 0.1 to 0.8 per cent, which is similar to the levels of natural glutamates found in food. Above these levels, MSG has no additional effect on flavour.

See also **Glutamates.**

Mushrooms

Mushrooms add a rich, deep savoury flavour for very few kilojoules and are almost as indispensable in cooking as onions. Think of the difference mushrooms make to stroganoff, risottos, omelettes, stir-fries and salads. It's all due to their high content of glutamate, the naturally occurring version of the flavour enhancer monosodium glutamate or MSG. They also have significant quantities of another key flavour compound—salicylate.

At only 96 kilojoules per 100 grams, mushrooms have what's called a low 'energy density'—this means they have few kilojoules for their weight or volume, a big plus when many of our snack and takeaway foods have a high energy density.

NUTRITIONAL VALUE

When it comes to nutrition, there are even more bonuses. They have no fat, but plenty of B vitamins, especially riboflavin, niacin and pantothenic acid. Combine this with some vitamin D following brief exposure to sunlight and this sets them apart from other vegetables. If they are farm-cultivated they also add a modest quantity of vitamin B_{12}, which is often difficult for strict vegetarians to obtain. It is the same type of bioavailable B_{12} as that found in meats and seafood. Being a fruit of a fungus and not a true vegetable, they have little vitamin C or beta-carotene, but are rich in the mineral potassium.

WEIGHT LOSS AND MUSHROOMS

A 2007 US study published in *Appetite* found mushrooms to be an ideal way to cut kilojoules without losing out on flavour or a sense of fullness. You eat well and you eat less! Researchers from Johns Hopkins Bloomberg School of Public Health found they could drop the kilojoule content of a lunch meal by half if they substituted ground (minced) white button mushrooms for beef mince in familiar dishes like lasagna, 'sloppy Joe' (a kind of savoury mince) and chilli con carne. When asked about palatability, appetite, satiation (post-meal fullness) and satiety (general fullness), the study participants didn't rate the mushroom meals any differently from the beef meals. And despite consuming fewer kilojoules with the mushroom meals, they didn't compensate by eating more later in the day.

NUMBER CRUNCH

A serve of 4–6 white cup mushrooms (75 grams) provides 3 grams of protein, a trace of fat, no starch, 1 gram of sugar, 1 gram of fibre and 32 kilojoules.

See also **Glutamates.**

N

Niacin (B3)

Also known as nicotinic acid and niacinamide, niacin is a B vitamin.

See also **Vitamins.**

Nigari

Nigari is a coagulant that's used to set soy milk to make tofu (similar to cheese-making, it separates the curd from the whey).

See also **Soy.**

Noni Juice

Noni (*Morinda citrifolia*) is an evergreen tree indigenous to India, South-East Asia and the Pacific. Its lumpy-looking fleshy fruit is very pungent when ripe, rather like strong cheese (it's also called vomit fruit). It is tough and not particularly palatable to eat unless processed, which gives you an idea why it is was generally regarded as 'famine food' throughout the Pacific.

These days, it's processed mainly into juice but also into pulp and capsules. The juices are either reconstituted from noni powder, or made from noni pulp diluted with water. Many contain only a small percentage of pure noni juice. It's often blended with grape juice, apple juice and other sweeter juices to mask its natural bitter, unpleasant taste.

Noni juice, often marketed as Tahitian noni juice, has been popular but also very controversial. It was one of the first exotic 'super fruits' and was marketed with all sorts of outlandish and unsubstantiated claims—'miracle fruit', 'increases stamina' and 'slows tumour growth'. It is often sold at inflated prices by multi-level marketing (MLM) schemes using distributors as slick salesmen. Coupled with the lack of decent trials and little supporting evidence, you can see why professionals have greeted noni with so much scepticism.

MY TAKE

There's nothing magical about commercial noni juice. Nutritionally, it's no better for you than orange juice. The hard-sell featuring pictures of palm trees and tropical islands make me even more suspicious. I may be proved wrong one day by a study which discovers something proving it has 'healing powers' but until then, I remain unconvinced.

NUTRITIONAL VALUE

The few laboratory tests done of pure noni juice show it's similar to any other fruit juice, perhaps even less nutritious. Noni does have some vitamin C, but only 6 mg per serving, which is much less than orange or grapefruit juice.

There are only miniscule amounts of any B vitamin, and virtually none of the beta-carotene, vitamin E, carotenoids and flavonoids antioxidants. Like all juice, there's not much fibre or protein. Potassium is there though, as you'd expect from any fruit. At only 4 per cent sugars, it's not sweet tasting, nor is it high in carbs. Like other juices, the noni blends can be high in sugar, so it's important to check the nutrition information panel.

Noni juice is promoted as being a rich source of the alkaloid xeronine, which its proponents claim is a powerful healing agent. Maybe eating the fruit fresh—as some Pacific Islanders do—is the key.

Nutrient Reference Values (NRVs)

Nutrient Reference Values (NRVs) list the recommended intakes for energy (kilojoules), protein, fats, carbohydrate, fibre, vitamins, minerals and fluid, based on age, sex and life stages. They are used by dietitians, nutritionists and other health professionals to assess the dietary needs of individuals and groups (such as residents of nursing home or pupils in boarding schools).

Australia and New Zealand have suggested figures for 33 essential nutrients, which were published in 2006 by the National Health and Medical Research Council (NHMRC). In place of the older single-figure values, the 2006 NRVs embrace five different values for each nutrient. These are:

ESTIMATED AVERAGE REQUIREMENT (EAR)

A daily nutrient intake level needed to meet the requirements of half the healthy individuals in a particular age, life stage or gender.

RECOMMENDED DIETARY INTAKE (RDI)

The average daily dietary intake level that is sufficient to meet the nutrient requirements of nearly all (97–98 per cent) healthy individuals in a particular life stage and gender group. The RDIs are derived from the EAR.

ADEQUATE INTAKE (AI)

This number is used when an RDI cannot be determined. It represents the average daily nutrient intake by a group of apparently healthy people known not to have a deficiency that we can assume is adequate.

UPPER LIMIT (UL)

This is the highest average daily intake likely to pose no adverse health effects to almost all individuals in the general population.

SUGGESTED DIETARY TARGETS (SDTS)

These are higher intakes that may prevent or reduce the risk of chronic disease such as heart disease, certain cancers or high blood pressure.

ESTIMATED ENERGY REQUIREMENT (EER)

This is the average amount of energy (kilojoules) predicted to maintain weight and good health for an adult for a given age, gender, weight, height and level of physical activity.

HOW IT WORKS

It looks complicated, I know, but here's an example of how it works in practice. The recommendations for daily iron intake (from food and supplements) for good health for women aged 19–50 look like this:

- RDI 18 milligrams—the average daily dietary intake to aim for
- EAR 8 milligrams—the bare minimum
- UL 45 milligrams—a safe maximum.

In contrast, we know a lot less about copper, a trace mineral. There is no EAR set and therefore no RDI. But there is an AI of 1.2 milligrams for women, based on the best research published.

Q

Are nutrients affected by food processing?

A

Processing has been carried out for centuries in the form of drying, salting, bottling, chilling, smoking and, more recently, freezing. In all processing there is usually some loss of nutrients—heat destroys some vitamins, with vitamins C, B_1 and folic acid being most sensitive, but it's no different from home cooking—you lose some vitamin C when you steam vegetables at home, too. Manufacturers pick produce at its peak and can or snap-freeze it, losing little in terms of quality and taste. Cooking and processing can actually improve certain nutrients. Lycopene is more readily available from canned tomatoes and pasta sauce than from fresh tomatoes, and cooking carrots raises their beta-carotene levels.

Nutraceutical

A nutraceutical is an ingredient (not a food) that has therapeutic benefits. Examples are vitamins, minerals and antioxidants that have a protective effect against cancer, high blood pressure and high cholesterol.

Nutrients

DID YOU KNOW?
No single food except breast milk for babies contains all the nutrients we need to maintain life and ensure growth.

Nutrients are the essential substances that provide the nourishment we require for health, growth and the maintenance of life. The seven essential nutrients our bodies need are carbohydrates, fibre, protein, fat, vitamins, minerals and water. We cannot do without these nutrients. They provide fuel in the form of kilojoules; they are the raw material for building new tissues, bones and teeth; they regulate the speed of metabolic reactions and help release energy from food—all of which keeps us functioning at top speed.

All food, however different in taste and appearance, can give us some or all of these seven nutrients. A salad sandwich is nutritionally equivalent to a bowl of vegetable and barley soup or rice with curried vegetables. Although vastly different in taste, they all contain starchy carbohydrates, fibre, B vitamins and protein. Thus, many combinations of different foods (in this case, grains plus vegetables) can supply all seven nutrients, explaining why people enjoy good health on very different diets.

Most foods are a combination of several nutrients and are not 'pure' in the nutritional sense (the exceptions are sugar, purified starches, oils and commercial fats). Bread is often labelled as a carbohydrate, yet the average loaf contains about 45 per cent carbohydrate, 9 per cent protein, 3 per cent fibre, 2 per cent fat, 1 per cent vitamins and minerals, and 40 per cent water.

With today's nutritional knowledge, scientists would easily be capable of formulating a powdered diet that contained all known nutrients. But there may be substances present in food that we don't even know about yet. For instance, until as late as the 1970s, fibre was a 'forgotten' nutrient. Now, many natural plant phytochemicals in vegetables and fruit, previously unknown, are emerging in research. Who knows how many other undiscovered nutrients would not be included in a synthetic diet? Also, such a 'space-food' diet doesn't take into account the pleasurable social aspects of eating; these alone are strong enough to ensure that our diet of the future will continue to be food.

See also **Carbohydrates; Fibre; Protein; Fats; Minerals; Vitamins; Water.**

Nutritional Supplements

Ideally, it's best to obtain your nutrients from food, not pills. Food provides vitamins and minerals in the most biologically available form, in the right amounts and combined with other complementary nutrients that work together as a team. For example, vitamin C increases the absorption of iron, vitamin E works with selenium and vitamin C as an antioxidant defence team, folate's biochemistry is intertwined with that of vitamins B_6 and B_{12} vitamins, and zinc is synergistic with vitamin A.

And of course, with food, there's little risk of overdose except under special circumstances.

But there are times when you can't eat a balanced diet or you have a health problem that may respond to higher intakes of one or more vitamins.

TIPS FOR TAKING SUPPLEMENTS

In recent years attitudes have changed, as numerous studies have emerged suggesting antioxidant supplements in particular are associated with better health profiles. If you choose to take a supplement there are some general rules you should follow.

- ✔ Take supplements with food or soon afterwards to help absorb them better.
- ✔ Think of them only as a top-up to your daily diet.
- ✔ Don't take more than the suggested dosage.

- ✔ Buy a reliable brand. Cheaper brands may not have the most biologically active form (for example, natural compared with synthetic vitamin E, calcium gluconate compared with carbonate) or they may have only tiny amounts.
- ✔ Check the amount of the pure vitamin or mineral you're getting—1500 milligrams calcium carbonate means 600 milligrams of pure calcium.
- ✔ Be wary of exaggerated claims made on packs and in advertising. Often the scientific evidence is scanty, preliminary or consists of anecdotes from 'satisfied' patients. A single study does not always prove the cause.
- ✔ Chewable vitamin C tablets are so acidic they can dissolve tooth enamel; if you take them, rinse your mouth well afterwards.
- ✔ Take an iron tablet with orange juice or a fruit rich in vitamin C to improve its absorption.
- ✔ Check the label if you have an allergy—most supplements are free of yeast, dairy, gluten and seafood.
- ✔ Distribute the dose over the day—two smaller tablets are usually better absorbed than one single one.

WHEN YOU MAY NEED EXTRA

There are times in our lives when we have higher needs for vitamins and minerals.

Before conception	A high intake of folate can protect against birth defects.
During pregnancy	Extra iron, iodine, folate and calcium are needed, as well as omega-3 fatty acids.
When breastfeeding	Extra calcium and omega-3 fatty acids are needed.
Vegans	Vegans may be short on vitamin B_{12}, iron, zinc, calcium and omega-3 fatty acids.
Smokers (and passive smokers)	Smokers have around double the vitamin C requirement and may need more zinc, folate, beta-carotene and other antioxidants.
Heavy drinkers	Excessive alcohol depletes B group vitamins such as thiamin and folate as well as zinc, potassium and vitamin E.
Athletes	Various vitamins and minerals are needed but generally the antioxidant vitamins C and E as well as iron.
People aged over 60	Absorption of nutrients declines in later years but requirements for vitamins B_6, B_{12}, calcium and vitamin D are increased.
Those on an elimination diet for allergy or food intolerance	The removal of whole food groups such as grains and/or dairy also eliminates related vitamins and minerals.
During illness and after surgery or burns	More vitamin C and protein are required for tissue synthesis.
Restricted weight-loss diet	Very low kilojoule intakes cannot provide sufficient vitamins and minerals—a multivitamin and mineral supplement are recommended.

GETTING THE DOSE RIGHT

When taking any supplement, more is not better. Large single doses of certain vitamins and minerals can have undesirable side effects and even potential dangers. At high doses, vitamins act as drugs. They may interact with each other or with medications such as diuretics, anti-inflammatories, antibiotics or the contraceptive pill.

VITAMIN OR MINERAL	SIDE EFFECTS OF HIGH DOSES
Vitamin A	Doses exceeding 3000 micrograms a day are dangerous for pregnant women—they can interfere with the development of the foetus or produce birth defects. Excess causes nausea, liver damage, dry itchy skin, hair loss, headaches and skin problems.
Beta-carotene	Turns the skin and whites of the eyes an orange-yellow colour (which slowly disappears once you cease consuming excess amounts). May also produce hair loss, nausea or blurred vision.
Vitamin D	More than 80 micrograms a day can lead to nausea, bone pain, liver damage, muscle weakness and lethargy. It also causes calcium to be deposited in soft tissues like the liver and kidneys.
Vitamin C	Not toxic, but doses greater than 2000 milligrams a day can cause upset stomach and diarrhoea. Increases the risk of iron overload.
Vitamin B_6	More than 50 milligrams a day can lead to neuritis, a painful numbness or tingling in the hands and feet due to damage to the nerves.
Niacin	Mild flushing reaction at over 1000 milligrams a day.
Iron	May cause gastrointestinal upset or constipation. Can produce iron overload in someone with haemochromatosis (iron-storage disease). May interfere with absorption of zinc. Major cause of death from accidental swallowing by toddlers.
Selenium	Hair and nail loss, irritability, nerve damage.
Calcium	Can interfere with iron absorption.

WHAT SUPPLEMENTS CAN'T DO

Supplements are not a magic cure-all, nor a short cut to better health. They can't:

- ✖ Guarantee you will get all 27 or so essential vitamins and minerals that you need
- ✖ Replace the huge number of natural phytochemicals in vegetables and fruit—over 600 carotenoids exist in plants, but you only get two or three of these in any pill (beta-carotene, lutein and zeaxanthin)
- ✖ Make up for a poor diet that's too high in fat, salt and sugar and too low in fibre
- ✖ Allow you to 'eat anything' knowing you've taken your vitamins and minerals
- ✖ Give you more energy when you're not getting enough sleep or are stressed or anxious
- ✖ Cure a cold or Alzheimer's.

Nuts

Nuts were once a dietary no-no, condemned to the same category as potato crisps and salty snacks. But today they're enjoying a new status as a heart-friendly health ingredient, thanks to dozens of recent studies on their nutritional benefits. As one of my favourite snack foods, it's something I'm in favour of.

More than 70 studies over the past two decades have found favourable effects on blood fats from almonds, Brazil nuts, hazelnuts, macadamias, pecans, pistachios and walnuts. It seems reasonable to assume other nuts would also offer the same protective effects. The other bonus is that this small amount of nuts doesn't cause weight gain.

NUTRITIONAL VALUE

Apart from chestnuts and coconut, all nuts have a similar composition.

- ✔ They are rich in unsaturated fats ('good' fats) along with generous amounts of vitamin E, vitamins B_1 and B_6, niacin and folate.

MY TAKE
I recommend one serve of nuts a day (30–50 g, which would be, for example, around 20 almonds). Be careful not to exceed this—while nutritious, nuts can pack a good punch in terms of fat. A handful of almonds adds up to about 18 g of fat and 840 kJ, which is about the same as 1½ slices of cheddar cheese or a tablespoon of butter.

- ✔ They offer 5–10 per cent fibre, so can make a useful contribution to your daily intake. If eaten raw, they have virtually no sodium (salt).
- ✔ They offer a range of essential minerals including magnesium, potassium, zinc, copper, manganese and selenium that, along with other antioxidants, help protect the fat in nuts from going rancid too quickly.
- ✔ Their protein varies from 7 per cent to 20 per cent, making them an important source for vegetarians.
- ✔ Nuts do not contain cholesterol.
- ✔ Most nuts are high in an amino acid called arginine, which is converted to nitric oxide in the body. Nitric oxide helps blood vessels dilate and, like aspirin, reduces the stickiness of the platelets in the bloodstream.

Try to eat a variety of nuts as you would fruits and vegetables, particularly those with reddish brown skins. The skins have been found to contain high levels of antioxidants and may even prove to be a food source for the healthy bacteria in our large colon.

ALMONDS

Almonds have been cultivated since ancient times and are a close relative of the plum and peach. Their fat is 72 per cent mono-unsaturated and they have the highest vitamin E content of all nuts—30 grams provides 80 per cent of an adult's recommended daily intake. Almonds are also notable for their high calcium content—⅓ cup (50 grams) offers 125 milligrams of calcium, as much as half a glass of milk. They also contain beta-sitosterol, a plant sterol that can block the absorption of cholesterol into the body. All these things combine to put them on the superfood list.

BRAZIL NUTS

Brazil nuts originated in the tropical forests of Brazil and South America, where they were a wild crop. Just two of these nuts provide the recommended daily intake of selenium, a key antioxidant depleted from many soils, as well as being high in magnesium and calcium. After macadamias, Brazils also have one of the highest fat contents of all nuts (62 per cent), though most of their fat is polyunsaturated.

CASHEW NUTS

A South American nut in origin, cashews are one of my weaknesses with their delicious flavour and crunch. They have the highest plant iron and zinc level of all nuts. Their fat is mainly mono-unsaturated, and they are also good for folate.

CHESTNUTS

Unlike other nuts, these large brown nuts are low in fat and kilojoules. More floury than nutty, an average 30 gram serve supplies only 215 kilojoules. They are a good source of fibre and are gluten free—ground nuts such as almond, chestnut or hazelnut meal can be used in baking in place of gluten-containing flours. Chestnuts are grown in cooler parts of Australia and have a short season over winter, although frozen chestnuts are available all year round.

DID YOU KNOW?

The nut revolution began in 1992 with the publication of a study of more than 314,000 Seventh Day Adventists in California. Their eating habits were tracked for six years by a team of researchers from the Loma Linda University. They found those who ate 30 g of nuts more than five times a week were 50 per cent less likely to experience fatal and non-fatal heart attacks, compared with those who ate nuts less than once a week. Those who ate nuts one to four times a week had a 27 per cent reduced risk.

COCONUT

The largest of the nut family, one-third of the fresh flesh is fat. Apart from a high fibre content, coconuts are not particularly high in many other nutrients. They are poor in vitamin E and most minerals apart from potassium and protein.

HAZELNUTS

Also known as filberts or cobnuts, hazelnuts are at the low end of the nut fat spectrum with only 36 per cent fat, but their fat is one of the most highly mono-unsaturated, close to macadamias. They are high in vitamin E and B_6 and offer good amounts of thiamin, niacin, folic acid and the mineral calcium.

MACADAMIAS

Native to Australia, macadamias were ignored by the early white settlers, but eventually became the only Australian native food plant to develop into a commercial crop internationally. Today South Africa is the number-two producer behind Australia. Macadamias have the highest fat content of all nuts—over 70 per cent—making them high in kilojoules and sometimes a little buttery to taste. Like other nuts, they contribute protein, vitamin E, B vitamins and minerals such as manganese. They have no cholesterol and of their fat, 80 per cent is in the healthy mono-unsaturated form with almost no polyunsaturated, and 13 per cent saturated.

PEANUTS

Also called groundnuts, peanuts are the most popular of all nuts. They are not a true nut, but belong to the legume family—the same botanic family as dried peas and beans. Nutritionally they are a blend of both nut and legume, having the high fat count of nuts (49 per cent), with the legume's high protein content (24 per cent). They also offer the legume's good content of thiamin and folic acid, as well as fair amounts of fibre and calcium. Like all nuts, they contain no cholesterol.

PECANS

A species of hickory native to the US, pecans resemble walnuts in appearance and nutritional value, but have a milder, sweeter flavour. Like walnuts, they are one of the few plant sources of alpha linolenic acid for omega-3s, and have a high count of flavonoids.

PINE NUTS

These are the edible seeds from various types of pine trees that grow in the Mediterranean region, notably Spain and Italy (where they're called *pignoli*), and the Middle East. Many pine nuts also come from China and other Asian countries. Nutritionally, pine nuts are closest to walnuts and pecans in food value.

PISTACHIOS

Vibrant green in colour, pistachios are an ancient nut native to the Middle East, Iran, Turkey and Syria and are mentioned in the Bible. They have a green oval-shaped kernel encased in a thick purple-pink and brown wrinkled skin. Pistachios are good for plant sterols that can block cholesterol absorption. Compared with other nuts, they have high amounts of protein, potassium and beta-carotene, which are converted into vitamin A in the body.

Growing bodies

Nuts are in the top eight allergy-provoking foods, particularly in babies and children. This applies to both tree nuts (including almonds, cashews and walnuts) and peanuts. Most people with a peanut allergy can still eat other nuts; however, one-third are also allergic to one or more tree nuts. If you have an allergic reaction, avoid all nuts completely until tested by your doctor.

WALNUTS

These were known to the classical Greek and Hebrew writers and were carried to many parts of Europe by the Romans. Over 60 per cent of their fat is polyunsaturated—the most of any nut. This explains why they can turn bitter if stored poorly. Walnuts (and pecans) are one of the few plant sources of an omega-3 fatty acid called alpha-linolenic acid, which keeps your blood flowing freely and your heart in good shape. The kernel is shaped like a brain and there is research underway into walnut compounds, which may protect brain function.

SHOPPER'S GUIDE

Buying fresh nuts makes the world of difference to me! According to Nuts for Life, the nut industry association, here's what to look for:

- ✔ Nuts in the shell—choose clean nuts free from cracks and holes. They should be heavy for their size, indicating a fresh, meaty kernel.
- ✔ Nut kernels—choose crisp, plump and meaty kernels indicating high quality.
- ✔ Once home, remove nuts from plastic bags and store them in an airtight container in the refrigerator or freezer. Nuts can be refrigerated for up to 4 months and frozen for up to 6 months.

NUMBER CRUNCH

One serve of mixed nuts (50 grams) provides 5 grams of protein, 30 grams of fat, 3 grams of fibre and 1040 kilojoules. Nut varieties vary slightly in their nutritional profiles; for example:

- 50 grams of walnuts provides 5 grams of protein, 27 grams of fat, 3 grams of fibre and 1040 kilojoules.
- 50 grams of macadamias provides 3 grams of protein, 38 grams of fat, 5 grams of fibre and 1050 kilojoules.
- 50 grams of peanuts provides 12 grams of protein, 25 grams of fat, 3 grams of fibre and 590 kilojoules.

NUT PASTES AND BUTTERS

I advocate eating nuts whole rather than as a nut butter or paste. Whole nuts have a more fibrous structure that traps some of the nut's natural oils and blocks the absorption of that oil into the body. Research shows that whole-nut eaters excrete more fat from the body, which helps manage weight gain.

Many nut pastes also have additional oil and sugar whipped into them, so they're not 100 per cent nuts. If this is what you're after, look for a peanut butter or almond paste that is 100 per cent nuts or labelled as no added sugar and salt. Alternatively, grind them into a paste yourself with a mixer.

MY TAKE

I like to think of nuts as small packages rich in essential nutrients that contribute to your health and wellbeing. They are in a class of their own.

A NOTE ABOUT NUTELLA

Nutella is marketed as a hazelnut spread, but has only 13 per cent hazelnuts and is 55 per cent sugar. That puts it on a par with chocolate. Its ingredients in order of most to least are sugar, vegetable oil, hazelnuts (13%), cocoa powder, non-fat milk solids, emulsifier (soy lecithin) and flavour (vanillin). Think of it as a chocolate spread rather than anything seriously nutty.

Nut and Seed Bars

Chock-full of sesame seeds, sunflower seeds, coconut and other nuts, oats and dried fruit, nut and seed bars line the counters of many health-food shops and juice bars. Compared with chocolate bars and lollies, they obviously offer more fibre, vitamins and minerals and thus are a more nutrient-rich snack. But be careful—what binds these ingredients together is honey, glucose or some form of sugar, which usually makes up about half the weight of the bar. Even sugar-free bars that are sweetened with dried fruit are high in natural sugars (drying fruit removes water and concentrates the remaining sugars—dates, raisins and sultanas are 75 per cent sugars).

O

Oats

Oats were first cultivated by Europeans in about 1000 BC, and were firmly established in Britain during the Bronze Age. They were primarily used as a feed for animals and have long been associated with colder climates such as Scotland, eastern Europe and Scandinavia. Their ability to grow in cold damp climates where other grains cannot survive has made them a valuable crop.

As with any grain, oats need some form of processing before they can be eaten. They are best known rolled into flakes to be cooked into rolled oats or porridge, but can also be milled into oatmeal or oat flour. Muesli is made up of around 50 per cent oats, while muesli bars have 25 per cent oats. Rolled oats also have a variety of uses in cooking and are used in biscuits, crumble toppings, puddings and cakes. Oat flour can be mixed with wheaten flour to make bread—alone it makes a poor loaf because it lacks gluten.

EASY WAYS TO ENJOY OATS

- Make porridge oats your warming winter breakfast! Add a finely sliced pear, a handful of sultanas or a grated apple (with the skin) halfway through cooking. Top with a sprinkle of cinnamon instead of sugar.
- Make your own natural museli by mixing 2 cups of raw rolled oats with ½ cup each of pumpkin seeds, slivered almonds, sunflower seeds and dried fruit (such as sultanas, or chopped dried apricots or apples).

NUTRITIONAL VALUE

Oats are a winner among all grains and one of my favourite superfoods.

- ✔ Their fibre is the soluble type of fibre and includes beta-glucans, which prevents breakdown products of cholesterol from re-entering the system via the intestine. The result is less cholesterol being made in the body.
- ✔ Traditional or rolled oats are also low GI, so their carbohydrate is slowly absorbed into your system.
- ✔ Oats have the highest fat content among grains (about 7 per cent compared with wheat at 2 per cent) and their fat is mainly mono- and polyunsaturated with important phytonutrients such as the tocotrienols. This gives oats a slightly higher kilojoule value over the other grains, but it is not significant in a day's total intake.
- ✔ They have double the calcium of other grains and are high in iron; however, the availability of these minerals is impaired by the presence of phytic acid and fibre, so they're not in the same class as milk or red meat.
- ✔ Oats are a good source of the B vitamins, especially thiamin and niacin, as well as vitamin E. They have one of the highest protein contents and virtually no sodium. They also top up your minerals like phosphorus, potassium and magnesium (which helps to steady the rhythm of the heart).
- ✔ Sprinkle oats over homemade muffins or banana bread just before baking.
- ✔ Substitute oats for one-third of the flour in any cake recipe.
- ✔ Top stewed fruit with an oat crumble. Mix equal quantities of oats and self-raising flour and, using your fingertips, rub together with a little butter or margarine. Spoon over stewed fruit and bake in a moderate oven for 10 minutes or until golden on top.

NUMBER CRUNCH

Half a cup of cooked porridge oats (130 grams) without milk or sugar provides 2 grams of protein, 1 gram of fat, 11 grams of carbohydrate, no sugar, 1 gram of fibre and 260 kilojoules.

See also
Cholesterol; Grains; Gluten.

Obesity

DID YOU KNOW?

20–30 per cent of children in Australia and New Zealand are currently too fat. Rates of obesity have doubled in just 10 years. Overweight children suffer psychologically as well as physically, and they don't grow out of it—about 80 per cent of obese teenagers will become obese adults.

The average weight of Australians is increasing, similar to trends in the US, UK, Canada and New Zealand. Despite all the diet books, light foods and fitness crazes, two out of three men and more than half of all women are overweight or obese. Sadly, the problem is more common in people with poor education, from a low socio-economic class and from some migrant groups.

Being overweight is linked to an increased risk of heart disease, type 2 diabetes, gallstones, hormone-dependent cancers (breast and endometrium), stroke, osteoarthritis, gout, fatty liver and sleep apnoea (a sleep disorder causing lack of oxygen to the brain and heart).

Growing bodies

How to help overweight kids

Health programs to help overweight and obese children have commonly targeted the kids themselves. But a two-year follow-up HIKCUPS study (Hunter Illawarra Kids Challenge Using Parent Support) published in 2011 shows it's mum and dad who make the difference. It found the most effective treatment for young children is to guide and support parents to help improve their family's food habits.

See also **Weight Loss; Exercise; Dietary Requirements.**

WHY WE'RE GETTING HEAVIER

We live in an obesogenic world—where everything is contrived to make you put on weight. We tend to drive more often than walk or ride, and do less daily exercise in general. Modern gadgets often reduce the amount of incidental exercise we get and many of us do not work in manual jobs. We watch a lot of TV and use the computer. Modern convenience foods have also impacted on our diets and we tend to eat refined, nutrient-poor foods that are packed with kilojoules. Our portion sizes have also become bigger.

FIVE WAYS TO MAKE A DIFFERENCE FOR YOUR FAMILY

- ✔ Set a good example. Eat the foods you would like your kids to eat. If your schedule is so busy that you often have to resort to high-fat takeaway dinners, you need to slow down. A home-cooked meal is better for everyone but it does take a little more time.
- ✔ Have regular family meals (including breakfast) with a small snack in between. Young kids need to eat small portions regularly, but that doesn't mean they should graze all day long. Children have higher nutrient requirements, so it's important snack foods are nutritious. This doesn't mean banning junk food, but keeping treat food for treats.
- ✔ Keep mealtimes happy—that means doing your utmost to avoid battles over what to eat and how much. Respect your child's appetite. It will vary so allow them to determine how much they need to eat. By forcing them to 'clean their plate', they lose the ability to listen to their appetite. Involving kids in food choice and preparation is a great way to raise food-smart kids.
- ✔ Make water the main family drink. Cordial, fruit juice and soft drink are high in sugar and too easy to have too much of.
- ✔ Get active. Turn off the TV and head outdoors to kick a ball in the back yard, go cycling or visit the park—anything to get everyone moving. Putting the older kids in charge of walking the dog every day is a good start.

Oils

Oils are extracted from seeds (sunflower, cottonseed, sesame, grape seed, palm oil), legumes (soy, peanut), fruit (olives, avocado), grains (maize, rice bran, wheat germ) and nuts (walnut, macadamia, almond, coconut). Each oil has different properties, nutritional profile and cooking uses.

Oils are extracted by several methods, the main one being a combination of expeller

OIL	% SATURATED FAT
Canola	8
Flaxseed	8
Walnut	10
Safflower	10
Sunflower	11
Grape seed	11
Avocado	13
Maize (corn)	13
Olive	14
Soy bean	15
Sesame	15
Peanut	18
Rice bran	20
Wheat germ	20
Cottonseed	27
Palm	51
Palm kernel	90
Coconut	92

Note: the Heart Foundation sets 20 per cent saturated (and trans) fat as its cut-off for approving a healthy oil.

pressing and solvent extraction—the seeds are first heated and pressed to squeeze out the oil, then the crushed seeds are mixed with solvent to dissolve out the remaining oil. The solvent is completely removed by evaporation and the two batches of oil mixed. Some oils, typically olive oil, are cold-pressed—hydraulic presses 'squeeze' out the oil with no heat being applied.

NUTRITIONAL VALUE

The greatest nutritional difference between oils is their degree of saturation—that is the proportion of saturated, mono-unsaturated and polyunsaturated fatty acids present. No oil is 100 per cent saturated or 100 per cent polyunsaturated—all are mixtures of the three types. It's the type occurring in the greatest proportion that gives the oil its classification.

Apart from coconut and palm oil, all oils are low in saturated fat but vary in the proportions of polyunsaturated and monounsaturated fats they contain. They are free of trans fats—occasionally you see low levels under 3 per cent, but this is often caused by heating to keep the oil stable, not hydrogenation.

All oils have vitamin E, but concentration varies. Wheat germ oil is the richest by a long way, followed by cottonseed, sunflower, safflower, maize and soy bean oil. Other oils are fair sources, except for coconut oil, which contains only a small amount.

Except for coconut, all oils are good sources of the essential fatty acid linoleic acid, which cannot be made by the body and must be obtained from food. Canola and soy bean also supply 7–10 per cent alpha-linolenic acid, which is another essential fatty acid and family member of the omega-3 polyunsaturated fats.

The choice of vegetable oils in the diet is often overlooked but very important, as it can determine the overall fat balance, shifting it from saturated to unsaturated.

OILS RICH IN POLYUNSATURATED FATS

Polyunsaturated fats are a good source of omega-6 fatty acids (and flaxseed has a high concentration of omega-3s) and tend to lower blood cholesterol, which makes them a recommended food by the Heart Foundation if you have high cholesterol. Safflower, grapeseed, sunflower, walnut, wheat germ and maize oil are the best sources.

SUNFLOWER OIL

An all-purpose oil with a clean neutral flavour, sunflower oil is low in saturated fat and rich in polyunsaturated fat. This can make it susceptible to oxidation (rancidity), which limits its use in restaurants and by food manufacturers who tend to prefer the more stable canola. It's often used to make polyunsaturated margarines and salad dressings. Some gourmet varieties of potato crisps are cooked in a variant of sunflower oil called high-oleic sunflower (Sunola), which has the same properties but is higher in mono-unsaturated fat. Regular crisps are cooked in palm oil, which is high in saturated fat.

RICE BRAN OIL

Made from the oil in the germ and outer hull of rice, rice bran oil is a very light, thin oil with not much flavour. This neutral taste makes it good for fish and delicate dishes and as a base for mayonnaise and white sauces. Its great advantage is its high smoke point, so it's handy to use in sautéing, stir-frying and roasting. Rice bran oil contains about half polyunsaturated and half mono-unsaturated fat, making it similar in composition to cottonseed or sesame oil.

GRAPE SEED OIL

Made from the seeds of grapes leftover after winemaking, grape seed oil is a light oil with a high smoke point. It's good for high-heat pan-frying and stir-frying at home. Along with safflower, it is one of the two oils highest in polyunsaturated fat with over 70 per cent as polyunsaturated fat.

FLAXSEED OIL

Made from flaxseeds (linseeds), this oil has an incredible 53 per cent omega-3 concentration as alpha-linolenic acid, one of the reasons it's often recommended for health. However, it oxidises easily and goes off more quickly than other oils. Store your flaxseed in the refrigerator in summer, and a cool dark place in winter.

BAD FAT

Saturated fat—mainly from animals, it raises blood cholesterol and is not recommended.

GOOD FATS

Mono-unsaturated fat—from seeds and vegetables, it lowers blood cholesterol although not as well as polyunsaturated fats.

Polyunsaturated fat—also from seeds and vegetables, it lowers blood cholesterol most effectively and is recommended by the Heart Foundation.

OILS RICH IN MONO-UNSATURATED FATS

Mono-unsaturated fats can also lower blood cholesterol. Olive, canola and peanut oils are the best sources.

CANOLA OIL

Canola oil is a good nutrition all-rounder. It has one of the lowest saturated fat contents of all oils, is a good source of heart-friendly omega-3 fatty acids and has a high mono-unsaturated content. It is derived from the seeds of the canola plant, which is a variety of rapeseed and part of the mustard family like cabbage and mustard seed. It was specifically bred in Canada in the 1980s to be low in erucic acid, a harmful fatty acid that limited the use of rapeseed (the word 'canola' is an acronym for 'Canadian Oil Low Acid').

MY TAKE

Whichever oil you use, remember that both polyunsaturated and mono-unsaturated oils are healthy. Your choice of oil depends on what you cook most often and your health goals. I like to use olive oil for general everyday cooking but have some peanut oil for Asian stir-fries and a local extra virgin olive oil for salads and dressing up vegetables.

OLIVE OIL

A key ingredient of the healthy Mediterranean diet, olive oil is low in saturated fats and high in mono-unsaturated fats, and has a great taste. Of all these oils, the extra-virgin cold-pressed oil has the richest antioxidant content (it's high in polyphenols, which gives it that sharp greenish taste). These oils oxidise quickly though, so store them in dark glass in the fridge and buy fresh olive oil each season.

PEANUT OIL

A favourite in Asian cuisine, peanut oil is fragrant with a high smoke point and can withstand high-temperature cooking. I keep a bottle of it in my cupboard just for stir-fries and wok cooking. Remember that any peanut product can be a potential risk to people with peanut allergy, but it's extremely low as almost no protein is present in the oil. Peanut oil has about half mono-unsaturated fats with some polyunsaturates.

OILS HIGH IN SATURATED FATS

Saturated fats raise blood cholesterol and are not recommended.

COCONUT OIL

At 92 per cent saturated fat, coconut oil has the highest level of saturated fat of all the oils. It has very little mono- or polyunsaturated fat, which puts it in a class with solid animal fats like ghee and lard, putting it on the list of things to avoid for anyone with

Q
Why do oils become rancid?
A
Some oils with a high proportion of polyunsaturated fat readily turn rancid when exposed to oxygen. The vitamin E in oil is a natural antioxidant and additives such as butylated hydroxy anisole (additive code 320) are also sometimes added to extend shelf life. Heating the oil causes the anti-oxidants to partly break down, and repeated heating (as in the re-use of oil for deep frying) not only reduces the amount of vitamin E but can also lead to the formation of harmful oxidised products.

Growing bodies
Useful sources of omega-3 foods containing more than 30 mg per serve include bread, milk and yoghurt. These aren't very rich sources but can be handy giving children a boost.

high cholesterol. Coconut oil has a different makeup from vegetable oils and animal fats, and is promoted as a natural oil that can suppress your appetite, prevent heart disease, kill germs, boost your immune system and turbo-charge your metabolism. If it weren't marketed with such hype, I'd feel more kindly disposed to it, but these outlandish claims do get my hackles up! There is inconclusive evidence about the value of the fat found in coconut oil. (Note that coconut oil is not the thin watery liquid found inside the coconut, which is referred to as coconut water.)

Omega-3 and Omega-6 Essential Fatty Acids

Not all polyunsaturated fats are equal. Research is revealing there are enormous benefits in increasing consumption of one type known as omega-3 fats. Just as vitamins are essential to good health, so are the essential omega-3 fatty acids and the related omega-6s.

The body is incapable of producing these and relies on food to obtain them. Omega-3s and omega-6s are converted into hormone-like compounds that control many key biochemical reactions. First though, a little chemistry to understand their differences.

OMEGA-3s

I've been a big fan of omega-3s ever since the 1980s when the first studies began trickling out flagging their usefulness in keeping the heart in good shape. I was working with an oil producer at the time and they were keen to promote the benefits of omega-3 in their new canola seeds and oil. There are three key omega-3 fatty acids.

ALPHA-LINOLENIC ACID (ALA)

ALA is the simplest omega-3 fatty acid. It occurs in flaxseed, chia, walnuts and pecans, a limited number of oils—canola, flaxseed and soy bean—and in a handful of green vegetables such as purslane, spinach, silverbeet, beans and broccoli.

EICOSAPENTAENOIC ACID (EPA)

EPA can be produced in the body by converting alpha-linolenic acid into this longer-chain omega-3 variant. In its natural state, EPA can be found in cod-liver oil, fish oils, fish and other seafood, and in small amounts in grass-fed lamb and beef. DPA is another related omega-3.

DOCOSAHEXAENOIC ACID (DHA)

DHA is concentrated in tuna oil while other fish oils, fish and seafood supply a smaller amount. Breast milk is rich in DHA and newborn babies utilise it to develop brain, nerve and eye tissue.

OMEGA-6s

Omega-6 fatty acids are competitors to omega-3s. While chemically similar, they act in very different ways and compete with each other for the same enzymes. There are three main omega-6 fatty acids.

LINOLEIC ACID (LA)

LA is the first member of the omega-6 family and is a major component of everyday vegetable oils like safflower, sunflower, soybean, corn (maize), peanut and grape seed. It is also present in grains, many nuts, seeds and wheat germ. Numerous studies have demonstrated how effective it is at lowering total and LDL cholesterol, one of the reasons polyunsaturated oils and spreads have proved so popular over the last 40 years.

GAMMA-LINOLENIC ACID (GLA)

GLA is derived from linoleic acid. It is the active component of evening primrose oil, borage or starflower oil (derived from the garden herb borage) and blackcurrant oil. Often recommended by alternative practitioners to help PMS, evening primrose oil is also used to treat eczema and to improve nerve function in patients with diabetes.

ARACHIDONIC ACID (AA)

AA is made from gamma-linolenic acid. It is a key component of the substances that regulate tissue function and inflammation and transmit messages between cells. Like DHA, it is found in human milk and in the tissues of vital organs such as the brain and eye, and it also helps to form and maintain nerve tissue.

EAT LIKE THE ESKIMOS

The omega-3 story began in the mid-1970s, when scientists were puzzled to discover that the Inuit people of Greenland had a much better health profile than Western populations, even though their diet of seal, oily fish and whale was high in fat. Their blood levels of cholesterol and triglycerides were very low and their blood also took a long time to clot—much longer than a similar group of Danish people who ate the typical high-fat Western diet based on full-cream dairy foods and fatty meat. The Inuit people were also much less likely to suffer from rheumatoid arthritis, psoriasis, asthma, heart disease, stroke and other diseases compared with their Danish counterparts.

GETTING YOUR OMEGA BALANCE RIGHT

Most of us currently consume too many omega-6 fatty acids and not enough omega-3s. While omega-6s are effective for lowering blood cholesterol, researchers now believe that an oversupply upsets the delicate balance of fats within our bodies and creates health problems. The most common cause of over-eating omega-6s comes from an excess of polyunsaturated vegetable oils in the diet.

Nutritionists used to suggest cutting back on oils rich in omega-6 and swapping to canola, flaxseed or olive oil to correct the balance, but they found it's not as effective as simply increasing your omega-3s. Essentially this means eating more fish and seafood or, for a clinical effect, taking fish oil capsules.

EIGHT WAYS OMEGA-3s HELP YOU STAY HEALTHY

HEART

The biggest area of influence, omega-3s slow the build-up of fatty material on the inner walls of blood vessels (atherosclerosis), allowing the blood to flow more freely, especially through small blood vessels. It prevents the platelets in the blood from clumping together and reduces the chances of blood clots (thrombosis), an effect similar to aspirin. Omega-3s work to counter irregular or chaotic beating of the heart, known as cardiac arrhythmia, which, if severe enough, can precipitate death. They drop the level of triglycerides, a blood fat, which, like cholesterol, is potentially dangerous if it gets too high. They make the arteries more elastic and thus more able to handle pressure, and they also reduce high blood pressure.

BRAIN

Omega-3s are in a key position to influence brain and nerve function, and work to keep you mentally sharp — fish truly is brain food! Fats make up more than 50 per cent of the brain and DHA, an omega-3 long-chain fatty acid, is the most abundant. DHA works to enhance nerve-signal transmission in the brain, and plays a key role in the development

SHOPPER'S GUIDE

Everybody should eat around 500 mg a day of the long-chain omega-3s. You'll get this by making sure you have two or three serves of oily fish in your trolley once a week. Alternatively, take two fish oil capsules a day. Fish oil is very safe even at high doses of 14 or more capsules a day. It is almost free of mercury and complements blood-thinning medications (Warfarin, Heparin) that many heart patients are taking.

Super sources
(more than 2000 mg per serve)

- ✔ Atlantic salmon (farmed)
- ✔ NZ King salmon (farmed)
- ✔ Salmon, red or pink, canned
- ✔ Sardines, canned or fresh
- ✔ Barramundi (farmed)
- ✔ Canned mackerel
- ✔ Rainbow trout
- ✔ Swordfish

Excellent sources
(200–2000 mg per serve)

- ✔ Blue-eye trevalla
- ✔ Silver perch
- ✔ Australian bass
- ✔ John dory
- ✔ Snapper
- ✔ Frozen fish fillets
- ✔ Tuna, canned (look for cans that say 'high in omega-3')
- ✔ Herrings
- ✔ Oysters
- ✔ Green- and blue-lipped mussels
- ✔ Omega-enriched eggs

Good sources
(more than 60 mg per serve)

- ✔ Grass-fed beef and lamb
- ✔ Game meats (like venison and kangaroo)
- ✔ Liver
- ✔ Kidney

of babies' brains and eyesight. It is abundant in breast milk and many primitive cultures have traditionally fed fish to new mothers to increase their milk levels.

MOOD

Omega-3 supplements are being increasingly recommended to assist with mental problems such as depression and schizophrenia, and to help children with learning difficulties such as dyslexia, dyspraxia and Attention Deficit Hyperactivity Disorder (ADHD). There have only been a few studies on this date, so their effectiveness is still uncertain. However, as omega-3 supplements don't produce any harmful side effects, talk to your doctor about giving your ADHD child a liquid fish oil capsule made for children.

AGEING

Studies show that higher intakes of omega-3s (EPA and DHA) lower the risk of age-related cognitive decline, including dementia and Alzheimer's.

EYES

Omega-3s are recommended for older persons to prevent macular degeneration and preserve eyesight. Eating more than two serves a week of oily fish was associated with a 39 per cent reduced risk of age-related macular degeneration in one US study.

RHEUMATOID ARTHRITIS

Studies of rheumatoid arthritis sufferers whose diets have been supplemented with fish oil have demonstrated improvements from the nagging symptoms of tender joints, morning stiffness, fatigue and poor grip strength. In some of these studies, the dose of anti-inflammatory drugs was decreased as a result of these improvements, which meant fewer side effects.

INFLAMMATION

Omega-3s can offer help to people suffering from illnesses with an inflammatory or immune component like psoriasis, eczema, asthma and inflammatory bowel disease. However, the doses needed are usually large and need to come from fish oil capsules in high doses (more than 12 per day) rather than fish. Not all the studies have been favourable, which makes it difficult to draw any firm conclusions at the moment.

DIABETES

Omega-3s can benefit people with diabetes, who often have raised blood triglyceride levels, high blood pressure, clotting and circulation problems. Omega-3 appears to offer protection against insulin resistance—the more there is incorporated into the cell membranes of our bodies' muscles, the lower the insulin resistance.

Oranges See Fruit.

Organic Food

No longer confined to health-food stores, organically grown food is now popular and stocked by local supermarkets. Retail sales of organic produce in Australia increased from about $28 million in 1990 to $350 million in 2006, and continue to grow at a 25 per cent rate each year. It's big business in the UK and Europe, with the UK market alone valued at around $2 billion thanks in part to food scares such as mad cow disease, and concern about genetically modified (GM) products.

Organic produce is not limited to fruit and vegetables. Organic meat, chicken, eggs and dairy products come from animals that are given no antibiotics or growth hormones and graze on land that is chemical-free. Even supplements, baby food, chocolate, beauty products, shampoo and wines are now on the shelves in organic form.

WHAT ORGANIC MEANS

Organic is a way of farming that eliminates synthetic chemicals. Producers do not use:

- ✖ Pesticides
- ✖ Herbicide sprays
- ✖ Growth hormones
- ✖ GM varieties.

Organic production is more holistic than this though; it is about farming using sustainable and environmentally sensitive practices that prevent soil erosion, promote biodiversity, allow crops and animals to grow at their natural pace and minimise the impact on local waterways. Organic farms feature:

- ✔ Crop rotation
- ✔ Composting
- ✔ Biological pest control.

MY TAKE

Buying organic gets my vote for a healthier, more sustainable environment. But it is more costly. Producing organic foods and materials is more labour intensive, it must be separated from non-organic products at all stages from farm to supermarket, and farms tend to be smaller and don't reap the economy of scale of larger agricultural productions.

TASTE

Some foods, like tomatoes or apples, often have a noticeably better flavour when produced organically. In other products, it makes no difference. What I have noticed is that many organic items like dairy foods and skin-care products are top-quality because the producer has put a lot of time and love them, and this is what makes the difference!

NUTRITIONAL VALUE

You don't have to buy organic to have a nutritious diet. To date, the bulk of studies show that vitamin and mineral levels in organic products are similar to those in standard produce, which is generally low in residues. Some studies have reported higher levels of antioxidants in organics, which makes sense because the plants have to produce more to defend themselves against attack. Other studies report higher mineral content thanks to improved soils containing mineral-bearing crushed rocks.

Whatever you choose to eat, make sure it's a wide variety of different types, which will minimise any likelihood of residues—and don't forget that simply washing or peeling produce will also reduce residues.

> **DID YOU KNOW?**
>
> Despite being free of synthetics and chemicals, organic is not necessarily any safer than non-organic food. Random testing by government agencies for pesticide residues in non-organic local produce reveals that more than 95 per cent have no detectable residue. It found those that do are well below the acceptable limits set by the World Health Organization. In fact one study comparing organic and non-organic grown produce showed that pesticide residues were still detectable in some organic produce. Again, the few samples that did have a trace of residue are well under safety limits.

READ THE LABEL

The only way you can be sure you are buying an organic product is if it has a recognised certification label from an accredited organic certifying organisation. This means the farmer or manufacturer is at a minimum operating in accordance with the Australian Standard for Organic and Biodynamic Products (AS 6000-2009) or a similar internationally recognised organic standard. The Australian Certified Organic Standard (2010) is the most prevalent and used standard in Australia, as is the organic 'Bud' logo that goes with it.

AUSTRALIAN CERTIFIED ORGANIC

Items carrying this label are guaranteed to arise from farms that have been organically managed for at least three years and are inspected regularly, and that contain a minimum 95 per cent of organic ingredients (excluding salt and water). (Up to 5 per cent non-organic ingredients are permitted to be present in organic produce where these cannot be sourced in sufficient commercial quantity, but not where they arise from GMOs, are irradiated or have known pesticide residues.)

Australian consumers are protected under Australian consumer law if there is a recognised certification logo, and related organic standard, that the product is claiming compliance to. Without reference to certification consumers should beware, and are less protected in terms of seeking redress if the product ends up not being the full organic article.

Oryzanol

Oryzanol (technically gamma-oryzanol) is a natural plant sterol unique to rice that reduces the absorption of cholesterol into the body and so lowers the 'bad' LDL cholesterol levels. It also acts as an antioxidant. Oryzanol has been suggested for conditions such as menopausal symptoms, mild anxiety and stomach upset, and as a sports supplement and conditioning supplement for horses. There is no real evidence that it works for any of these.

Osteoporosis and Diet

Osteoporosis is a condition in which the bones lose calcium, become fragile and break more easily. The term osteoporosis literally means 'holes in the bones'. It affects one in two women and one in three men over the age of 60.

Calcium is essential for building and maintaining bones and teeth. In fact, almost all the body's calcium (about 99 per cent) is found in the bones. It combines with other minerals such as phosphorus, potassium, magnesium and zinc to form the hard crystals that give bone its strength. The skeleton is not inert. It's a living tissue and acts like a mineral reservoir, which must be topped up. When your diet is insufficient, some of the minerals in bones dissolve and give their store back to the bloodstream. If your mineral intake is too low and there are more withdrawals than deposits from your bone bank, you risk losing bone strength.

The hormonal changes that begin in the forties and accompany menopause accelerate the loss of calcium and other minerals. When osteoporosis develops, the outer bone (the hard outer shell) becomes weak and thin. Replacement of lost bone is not usually possible, as often it is not noticeable until a sizeable portion of the bone mass has gone.

Osteoporosis affects one in two women and one in three men over the age of 60.

PREVENTION

The best protection is to build strong healthy bones by your adult years as our bone density peaks in the late teens. Here's what else you can do:

- ✔ As you get older, have your bone density tested, especially if you come from a family with a small build or a history of weak bones, or hip or wrist fractures later in life.
- ✔ Vitamin D is needed to absorb the calcium properly. Make sure you get around 15–20 minutes of exposure outdoors a couple of times a week to generate our own vitamin D from sunlight on the skin.
- ✔ Maintain regular exercise, particularly weight-bearing (or resistance) exercise such as walking, weights, jogging/running, dancing, aerobics, jumping rope, climbing stairs or tennis. Just as muscles become stronger when used, bones develop strength when muscles pull on the skeleton.
- ✔ Drop your salt intake. A diet high in salt can accelerate bone loss. Every 2000 milligrams of sodium removed by the kidneys in the urine (a reflection of the average salt intake) takes with it 60 milligrams of calcium. Over 10 years, the job of eliminating this salt load from the body would remove 150–200 grams of bone calcium, an amount equal to 15 per cent of the skeleton.
- ✔ Fizzy or carbonated drinks are associated with softer bones in teenagers. A Harvard University study reported that physically active girls in years 9 and 10 at school who drank soft drink were five times more likely to have a fracture than active girls who didn't drink soft drinks.
- ✔ Even though they're not rich in calcium, fruit and vegetables provide a 'mineralising' effect on bones which means they counteract the calcium drain, as well as topping up vital minerals such as potassium and magnesium. So it pays to up your intake of vegetables and salad and snack on more fruit.

TREATMENT

Hormone replacement therapy (HRT) is one of the most effective ways of stopping and partially reversing the bone loss that occurs when a woman's hormone levels start to dwindle in menopause. A combination of oestrogen and progesterone is usually taken cyclically. This produces monthly bleeding similar to a menstrual cycle.

Calcium and vitamin D supplements are usually combined with hormone replacement to stop further bone loss, as even as much as 2000 milligrams of calcium a day can't slow bone loss without the corresponding hormones. Aluminium interferes with calcium absorption, so be wary of antacids containing this element if you have indigestion.

See also **Calcium; Menopause; Minerals.**

Overweight *See* **Obesity; Weight Loss.**

Oxalic Acid

This is a compound present in sorrel, spinach, rhubarb leaves and strawberries that is toxic if eaten in large quantities.

P

Paleolithic Diet

The diet that sustained our hunter-gatherer ancestors throughout two million years of evolution has long intrigued scientists. Led by a group of paleobiologists, nutritionists and archaeologists, we now have a fairly accurate picture of what early hominids ate—fruits, nuts, vegetables, insects, fish, seafood, lean meat, eggs and not much grain food. This early diet is called the 'paleolithic diet'. It is important because scientists believe that modern humans still have the same ancient genes, which can't handle our rapidly growing intake of refined carbs, refined oils and junk food in general.

Using fossil records, bone mineral studies and dental reconstructions, they have studied 229 different traditional societies and deduced that the majority of them derived more than half of their food from animals—including reptiles and insects. No society relied entirely on plants, as it was more energy efficient to eat animals. In other words, by eating meat, they would gain the most energy for the least effort. In contrast, if they lived on vegetables and berries (which are generally low in kilojoules), they would have to expend more energy searching and gathering these foods than they got in kilojoule return. All this was long before modern grains were consumed and before farming cereals had begun. Milk and dairy foods were not part of the diet either. Eggs were the odd treat if they were lucky enough to stumble over a nest, while the honey from wild bees was much prized (and worth the risk of being stung).

Interestingly hunter-gatherers ate not just the lean muscle, but also the whole carcass. The preferred parts were the organs (kidney, liver and heart), any tissues of the head (like the eyes or tongue) and the fat. These were easier to chew and digest. Of course, the muscle meat they ate was lean, more like game (venison, kangaroo and emu, for example) than our grain-fed beef that's specifically produced to be finely marbled with fat.

There is little doubt about the health potential of such a diet; however, adoption in its entirety today is probably a little unrealistic. But there is nothing wrong with increasing fruit and vegetable intake, reducing processed and refined carbohydrates, eating more fish and lean meat including healthy game meats, and increasing physical activity—all aspects of the diet of hunters and gatherers that nutritionists recommend.

Pasta and Noodles

It's said that pasta (Italian for 'dough') comes in more shapes and sizes than there are days of the year. Whatever the shape, it's perfect for quick meals and scores well nutritionally.

Marco Polo is widely credited with having introduced spaghetti to Italy following travel to China in the 13th century where he discovered the Asian staple, noodles. But in fact there is plenty of evidence to show pasta was around long before this, and possibly even in the times of the Etruscans.

Pasta and noodles are made from flour and water, which is mixed to a stiff dough and extruded under pressure. Eggs are sometimes added and this gives a yellower colour and firmer texture.

Traditional Italian pasta is made from semolina, a coarse flour derived from hard durum wheat, which is considered of superior quality, holding its shape well after cooking and having the best texture. These days a wide range of grains are used including kamut, spelt and gluten-free grains such as rice, corn and quinoa.

DID YOU KNOW?

Couscous is a type of pasta. While most couscous has a moderate GI, pearl or Israeli couscous, which is like a toasted pasta, has a low GI (52).

Wholemeal pasta is also available, but it hasn't really caught on with consumers despite being a nutritionally superior option. I can understand this—in my experience wholemeal pastas don't have the same texture and mouth feel as traditional ones and it's been a hard sell in my own household. Sometimes you just have to stick with tradition and get your wholegrains from other foods!

Noodles are made from a wide variety of flours including wheat, buckwheat, mung beans, soy beans, rice and even sweet potato flour.

NUTRITIONAL VALUE

Pasta and noodles are winners with nutritionists.

- ✔ Pasta and noodles contain a good helping of protein, B vitamins (notably vitamin B_1, needed to release energy from food) plus a little iron and calcium. Quantities depend on the grain that was used. Compared with its starchy competitor, the potato, pasta and noodles are higher in carbohydrate, protein, B vitamins and minerals, but have no vitamin C.
- ✔ They are low in fat, with no added salt, and are high in starchy carbohydrate, the type that can fuel the muscles of endurance athletes (and weekend warriors too).
- ✔ When cooked *al dente*, pasta has a low GI and will help to keep blood-glucose levels on an even keel. Be aware that canned spaghetti has a moderate GI value.
- ✔ Most noodles have low or moderate GI values.

PASTA

There are over 300 different shapes of pasta, but they can be divided into five categories:

- Penne, fusilli, rigatoni and other short pastas go best with thick, chunky sauces.
- Fettuccine, spaghetti and linguini are long strands that team well with creamy sauces.
- Macaroni, lasagne and cannelloni are great for baking.
- Pasta with pouches and pockets—such as ravioli, tortellini and agnolotti—are used with stuffing.
- Very small pasta, such as alphabet macaroni, is best in soups.

MY TAKE

Instant noodles are a great standby in the cupboard, but some can be high in fat (around 17 per cent) and on the salty side. Keep them as an occasional food or buy packs labelled 'low fat' or '97 per cent fat free'.

NOODLES

Despite being an Asian staple, the word 'noodle' actually comes from the German '*Nudel*'. Thin or thick, fresh or dried, the variety available today is endless, and they can be made from any starchy staple that can be ground into a flour. Here's a simple summary of the main ones you'll come across in your supermarket or favourite Asian restaurant:

- Buckwheat or soba noodles (these are sometimes a combination of buckwheat and wheat flours)
- Egg noodles
- Mung bean noodles (also called cellophane, bean thread, transparent or glass noodles)
- Rice vermicelli and rice stick noodles
- Wheat flour noodles including somen and udon noodles.

PORTIONS

Pasta and noodles make a quick and easy meal with many prepared sauces on the market (although it's very easy to make your own). It's perfect for people with busy lives and a delicious way to create healthy meals for active families. However, as it's all too easy to slurp, gulp, twirl and overeat pasta noodles, be sure to keep those portions

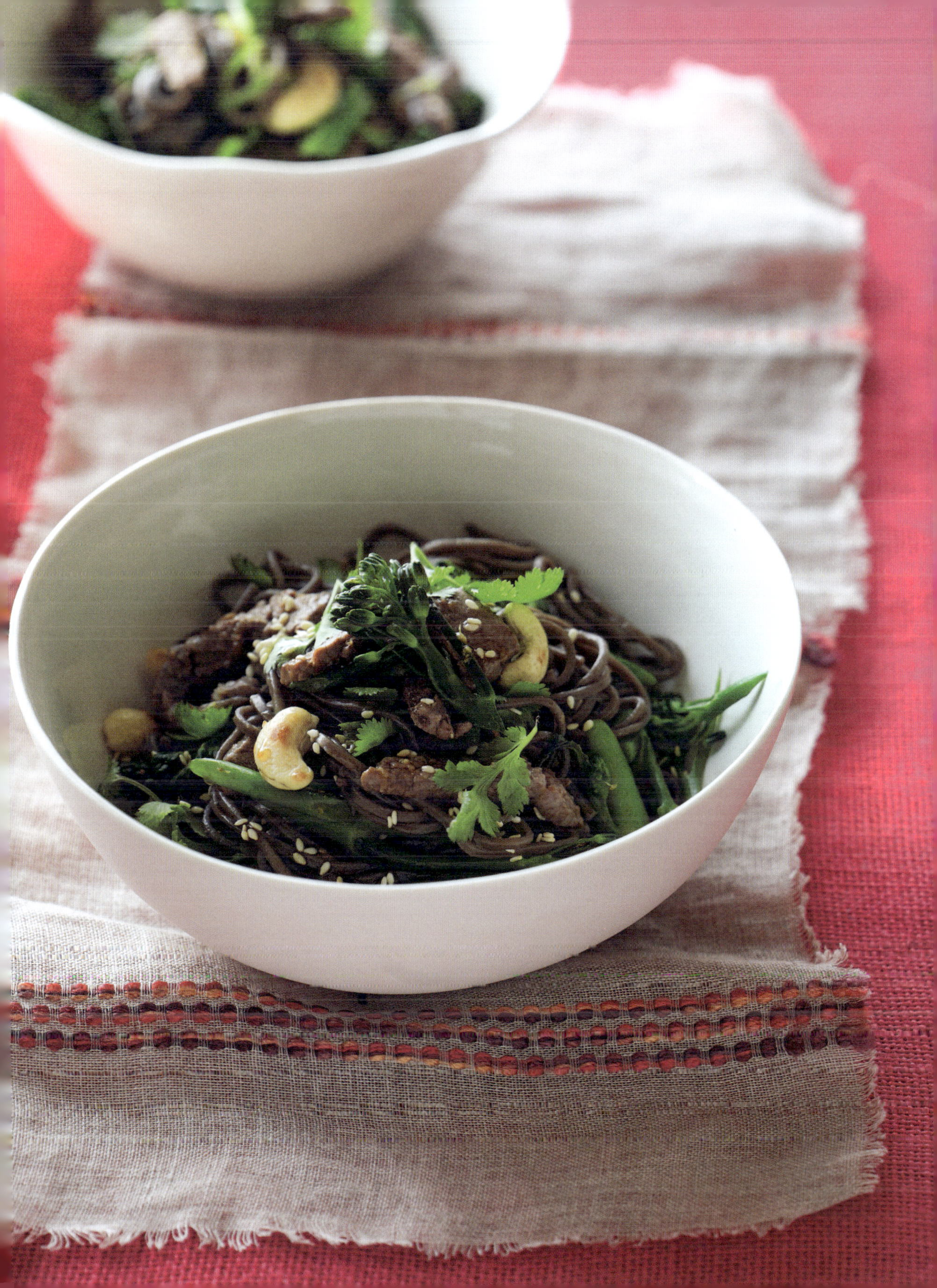

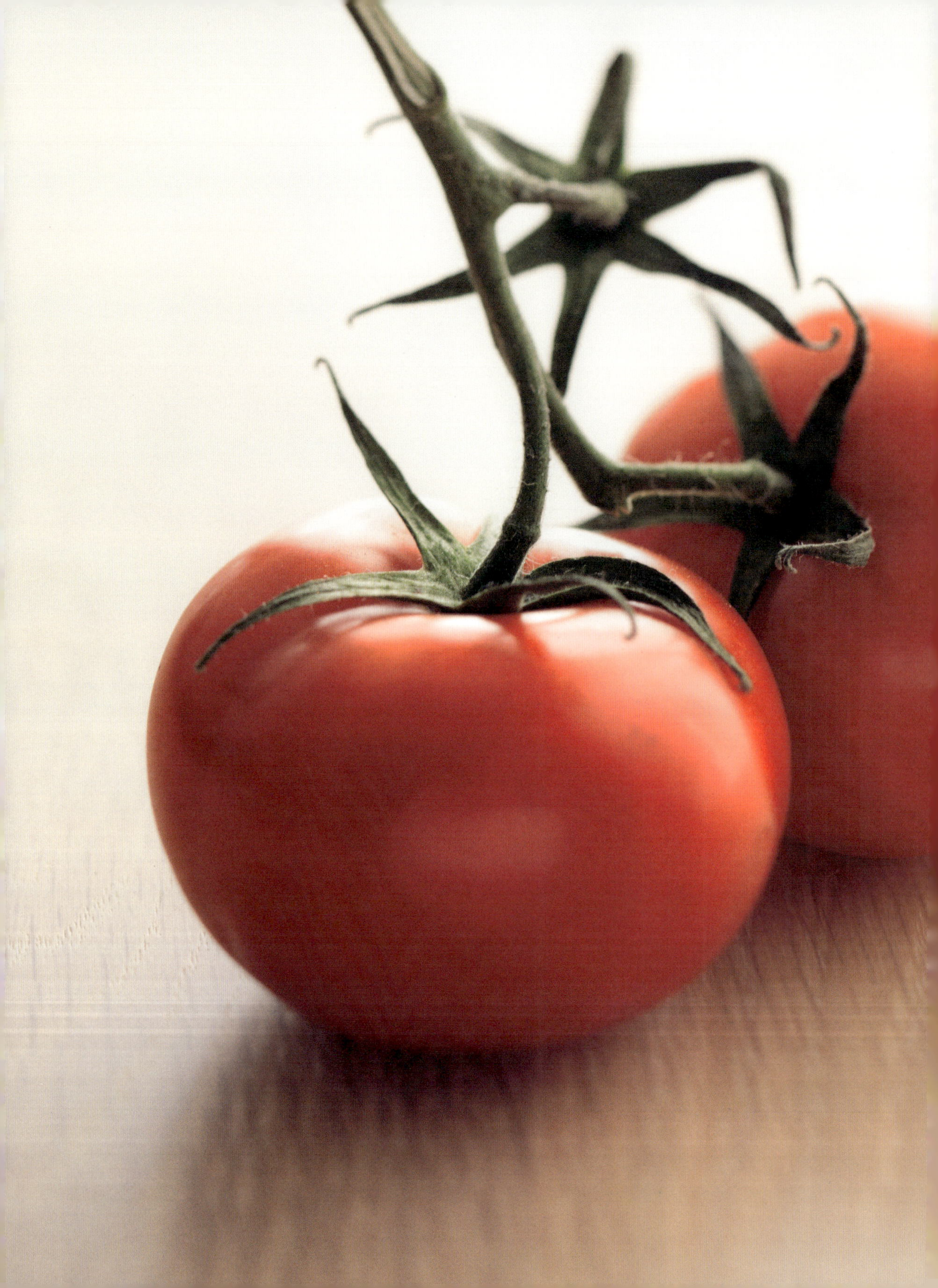

moderate (around a cup of cooked pasta or noodles is plenty for most of us). So, instead of piling your plate with pasta or noodles, serve plenty of vegetables and a little fish, chicken, tofu or lean meat. If dining out, ask for an entrée-size pasta dish.

SAUCE

Remember when planning meals that the sauces you serve with them can provide a lot more kilojoules than the pasta and noodles themselves. For example, if you cook a simple herb and tomato sauce, it keeps a bowl of fettucine light and low-fat, with under 5 grams of fat, due to any olive oil used. But if you go for a creamy sauce like carbonara, these will provide a whopping 30–40 grams of fat, largely saturated fat. With their cream, eggs, bacon and cheese, such pasta dishes have been described as a 'heart attack on a plate'. Pesto sauce is also high in fat with around 30 grams, thanks to its oil, pine nuts and cheese content, but at least it's mainly 'healthy' fat that's kind to your heart.

NUMBER CRUNCH

One serve of cooked pasta or noodles (¼ cup or 90 grams cooked weight) provides 4 grams of protein, less than 1 gram of fat, no sugar, 25 grams of starch, 2 grams of dietary fibre and 525 kilojoules.

See also **Grains and Cereals.**

Pectin

This is a gelling substance found in fruit and vegetables and extracted from apples, plums and orange pith used to set jam. It is a component of fibre. Its additive code is 440.

Phenylalanine

This is an amino acid (component of protein) classified as essential as it cannot be made in the body and so must be obtained from food. It is abundant in the protein of milk and eggs. Treatment of the inherited disorder phenylketonuria (PKU) is via a diet free of the amino acid phenylalanine.

See also **Phenylketonuria.**

Phenylketonuria (PKU)

PKU is an inherited defect of metabolism where an essential enzyme is not made by the body. This causes accumulation of phenylpyruvic acid, which leads to retardation. Affecting one in 10,000 infants, the condition is tested for after birth and can be minimised by a low-phenylalanine diet, which aims to eliminate phenylalanine from protein foods.

Phosphorus *See* **Minerals.**

Phytate

This is a phosphorus-based compound of bran, wholegrains, beans and nuts, which complexes with calcium, iron and zinc, making them unavailable for absorption into the body. Yeast fermentation during bread baking breaks down much of the phytate.

PHYTOCHEMICAL	BEST FOOD SOURCES	NUTRITIONAL VALUE
Carotenoids (includes beta-carotene, lycopene, alpha-carotene, lutein, zeaxanthin and beta-cryptoxanthin)	Yellow-orange fruit and vegetables—pumpkin, carrot, sweet potato, orange, apricot, rock melon. Green vegetables—spinach, silverbeet and Asian greens.	Acts as antioxidant Protects against cancer Enhances immune function.
Lycopene (a carotenoid)	Tomatoes and tomato products, ruby grapefruit, watermelon.	Decreases risk of prostate cancer.
Lutein and zeaxanthin (two carotenoids)	Occur together in spinach, silverbeet, dark-green lettuces and other yellow-orange and green fruit and vegetables.	Protects the macula of the eye from degeneration, a leading cause of vision loss in older adults.
Flavonoids (includes catechins, quercetin, kaempferol)	Wine, grapes, apples, tea, onions and berries, as well as small amounts in most fruits and vegetables.	Acts as antioxidant Reduces the risk of heart disease by minimising the oxidation of LDL cholesterol.
Catechins	Green and black tea.	Powerful antioxidant May help protect against heart disease, skin cancer and stomach cancer.
Isoflavones (phytoestrogen; includes genistein, diadzein and biochanin)	Soy beans, lentils and other beans, tofu, soy milk and peas.	Helps prevent osteoporosis Can interfere with oestrogen synthesis and may cut the risk of breast cancer.
Lignans	Flaxseeds, sesame seeds, most oil seeds (but not in the oil itself), seaweed, brans, wholegrains, beans, fruit and vegetables.	Similar benefits to isoflavones.
Anthocyanins	Blue and purple plants such as cranberries, raspberries, blueberries, blackberries, grapes, eggplant and cocoa.	Powerful antioxidant Has a mild antibacterial effect.
Indoles and isothiocyanates (such as sulphorophane)	Cruciferous vegetables—broccoli, cabbage, cauliflower, Brussels sprouts and turnips.	Triggers the appearance of enzymes which block carcinogens from working Reduces tumour development.
Allicin and related sulfur-compounds	Garlic, onion, leeks and chives.	Antibacterial and anti-viral effects Helps neutralise carcinogens Stimulates enzymes such as glutathione transferase Thins the blood, which may protect against heart disease.
Terpenes (such as limonene)	Citrus fruit—orange, lemon and grapefruit, as well as mushrooms, caraway seeds, ginger, cumin seed and cruciferous vegetables.	Blocks development of cancer tumours in mammary tissues in animals Reduces the size of skin cancers in animals.
Saponins	Soy beans, chickpeas, lentils, alfalfa sprouts, peanuts, oats, liquorice and spinach.	May slow DNA replication in cancer cells that are multiplying.
Curcumin	Turmeric and mustard.	Anti-inflammatory agent May block cancer-causing substances.
Ellagic acid	Grapes, strawberries, raspberries and apples.	Reduces the activity of carcinogens.
Phytates	Dried beans, brans and wholegrains.	Anti-cancer agent.
Coumarins	Parsley, parsnip, cucumber, angelica, carrot, celery, liquorice root, wholegrains, brans and citrus fruit.	Inhibits the growth of cancers.

Phytochemicals

Over the last few years, researchers have discovered a huge number of naturally occurring substances, which nutritionists had previously ignored or dismissed as having no real purpose. The term 'phytochemicals' was coined to cover these numerous plant chemicals, which are biologically active, yet you won't find many of them in supplements. They are another class of protective compounds, just like vitamins and minerals, that may slow the ageing process and protect against cancer or heart disease.

The old saying 'eat by the rainbow' is still a good guide to getting plenty of different types of phytochemicals.

NUTRITIONAL VALUE

Initially, many of these phytochemicals were called antioxidants as researchers believed that they worked their magic by scavenging up free radicals and slowing the damage to cells from oxidation. Some do have antioxidant activity—such as vitamin C and E, and the flavonoids in tea, apples and onions—but not all. Recently we've had to shift thinking for two reasons:

- Phytochemicals work very well in the test tube but not necessarily in the body. So just measuring the antioxidant content of individual foods does not take into account bioavailability or physiological effect, which explains the variations you find in those comparisons of how much antioxidant there is in this berry or that drink.
- They work by different mechanisms or a direct action on one part of the body—at least as far as we can measure. For instance, the catechins or flavonoids are believed to have an impact on blood vessels, helping them stay elastic and flexible to transport blood around the body.

BEST FOOD SOURCES

Phytochemicals occur naturally in all plants, so you'll find them in a wide range of vegetables, fruits, nuts, seeds and cereal grains. They are concentrated in brightly coloured produce, in the bran layer of grain and in the skins of nuts and seeds. The old saying 'eat by the rainbow' is still a good guide to getting plenty of different types of phytochemicals. Certain foods have very high concentrations and are often singled out in studies. Sometimes known as superfoods, these are spices, herbs, most berries, citrus fruit, wine, tea, onions and garlic, cruciferous vegetables, flaxseed, brans and wholegrains.

MY TAKE
The bottom line is that phytochemicals are important but they do not necessarily work as antioxidants—they do other good things.

RECOMMENDED DAILY INTAKE

There are no standard recommended intakes for phytochemicals as there are for vitamins—yet. There may well be set quantities in the future as research progresses. For instance, with the lycopene in tomatoes, early studies showed that somewhere in the order of 6–15 milligrams a day worked to reduce the incidence or severity of prostate cancer. But not all later studies have not been able to confirm this figure.

In contrast, around 200–300 milligrams of flavonoids from tea (3 to 4 cups a day) have been found to be enough to reduce the risk of heart disease. Good advice at the moment is simply to eat a variety of different vegetables and fruits, as well as some tea, wine, dark chocolate and wholegrains.

Phytoestrogens

These are substances present in plants with a chemical structure close to that of the human female hormone oestrogen. Although not as strong, they are able to mimic the effect of oestrogen and may protect against cancer of the breast and cervix as well as heart disease. They were also originally believed to alleviate symptoms of menopause such as hot flushes and vaginal dryness, but to date this has not been supported by clinical trials. The best known types are isoflavones (genistein, diadzein and biochanin), lignans and coumestrans. These are found in soy beans and other legumes as well as flaxseed and rye.

See also **Phytochemicals.**

Pica

Pica is a disorder that includes behaviours such as eating soil, sand, paper or other non-food items. It is thought that it is possibly due to a deficiency of minerals.

Plant Sterols (Phytosterols) *See* **Sterols.**

Polycystic Ovarian Syndrome (PCOS) and Diet

PCOS is the most common endocrine disorder among women of reproductive age. It is a hormonal imbalance thought to affect up to 10 per cent of women. Symptoms include irregular or absent periods, infertility or reduced fertility, hirsutism (excess hair growth on the face, chest and abdomen), alopecia (scalp hair loss), acne, obesity and difficulty losing weight and increased risk of miscarriage. Many women also complain of excessive tiredness and fatigue, hypoglycaemia (low blood sugar), and poor memory and concentration.

We don't know why PCOS develops, but we do know that there are a number of different causes and that most women with PCOS are insulin resistant and thus at risk of heart disease and diabetes. Reducing insulin resistance is not only vital for improving PCOS symptoms, but also for reducing complications that often follow, including heart disease and diabetes.

A DAY ON A PCOS DIET

- BREAKFAST—Natural muesli with yoghurt and sliced peach or canned pears; tea or coffee with low-fat milk.
- MORNING SNACK—Raisin toast with a thin spread of margarine or 2 tablespoons ricotta; tea or herbal tea.
- LUNCH—Open sandwich with ham, cheddar cheese and tomato; tossed green salad; mineral water or diet soft drink.
- AFTERNOON SNACK—Tub of passionfruit yoghurt.
- DINNER—Barbecued or steamed fish fillet with lemon juice and dill; lentil and brown rice risotto; steamed broccoli and green beans; glass of red wine (optional—limit it to three glasses per week if overweight).
- BEFORE BED—Mug of hot low-fat milk with a little honey or Milo.

MANAGING THE SYMPTOMS

Managing PCOS requires an integrated program of lifestyle change and medication to achieve your treatment goals, which might include weight loss, control of acne, regular periods and becoming pregnant.

This generally involves taking metformin, a diabetes drug that also improves ovulation, improves regulation of glucose, decreases risk of miscarriage and turns off the androgens (male hormones). Other drugs may be given that make the body more sensitive to insulin. Fish oil also helps.

Your diet should be low GI to improve insulin sensitivity, and be high in fibre and wholegrains, moderate in salt and sugar, and low in saturated fats.

It should incorporate a variety of vegetables, fruits, nuts, legumes, lean meats, fish and low-fat dairy foods. A diet rich in omega-3s also helps.

REDUCING INSULIN LEVELS

When you have PCOS, reducing insulin levels is important. When it comes to what you eat, the key is reducing the overall glycemic load of your diet. There are two ways you can do this. You can reduce the GI of your diet overall, or reduce your carbohydrate intake. Many women try the second option because it sounds easy to simply cut out the carbs. While this may help short term, it's not the answer for long-term good health and managing your PCOS. The reason for this is that low-carb diets can worsen insulin resistance and they eliminate many of the foods we know are important for good health and reducing the risk of diseases such as cancer, heart disease and diabetes. However, if weight loss is one of your goals, a high-carbohydrate diet is probably not the answer for you either. I suggest a combination of lower carbs emphasising the less-refined, low-GI carbs that trickle glucose into the bloodstream and stabilise blood glucose and insulin levels. These will help keep you feeling fuller for longer and help you maintain a healthy weight.

See also **Glycemic Index; Weight Loss.**

Polydextrose

This is a humectant and bulking agent that's often used as a replacement compound for sugar or fat, adding bulk and texture to low-kilojoule foods. It is only partially digested and so provides only one-quarter of the kilojoules of sugar, i.e. only 4 kilojoules per gram. Very high doses may have a laxative effect. Its additive code is 1200.

Polyphenols

Polyphenols (phenolic compounds) are a diverse group of thousands of compounds all related by their chemical structure. Their chemical structure consists of a number of aromatic rings with each containing at least one hydroxyl group. They are usually divided into flavonoids, non-flavonoid polyphenols such as ellagic acid, and phenolic acids such as chlorogenic acid and hydroxy benzoate. Many are potent antioxidants and can protect the body's tissues from oxidation but they can work by other mechanisms too.

See also **Antioxidants.**

Polysaccharides

Large molecules containing from tens to many thousands of monosaccharides (single units of glucose or other sugars) joined together. Amylose and amylopectin are polysaccharides that are present in starches. Gums and most types of fibre are also polysaccharides.

See also **Carbohydrates; Fibre.**

Portion Sizes

Portion sizes have been getting bigger and bigger over the past 20 years and it's now clear that they've been a major contributor to the obesity problem. There's a name for it—portion creep. The portion on your plate may be as many as eight times the amount that represents a standard serve. The problem is that the bigger the portion in front of you, the more you tend to eat. But if you know to look out for

> US researchers have tracked this upward trend in serve sizes. They report that from 1991 to 1996, the size of juices increased by 30 per cent, and wine and soft drink rose by 50 per cent.

portion distortion, you can enjoy a favourite treat without the ever-present danger of overeating.

US researchers have tracked this upward trend in serve sizes. They report that from 1991 to 1996, the size of juices increased by 30 per cent, and wine and soft drink rose by 50 per cent.

Look again at what you buy. What used to be considered a family-size block of chocolate is now the standard size. Fizzy drinks come in huge 1.5 litre bottles (25 per cent more for free; but you also get to keep the fat the extra kilojoules add). Movie popcorn is sold in buckets, muffins balloon out of their paper cases and fresh juice comes in a 650 millilitre cup—equal to six or seven pieces of whole fruit. Fast-food operators are the masters at upsizing. Supersized serves and two-for-one meal deals may be great value for money, but it's a bargain that our waistlines don't need.

USE YOUR HANDS

Meat, chicken, fish (cooked)	75 to 100 g	The palm of your hand or a deck of cards.
Pasta, rice (cooked)	½ cup	The size of your fist or a computer mouse.
Vegetables	½ cup	The size of your fist or a computer mouse.
Fruit	½ cup	A medium apple, pear or orange is the size of a tennis ball.
Cheese (hard)	45 g	Your thumb or a C-size battery.

TIPS FOR PREVENTING PORTION CREEP

- Serve meals on smaller plates in the kitchen rather than at the table.
- With main meals, make sure half your plate is green or salad veggies (not including starchy ones like potatoes).
- Don't go back for seconds.
- You don't have to clean your plate; stop when you feel full.
- Women generally need smaller portions than men; if you eat together as a couple, don't eat the same-sized serves.
- When eating out, if there's a choice, opt for the smaller size.
- Ask for a 'doggie bag' to take leftovers home for later.
- When it comes to treats, indulge in the real thing, but be satisfied with less.

SNACKS AND CONFECTIONERY

Most popular snacks are more than a just a quick bite—they're really a mini-meal. Take doughnuts as an example. At 20 grams of fat and more than 2000 kilojoules, two cinnamon doughnuts pile on one-third of the day's recommended intake of fat and kilojoules for a sedentary woman. Most of this fat is saturated and trans—the type that clogs arteries and thickens waistlines. Ditto for pastries, a bucket of hot chips or a large slice of banana bread.

HEALTHY SNACKS UNDER 600 KILOJOULES

Try to keep snacks in their proper proportion compared to meals. For example, snack on:

- ✔ Ready-prepared fresh fruit salad—it's light, fresh and the lowest in kilojoules of all the snacks at around 300 kilojoules
- ✔ A handful of almonds (about 20)—rich in good unsaturated fats, nuts make a healthy snack and give your heart a health bonus, 600 kilojoules
- ✔ One slice of raisin toast with a light spread of butter or margarine—low in GI, this warming snack will help keep hunger pangs away until your next meal, 565 kilojoules

- ✔ Small tub (150 grams) of diet fruit yoghurt—a light, high-calcium snack, 580 kilojoules
- ✔ Snack-box (40 grams) of sultanas—this is about 100 sultanas if you want to count them! 510 kilojoules
- ✔ Thin slice (45 grams) banana bread, no spread—this is around a third of your average café slice, 590 kilojoules
- ✔ Nineteen rice crackers—count them out then put away the packet. Once you start munching, it's hard to stop, 585 kilojoules.

TREATS UNDER 600 KILOJOULES

- ✔ Fun-size (25 g) Mars bar—it's only one mouthful, but it may satisfy that chocolate craving.
- ✔ Small packet (25 g) of potato crisps—this is the smallest pack available, the same size as those in the multi-packs to put in the kids' lunch box. It is half the size of what's on offer in vending machines or petrol stations.
- ✔ 375 ml can of beer—great to drink after a hard day, but stick to one if you're serious about weight loss.
- ✔ One glass of white wine (200 ml)—this is the size of wine generally poured these days—but it is actually equivalent to two standard drinks, not one.
- ✔ Twelve jelly babies—for when you want a sugar fix without fat!
- ✔ One Tim Tam biscuit—yes, just one!
- ✔ Small (25 g) pack of smarties—stick to the small pack and you'll be OK.

See also Weight Loss; Junk Food; Fast Food.

Potassium

Potassium is the predominant mineral in all body cells. Together with sodium, it maintains the electrical differential of the cell membrane and so controls the working of muscles and nerves. Potassium is a complementary mineral to sodium and plays a major role in normalising blood pressure and overcoming a high salt intake. Along with magnesium, potassium helps preserve bone calcium. Potassium is believed to act in place of calcium to neutralise acids in the body. Magnesium helps transport potassium into bones, so it is able to carry out this task and contribute to the mineral content of the skeleton. Diets high in fruits and vegetables are rich in both these minerals.

FOOD	POTASSIUM (mg)	SODIUM (mg)	RATIO*
Tomatoes, fresh	200	6	33 to 1
Tomatoes, canned	184	62	3 to 1
Tomato soup	224	342	0.7 to 1
Potatoes, boiled	430	3	143 to 1
Potato chips	540	180	3 to 1
Potato crisps	1200	640	2 to 1
Beetroot, fresh	290	54	6 to 1
Beetroot, canned	140	300	0.5 to 1

*The higher the ratio of potassium to sodium, the better for your health.

DAILY REQUIREMENTS

Requirements are 2800 milligrams or 72 millimoles (women) and 3800 milligrams or 97 millimoles (men).

SAFE UPPER LIMIT

There is no firm data, but over 10,000 milligrams (10 grams) in a single dose may cause cardiac arrest.

BEST FOOD SOURCES

Potassium is widely distributed in nuts, yeast extract, dried fruit, coffee, bran, wheat germ, raw vegetables, lean meat, fish and fruit (fruit juice in particular). In natural, unsalted foods at least twice as much potassium as sodium is present, which is an ideal ratio to aim for. For example, fresh tomatoes have a potassium-to-sodium ratio of 33 to 1. Canned tomatoes, on the other hand, have salt added and so have a ratio of 3 to 1—just three times more potassium than sodium. Tomato sauce rates even worse at 0.2 to 1, while tomato soup is so salty it comes out at 0.7 to 1.

See also **Minerals.**

Potassium Chloride

Potassium chloride is a white crystalline powder commonly used as a salt substitute (table salt is sodium chloride), although it leaves a bitter metallic aftertaste when added in large amounts. Care must be taken to avoid overuse, especially by people with heart problems, as excess potassium can cause heart irregularities. Used as a mineral salt in food manufacture. Its additive code is 508.

Potatoes *See* **Vegetables.**

Poultry

Poultry (chicken, turkey, duck, goose, quail and spatchcock) used to be fare for a special occasion, but over the past 50 years its consumption has been steadily increasing. Changes to farm production, concentration of ownership with high vertical integration and intense competition have all played a part in making poultry affordable and consistent in quality.

MY TAKE
I like chicken shops because there are always salads to team up with your chicken, unlike other fast food. So please, order two salads with your chicken and you'll raise your dinner to a new level of nutrition stardom! I like a tabbouli plus a tangy Greek salad—it just seems to hit the spot.

CHICKEN

Chicken consumption has risen steadily over the last 50 years, and it is now a staple meat—a far cry from the expensive, once-a-year bird of the 1950s. In terms of volumes consumed, chicken meat is close to replacing beef as Australia's preferred meat. Chicken's low price and consistent quality have played a large role in this change. Its use by fast-food producers—unfortunately usually in deep-fried form—has also helped.

Chicken's versatility is a key to its growing popularity. There are countless chicken products, from whole birds to deboned cuts (breasts, thigh fillets and mince) and, lately, a whole range of ready-to-cook kebabs, half drumsticks and marinated, crumbed or stuffed pieces. It is the most popular of all poultry, accounting for 90 per cent of poultry production. Turkey is next in line and is growing in volume while duck, goose, quail and spatchcock are minor products by comparison.

NUTRITIONAL VALUE

Considered a 'white meat', chicken is favoured by consumers wanting a meat that is low in fat and cholesterol. However, recent university tests of Australian meat and poultry reveal that there is little difference between skinless chicken and lean cuts of red meat such as topside, rump and chuck steak. Chicken's cholesterol count is higher than beef's, and its fat level can be high if the skin is eaten. Most of the fat lies in the skin—a skinless chicken breast has only 5 per cent fat after cooking, but if roasted with the skin on, it contains 13 per cent. On the plus side, serving sizes of chicken tend to be smaller, so the total intake of fat, cholesterol and kilojoules can be less than from beef.

Chicken is a nutritious food and contributes essential protein, B vitamins and minerals like iron and zinc. It has around one-third of the iron content of red meat, but it is well absorbed. The light meat from the breast is lower in fat than the dark meat on the thigh and drumstick.

NUMBER CRUNCH

A 125 gram serve of roast chicken (cooked without the skin) provides 19 grams of protein, 15 grams of fat, 3 grams of carbohydrate, 3 grams of sugar, zero fibre and 925 kilojoules.

THE GIANT CHICKEN MYTH

Does your local shop advertise 'hormone-free' chickens? If so, their chickens are just the same as everywhere else. The use of growth hormones was banned back in the 1960s (historically, oestrogen was once fed to young male chickens as an alternative to castration). Knowing consumers want to be confident that producers abide by this ban, the government's National Residue Survey tests chicken (and all other produce) for hormonal growth promoters and to date, no residues have been detected since the ban, which means that all chicken meat on the market is hormone free. Hormones are often confused with antimicrobials, which are given to animals to enhance digestion and kill off any bad bacteria that would otherwise cause disease (similar to the friendly probiotic bacteria in yoghurt). Only antimicrobials not absorbed from the gut can be used, and all are thoroughly assessed and approved by the regulatory authorities. Chickens are bigger than they used to be due to selective breeding (mating big birds with big birds over a period of time), a better diet, and improved healthcare and animal husbandry practices.

TURKEY

Turkey sales are increasing. Well priced, easy turkey cuts including breasts, steaks, wings, drumsticks, schnitzel and mince are making it easy for consumers to use it as a substitute for chicken in a wide range of recipes. I have even seen the drumsticks suggested as a substitute for pricy lamb shanks.

NUTRITIONAL VALUE

Like chicken, turkey is a nutritious food contributing essential protein, B vitamins and minerals like iron and zinc. Overall it's slightly lower in fat than chicken, though they are the same in that the light meat from the breast is lower in fat than the dark meat on the thigh and drumstick.

DUCK

Duck seems to be one of those foods (like fish and seafood) that most of us enjoy more often when eating out than cooking at home—except perhaps over the Christmas festive season. At least that was until the MasterChef recipes like sweet and sour duck, duck tortellini, grilled duck breast and confit duck came along, making consumers more interested in giving it a go. Whole duck or breasts, legs and marylands and other cuts are available in specialty poultry shops and larger supermarkets.

SHOPPER'S GUIDE

The charcoaled chook is hard to make a nutritional judgement on. Individual chicken shops serve it differently with some giving it an extra basting of oil during cooking, while others let the fat drip away. If you're lucky enough to live near a proper Portuguese char-grilled chicken outlet, you'll be able to get those crispy, flattened semi-boned chickens that are delightful to eat and usually a lot less fatty than the standard barbecued chooks. Whichever chicken you buy, the one big advantage is that you can pull away the skin (yes—be strong!) removing most of the salt and a lot of the fat. Sucking the chicken meat off the bones is surely one of life's great joys—even if char-grilling at high temperatures creates nasty carcinogens that are associated with cancer.

NUTRITIONAL VALUE

Like other poultry, it is a nutritious food, contributing essential protein, B vitamins and minerals like iron and zinc. Skin on, they are fattier than chickens and turkey. This is because they swim, so have a fat layer beneath the skin to help keep them afloat. That's why before cooking a whole bird, you need to prick the skin all over with a fork to render out the fat during cooking.

Prebiotics

This is a non-digestible food component that stimulates the growth or activity of the friendly bacteria in the large bowel. The best studied are inulin (fructo-oligo-fructose) extracted from chicory, high-amylose starch (Hi-Maize) and polydextrose. These are often added to foods to provide a food source for the bacteria during storage and listed as 'fibre' on the ingredient list. Natural prebiotics are found in almost all high-fibre foods but especially in onions, garlic, legumes, asparagus and wholegrains—particularly rye.

Pregnancy, Breastfeeding and Diet

A nutritious diet is always important for your health, but it's vital when you are pregnant. Your baby depends entirely on you for all the nutrients it needs to grow and develop. A healthy diet will also help you enjoy a healthy pregnancy with plenty of energy, glowing skin and shiny hair. The good news is that it's never too late in your pregnancy to improve your diet, and these changes will help you set a healthy example for your family for a lifetime.

EAT FOR YOU, NOT FOR TWO

While it's important to gain the right amount of weight during pregnancy, the old advice of eating for two is not the way to do it. The extra kilojoules needed don't really become significant until the second trimester, when they add another 1400 kilojoules extra a day, rising to 1900 extra in the third trimester—if you are a healthy weight to start with. Overweight women do not need as much as underweight women, thus requiring fewer additional kilojoules.

This does not mean you should diet in pregnancy, though. While you should eat nutritious foods and limit things like chips, pastries, takeaways, biscuits, chocolate and soft drinks, now is not the time to skimp on kilojoules. Gaining anywhere from 9 to 14 kilograms is vital for your baby's growth and development—count the weeks, not the kilojoules!

If you are breastfeeding, you may feel more hungry than usual and require more energy—up to about 2000 kilojoules more if you are fully breastfeeding for 6 months. Again, eat nutritious foods including additional serves of milk, yoghurt or cheese, fruit, nuts or some avocado, grainy bread or fish for omega-3s.

KEEP THE BOWELS REGULAR

Constipation is a common complaint during pregnancy, so keep your fibre and fluid intake high. Best foods for regularity include bran cereals, legumes (baked beans are easy), wholegrain breads, dried fruit and vegetables. Plenty of water and a daily walk also help.

BONE BUILDING

If you don't have enough calcium during pregnancy, the store of calcium in your own bones will be drained to support your baby's developing bones and teeth. Keep your bones safe from osteoporosis by making sure you get four serves of calcium-rich foods a day from low-fat milk, yoghurt and cheeses. Alternatively, opt for a calcium supplement.

BRAIN FOOD

Essential omega-3 fats are vital to your baby's brain, nervous tissues and eyes. So include fish and seafood, lean meats and omega-enriched eggs regularly in your diet. Eat two to three serves of fish a week but avoid fish with high mercury levels such as shark, broadbill, marlin, swordfish and orange roughy (sometimes called ocean or deep sea perch).

Iodine is also critical during pregnancy because even mild deficiencies can cause learning and developmental difficulties in toddlers. Iodised salt is now added to bread and some comes from iodine-rich foods (such as seafood and seaweed), but it's a good idea to take a supplement of 150 mg daily during pregnancy and breastfeeding.

FOODS TO AVOID

Listeriosis is an illness that can be picked up from the common foods we all eat. It causes few symptoms in healthy people, but can lead to serious illness or miscarriage in the unborn child. Risk of infection can be greatly reduced by good hygiene practices at home and taking care with ready-to-eat foods when out. Foods to avoid include:

- Paté
- Smoked seafood
- Soft cheeses such as brie, camembert, ricotta, blue vein and feta
- Cold deli meats
- Salads that are prepared, pre-packaged or served from smorgasbords or salad bars
- Chilled seafood such as oysters and sashimi
- Pre-prepared sandwiches with cold meat fillings
- Foods that are not kept very hot
- Soft-serve ice-cream
- Unpasteurised milk and any dairy products made from it
- Raw or lightly cooked eggs
- Raw sprouts, especially alfalfa sprouts
- Unpasteurised juices.

ALCOHOL AND CAFFEINE

As soon as you suspect you are pregnant or your pregnancy is confirmed, cut out alcohol. It's not known exactly how much is safe to drink when you are expecting, so it's best to stop it altogether as it can cause physical defects and learning disabilities in children. You might want to keep your caffeine intake to a minimum too—no more than about two cups of instant coffee, one cappuccino, or three cups of tea a day.

Not drinking alcohol is the safest option when breastfeeding also. If you wish to drink alcohol you should avoid it in the first month after delivery until breastfeeding is well established. After that, limit your alcohol intake to no more than two standard drinks a day and you should avoid drinking immediately before breastfeeding. You should also consider expressing milk in advance as alcohol is concentrated in breast milk.

MY TAKE

Throughout your pregnancy, make sure you eat regular meals and snacks and avoid getting overly hungry. Skipping breakfast is a no-no!

FOLATE

Folate is a B vitamin required for baby's neural tube and spinal cord development. You need more folate in the first 3 months of pregnancy to reduce the risk of neural tube defects such as spina bifida. This can be met with naturally folate-rich foods such as leafy vegetables, avocados, wholemeal bread, nuts (almonds, hazelnuts, peanuts and walnuts), yeast extract (Vegemite, Marmite), oranges and orange juice. Folate is also added to cereals, breads and many juices. In addition, a supplement of 400 micrograms daily is recommended.

See also Calcium; Fibre; Folate; Gestational Diabetes; Iodine; Iron; Omega-3 and Omega-6 Essential Fatty Acids.

IRON

Pregnant women need plenty of iron—women normally require 18 milligrams a day throughout their adult lives, and this jumps to 27 milligrams during pregnancy. It is hard to meet these needs without red meat or an iron tablet. For breastfeeding mums, it drops back to 18 milligrams a day. Iron-rich foods will keep your energy levels up and help build baby's iron stores. Red meat is the best source of easily absorbed iron, with lesser amounts found in chicken and fish.

Preservatives

Preservatives are substances able to slow the spoilage of food by preventing the growth of mould and bad bacteria. Some act as antioxidants to prevent food from oxidising or going rancid.

The earliest preservatives were ingredients already in the pantry—salt, vinegar, alcohol and sugar. Foods that are made with high levels of these ingredients (like jam) do not need preservatives. Chemical preservatives act in a similar fashion to these pantry ingredients such as sugar and salt. The most commonly used preservatives are sorbates, benzoates, sulphur dioxide and sulphites, and propionates.

CULPRIT CHEMICALS

Preservatives can cause problems for some people.

PRESERVATIVE GROUP	DETAILS	CHEMICAL NAME AND CODE NUMBER
BENZOATES	Benzoates occur in cranberries, bilberries and other fruit, vegetables, pepper, herbs, spices, peppermint and honey. Sodium benzoate and potassium benzoate are used as preservatives in soft drinks, cordials and fruit drinks. Both must be avoided by sensitive people who can experience general symptoms of intolerance such as an upset tummy, migraine, fatigue and skin rash.	Benzoic acid 210 Sodium benzoate 211 Potassium benzoate 212 Calcium benzoate 213
SULPHITES	The early Greeks used sulphur to preserve wine. Sulphur and its related compounds of sulphur dioxide and sulphites destroy undesirable bacteria in wine storage vats, prevent the darkening of dried fruit (in particular apricots and apples) and juices, and are used to preserve soft drinks, pickled onions and sausages. In sensitive asthma patients they can trigger wheezing and throat tightening, often within one or two minutes of consumption.	Sulphur dioxide 220 Sodium sulphite 221 Sodium bisulphite 222 Sodium metabisulphite 223 Potassium metabisulphite 224 Potassium sulphite 225 Potassium bisulphite 228
PROPIONATES	Propionates are used to inhibit the growth of mould, particularly in baked goods like breads and cakes. They also occur naturally in many foods, such as Swiss cheese.	Propionic acid 280 Sodium propionate 281 Calcium propionate 282 Potassium propionate 283
NITRITES	Nitrates are used to preserve meats such as ham, bacon, corned beef, salamis, hot dogs, frankfurters and luncheon meats. They can be converted into nitrosamines in the body, which may cause cancer.	Potassium nitrite 249 Sodium nitrite 250 Sodium nitrate 251 Potassium nitrate 252

PRESERVING FOOD WITHOUT ADDITIVES

There are many shoppers, like me, who want to buy foods that are safe to eat, but contain the minimum amount of additives, or are additive free. Traditional ways of preserving the bounty of the harvest for use throughout the year were bottling, pickling, drying and smoking. Of course, many foods are still preserved this way. In addition to these, today there are a number of other ways food can be preserved and made shelf-stable without any additives. Of these, canning, ultra high-temperature (UHT) processing and freezing are the most common.

Canned foods are prepared from fresh ingredients, without the addition of preservatives. It involves heat treatment—pretty much as you would cook them yourself.

UHT stands for 'ultra heat treated' and is often just called 'longlife' milk. It involves a higher temperature treatment of milk or juice, which inactivates all bacteria and enzymes but does not harm the protein or vitamins. It is then maintained in aseptic packing, which means the drink, if unopened, keeps for about 5 months unrefrigerated, a great help when refrigeration is limited.

Freezing is better than canning as frozen vegetables retain a lot more of the heat-sensitive nutrients (particularly vitamin C, thiamin and folate), and have a better texture. Also, there's little additional salt, which is a big drawback with canned vegetables.

See also **Additives; Allergies; Food Processing.**

Preschool-aged Children and Diet

4–6 years

A good rule of thumb to guide parents through this stage is to remember that parents decide what children eat; children decide how much and when. As the parent, it's up to you as to what foods to have in your pantry. Have strong boundaries. If you have a healthy selection for the child to choose from, this will make your job easier! Involve the kids in food shopping and preparation so it teaches them about foods and gives them a sense of responsibility and ownership.

YOU VERSUS ADVERTISING

Pre-packaged foods aimed at this age group are often promoted using bright colours, fun cartoon characters and the offer of free toys, creating an experience that leads preschoolers down the 'pester power' path. They develop a strong desire for processed, unhealthy foods and drinks, and badger their parents for them. When our children were little, I had a rule that I never bought fizzy drinks or potato chips. While they whinged about it, the kids knew there simply weren't any in the house. They were 'party foods' that were only around for treats or birthdays, not after school or as a lunchbox extra.

> **RECOMMENDED DAILY INTAKE**
> Ranges from 5500 kJ for a sedentary, inactive girl to 8200 kJ for a sporty, active boy.

Primary School–aged Children and Diet

7–12 years

Primary-school children should be eating at least five serves of vegetables and two pieces of fruit every day. Creativity becomes a key ingredient in ensuring lunchboxes are filled with fun, colourful, nutritious foods that appeal to the child and are easy to eat when there's lot to distract them in the playground.

BREAKFAST

Creating a pattern of making time for a good breakfast every day is also extremely important at this age. Breakfast provides the fuel to help children concentrate and sustain their learning, and the energy for them to play. Set up good eating habits early. Teachers often schedule complex maths classes in the morning periods so fuel for the brain early in the day is critical. Having breakfast also makes it less likely your kids will have an attack of the mid-morning munchies.

EAT TOGETHER

Aim to eat together as a family as often as you can. It's not only important for encouraging good manners and conversation, but leads to better-quality diets for children, according to a number of recent studies. Turn the television off and talk about your day. Busy schedules and work commitments often mean that families eat together on average only three nights of the week.

RECOMMENDED DAILY INTAKE

Ranges from 6500 kJ for a sedentary, inactive girl, to 11 600 kJ for a sporty, active boy.

SNACKS

I've always believed that children need snacks! With their small stomach capacity, they can't survive on just three meals a day, so top up their intake with something in between. But avoid those colourfully packaged snack foods and include nutritious foods that contain calcium, vitamins or wholegrains.

See also **Snacks.**

Probiotics

We've all seen those little bottles of milky drinks in the dairy cabinet at the supermarket, the ones that claim to keep you 'healthy on the inside'. And then there are the yoghurts with *Lactobacillus acidophilus* or ABC cultures, which are marketed as the way to digestive health. Probiotics, or friendly bacteria, are a health trend, but do they work, and if so, how often do you need to take them?

LONG-LIVING BULGARIANS

The idea of consuming good bacteria for health is not new. It dates back to the early 20th century when a Russian scientist, Dr Élie Metchnikoff (1845–1919), suggested that the long lifespan of Bulgarian peasants was due to their consumption of yoghurt fermented with *Lactobacillus* (the bacteria used in yoghurt). Metchnikoff believed the lactobacillus exerted an important influence on intestinal health. The word probiotic was later coined to describe these 'good bacteria'. Derived from Greek, it simply means 'for life' or 'for health'. Probiotics were initially applied to yoghurt bacteria because scientists were trying to test Metchnikoff's theory.

INNER BALANCE

Our intestine is host to more than 500 species and sub-species of bacteria, collectively known as gut flora. They are most important for health and among other things, they produce vitamin K, vitamin B_{12} and folate. This flora is typically made up of a healthy balance of good and bad bugs. If the balance tips and the bad bugs start to multiply (due to things such as stress, infection or antibiotics), our digestive system suffers and so do we.

In contrast, probiotics are those friendly bacteria or live microbes that, when consumed, can stabilise the intestine's resident bacteria, restoring our natural balance in the digestive system. Beneficial in a number of ways, they can:

- ✔ Replace normal bacteria that have been killed off by a course of antibiotics
- ✔ Produce substances that make your internal environment unwelcoming for salmonella, rotavirus and other harmful bugs
- ✔ Shorten episodes of diarrhoea, including traveller's and toddler diarrhoea
- ✔ Aid digestion
- ✔ Prevent 'leaky gut' so the internal lining of your intestine is less likely to let allergens through
- ✔ Stimulate the immune system
- ✔ Regulate your bowel movements and ease constipation and flatulence
- ✔ Ease irritable bowel syndrome and Crohn's disease
- ✔ Digest the lactose from milk
- ✔ Induce anti-cancer activity
- ✔ De-activate harmful enzymes in the intestine.

DID YOU KNOW?

Probiotics that are past their use-by date or not kept cold simply won't have the number of viable bacteria present. It's best to:

- ✔ Store the probiotic correctly—keep it chilled at all times, especially during the trip home from the supermarket.
- ✔ Buy from a large supermarket with fast turnover so the probiotic is fresh.
- ✔ Consume it within a couple of days.

WHO AND HOW MUCH

As a general rule, a probiotic two or three times a week is good for overall health, but if you are ill or need to correct bacterial imbalance, then aim to consume it twice a day. This could include those who:

- ✔ Have just finished a course of antibiotics
- ✔ Are recovering from a bout of gastro
- ✔ Have diarrhoea
- ✔ Need to undergo bowel decontamination before surgery
- ✔ Require a major diet change
- ✔ Are stressed
- ✔ Will be travelling where the water or food may not be safe.

FERMENTED FOODS

Live bacteria are found in a number of different sources:

- Fermented dairy foods such as kefir, lassi and yoghurts, but particularly those with added probiotic strains (such as L66 or HOWARU)
- Low levels in fresh sauerkraut (not canned or bottled, which have been heat-treated), olives in brine, pickled cucumbers, camembert, blue vein and other mould-containing cheeses, tempeh and sourdough bread
- Capsules and powders of lactic acid or acidophilus or bifidus strains—ideally freeze-dried and stored in the refrigerator (such as VSL#3 or Forbiotic)
- Milk drinks with added bacteria (such as Yakult)
- Human breast milk.

CHOOSING THE RIGHT YOGHURT

Most yoghurt sold in supermarkets today is made with a starter culture, so you know you're getting some probiotics. But the level of lactic acid bacteria (such as *Lactobacillus acidophilus*, *Bifidobacterium* and *Lactobacillus casei*) is not sufficient in all yoghurts to give you the digestive benefits I'm talking about.

You need to look for yoghurts that contain both a starter bacteria as well as an added probiotic. These are special strains of clinically tested bacteria such as the Shirota strain in Yakult and the *Lactobacillus* GG in Vaalia or *L. casei* DN–114 001 in Actimel, which are added after the yoghurt or drink has been made. To

> As a general rule, a probiotic two or three times a week is good for overall health, but if you are ill or need to correct bacterial imbalance, then aim to consume it twice a day.

be classified as a probiotic, the strain must be present in sufficient numbers in the product. Most importantly, it must be able to survive the gastric juices and bile acids to arrive at the small or large intestine, where it can grow and multiply.

Not all bacteria can manage this. Only those tested and proven can claim to be genuine probiotics. This doesn't mean ordinary yoghurt isn't an excellent food, but if you're seeking help for a medical problem (to recover from diarrhoea, for example), you need to buy those specific brands.

PREBIOTIC BOOSTERS

Most probiotic yoghurts contain fibre booster substances called prebiotics, which aid the delivery of active cultures to the digestive system. In other words, the booster acts as food for the friendly bacteria so they can grow and multiply inside you and do their good work.

See also Prebiotics.

Processed Food

Processing food duplicates practices that have been done for centuries—drying, salting, bottling, chilling, smoking and, more recently, freezing and canning. To make food available all year round, some processing is essential. Manufacturers pick produce at its peak and can or snap-freeze it, usually losing little in terms of quality and taste.

BEST	Chilled
	Frozen
	Canned
	UHT
	Dried/dehydrated
	Smoked
	Salted
WORST	Pickled

In all these processes, there is always some loss of nutrients. Heat destroys some vitamins—with vitamins C, B_1 and folic acid being most sensitive—but it's no different from home cooking; for example, you lose some vitamin C when you steam vegetables. Cooking and processing can actually improve certain nutrients. Lycopene is more readily available from canned tomatoes and pasta sauce than from fresh tomatoes, and cooking carrots raises their beta-carotene levels. It's all a matter of balance between processed and fresh fare.

See also Additives; Preservatives.

Protein

Protein is required throughout life to create, maintain and renew our body cells. Enzymes, antibodies, haemoglobin and other blood compounds are assembled from proteins or are proteins themselves.

AMINO ACIDS—THE BUILDING BLOCKS

Proteins are made up of chains of amino acids. There are only around 20 amino acids occurring in food, but the number of combinations in which they are arranged is infinite. Eight of these amino acids are essential, even though they cannot be made by the body and must be provided by food. These are isoleucine, leucine, lysine, methionine,

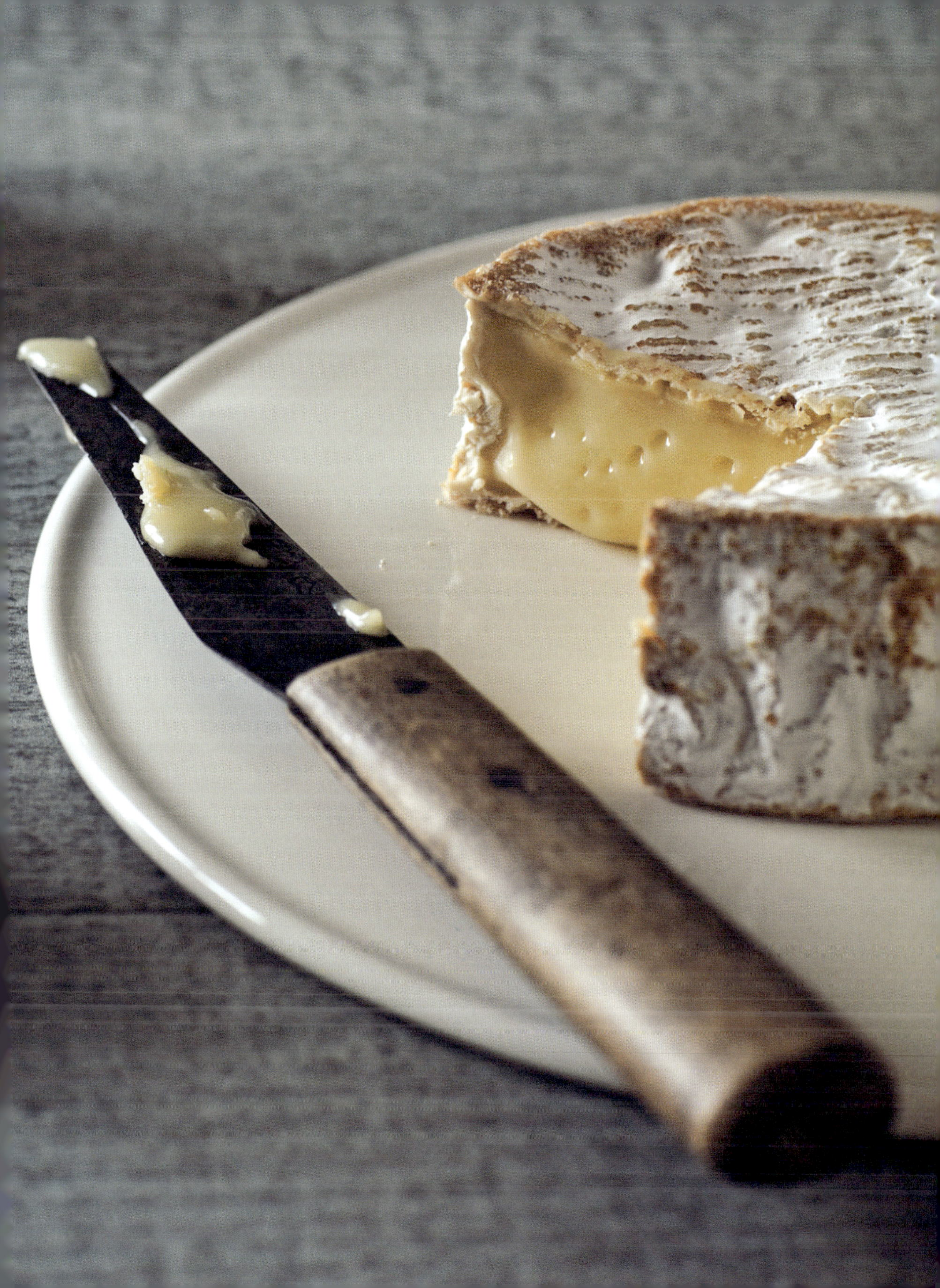

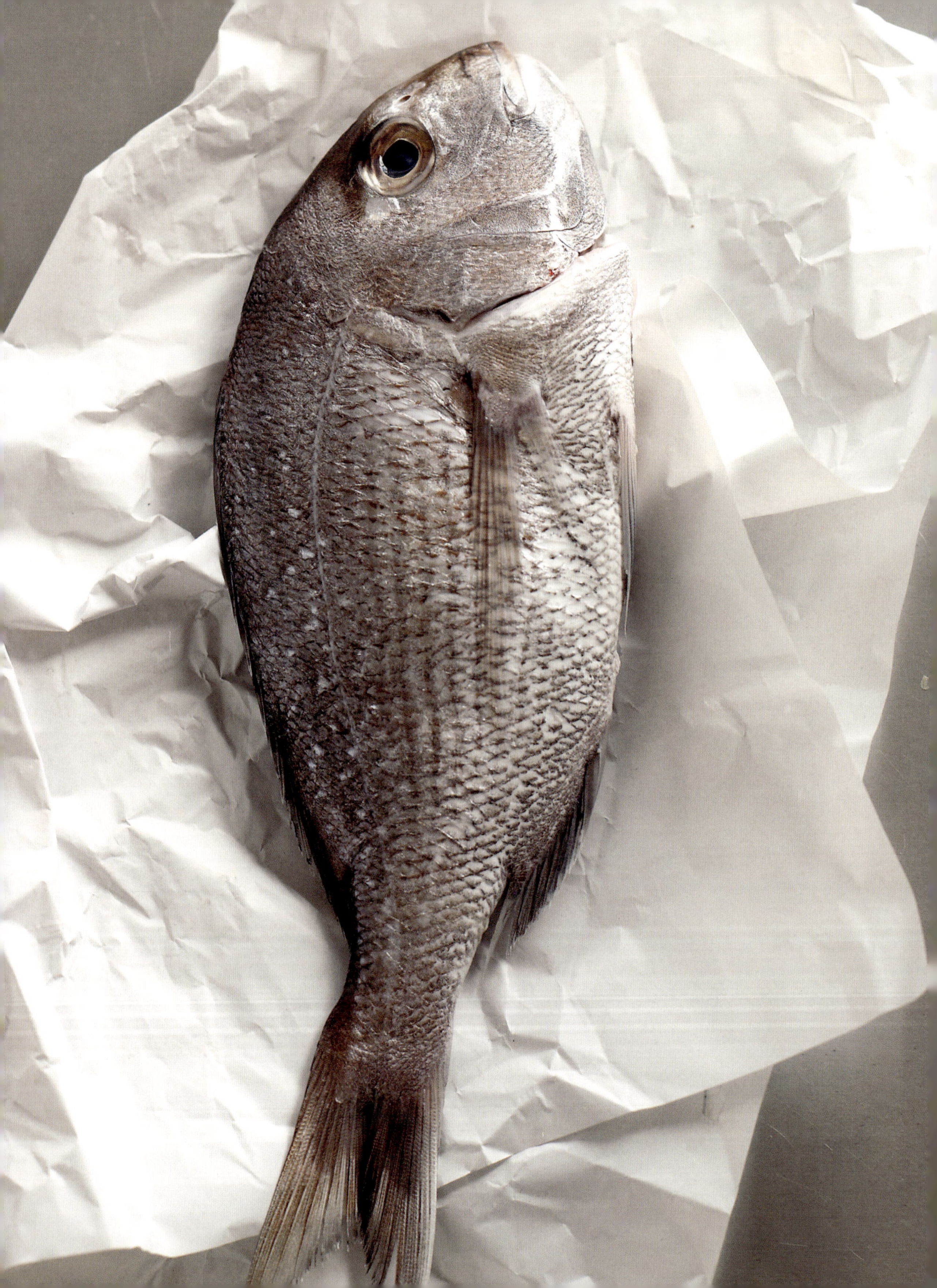

ANIMAL PROTEIN	% PROTEIN
Milk powder, non-fat	36
Chicken, roasted	28
Liver or lamb, fried	27
Milk powder, full-cream	27
Beef (lean), roasted	27
Cheddar cheese	26
Pork (lean), grilled	26
Tuna, canned in brine	22
Prawns	20
Fish (white), steamed	18–26
Cottage cheese	16
Devon and other lunch meats	15
Eggs	13
Yoghurt, plain low-fat	7
Milk, full-cream and low-fat	3–4

PLANT PROTEIN	% PROTEIN
Yeast spread	24
Wheat germ	24
Sesame seeds	22
Cocoa powder	19
Wheat bran	17
Soy beans, boiled	14
Nuts	13–25
Flour, wholemeal and white	10–12
Bread, wholemeal and white	8–10
Cracker biscuits	8–10
Lentils, boiled	7
Beans, boiled	6–8
Breakfast cereals	5–20

phenylalanine, threonine, tryptophan and valine. A ninth, histidine, is essential for infants. The remaining amino acids are interconvertible and can be made from these eight or from each other. When food proteins are digested, our bodies split them to their individual amino acids and then reassemble them into the types of human protein we require.

Growing bodies

Because they are synthesising new tissues, children, adolescents, pregnant and breastfeeding women require more protein in relation to their body weight than the average adult.

RECOMMENDED DAILY INTAKE

We need as little as 40–50 grams of protein per day (one average-sized piece of steak and a wedge of cheese or 100 grams of cooked lentils), for turnover or repair of muscles, skin, enzymes and hormones. Any more than is required will be diverted into kilojoules and, unless they are burned up by physical exertion, are stored as body fat. Most people eating a meat- or dairy-based diet have no difficulty in obtaining sufficient protein. In fact, most of us consume more than we need with the average protein intake at around 100 grams per day for men and 75 grams for women.

BEST FOOD SOURCES

No food is entirely protein, although we may talk of protein foods or protein powder. Dried skim milk contains only 36 per cent protein, while cheese and fish rank lower at 18–30 per cent. Milk (because it is mostly water) contains a mere 4 per cent.

VEGANS AND PROTEIN

The balance of amino acids is particularly important for vegans. Plant proteins from grains, legumes and nuts are limited in one or two of the eight essential amino acids. Protein from wheat, for example, contains 2.9 grams of lysine (per 16 grams of

MY TAKE
The original Healthy Eating Pyramid offered a simple, at-a-glance guide to getting the right proportions of the basic foods for the average person. It was flexible enough to be adapted yet memorable enough to catch your imagination. I still use it as an easy teaching tool, particularly for school children and adults with low literacy. However, I prefer to show vegetables, fruits and legumes in the 'eat more' base, with bread and cereals in the moderate level. The Plate has now taken over the Pyramid (both in the US and in Australia) as a healthy eating icon, but in my opinion, it is not as flexible as the Pyramid.

See also **Dietary Guidelines; Weight Loss.**

A DAY ON A PROTEIN-RICH DIET

This meal plan allows for more protein from meat, fish, chicken and eggs. It's correspondingly lower in carbohydrates (bread, cereal, potato) but doesn't eliminate them altogether. It's a good diet to follow for weight loss, or if you need a high intake of iron and zinc.

- BREAKFAST—Egg, poached or boiled, with grilled tomato halves or mushrooms, served on 1 slice wholemeal toast
- LUNCH—Large salad plate with mixed leaves, cucumber, grated carrot, tossed with vinaigrette dressing and topped with canned salmon and white beans
- SNACK—½ avocado
- DINNER—Grilled lean lamb cutlets with pesto sauce served with green peas, carrots and beans; fresh fruit salad with low-fat yoghurt.

nitrogen), which is insufficient to meet our daily lysine needs of 5.5 grams. By contrast, beef contains 8.9 grams of lysine, which well and truly covers the daily requirements for lysine.

That said, mixtures of two plant proteins can complement each other, with one making good any deficiency of the other. For example, a dish of grains, barley, couscous or rice (which is low in lysine) served with dried beans like chickpeas, soy beans or lentils (rich in lysine, but limited in methionine) can provide the correct balance of all essential amino acids.

Pyramid and Healthy Eating

The Healthy Eating Pyramid is a food selection guide that groups foods into a semi-quantitative pictorial triangle. Divided into three segments, the base of the pyramid shows which foods you are meant to eat the most of—vegetables, fruit, breads and grains; the middle layer has those meant to be eaten in moderation—lean meat, fish and dairy; and at the apex are those to be eaten in small amounts—sugar, butter, margarine and oils. It is a simple, clear guide and one that I often use myself.

The first Pyramid was created in 1982 by the Australian Nutrition Foundation (now Nutrition Australia) and has since been used in various formats in many countries. For example, there are now Pyramids for vegetarians, and the Asian, Mediterranean and Pacific Rim diets, each reflecting particular food preferences.

Simplified Healthy Eating Pyramid

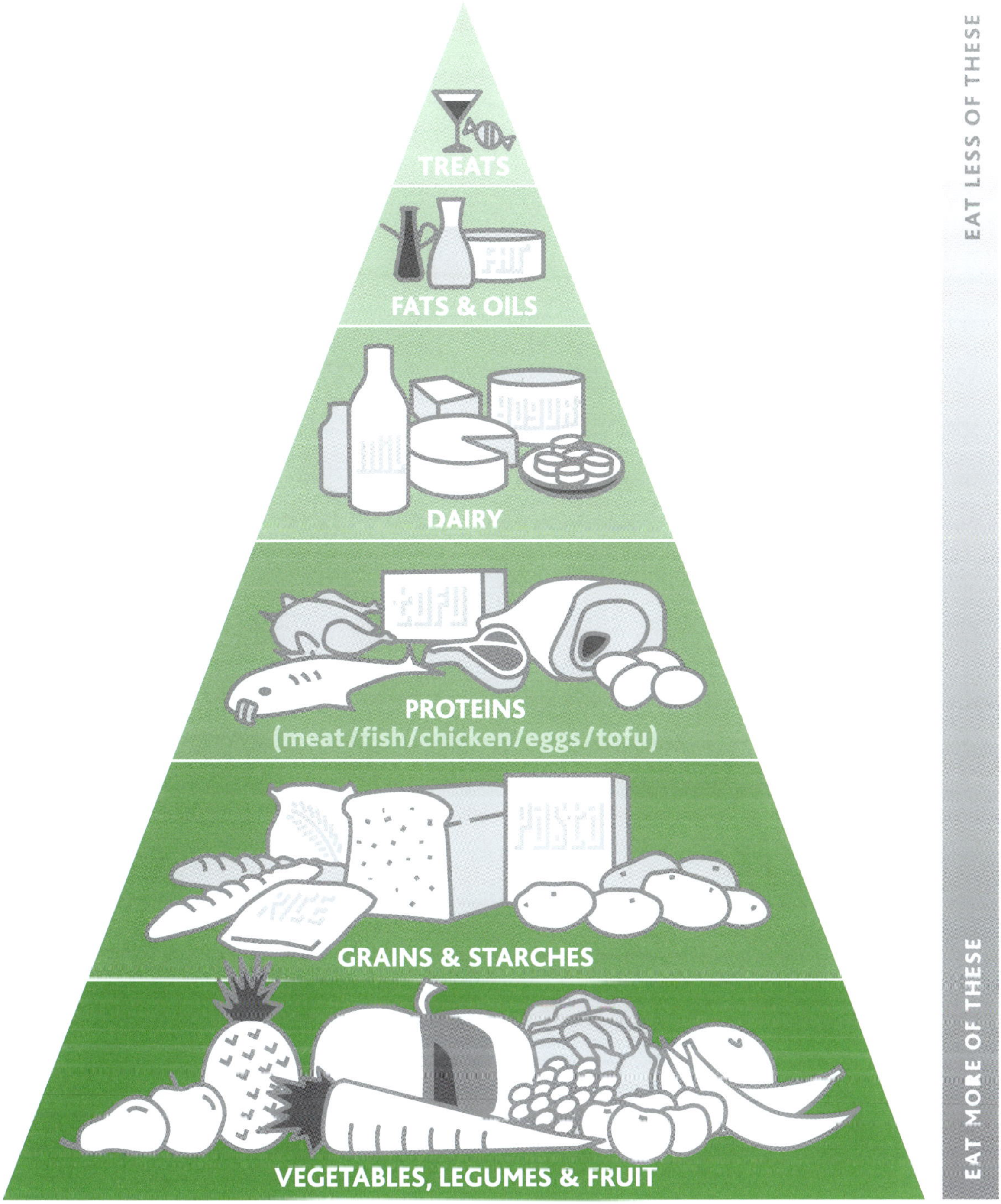

QR

Quetelet's Index

This is an index of body fatness, based on weight and height and devised in 1835 by a Belgian astronomer and statistician named Lambert Quetelet (1796–1874). Now known as the Body Mass Index or BMI, it is used as a convenient method to estimate a person's relative weight.

See also **Body Mass Index.**

Quinoa

An ancient grain from South America, quinoa has become so popular in recent years that there's scarcely enough left in Peru, Bolivia and Chile to feed the locals.

White quinoa is most popular, and looks much like couscous in size (it is cooked using a similar method). Grey, black and red varieties are also available.

NUTRITIONAL VALUE

A nutritionally impressive grain, quinoa is an excellent source of minerals (magnesium, manganese, copper, phosphorus, potassium, zinc) and vitamins (vitamin E and B-complex vitamins). It has double the protein of most grains and an impressive amount of fibre, with three times the amount contained in brown rice. It's also rich in iron, which is unusual for grains.

With a low GI of 53, it's near the max for slow carbs but is still good for anyone with diabetes. It is also gluten-free—ideal for anyone with a wheat intolerance or coeliac disease.

See also **Grains and Cereals.**

Quorn (mycoprotein)

Mycoprotein is a meat substitute. It is manufactured from the mould *Fusarium venenatum*, which is grown in large sterile fermentation tanks. It contains glucose (as a food for the fungus) and various vitamins and minerals (to improve the product's food value). After harvesting, it is heat-treated and then mixed with egg albumen, which acts as a binder. The final product has a chicken-like texture, and is pressed into a mince, patties or dice, ready for home cooking or for use in ready-prepared meals. It can be grilled, sauteed, baked or added to casseroles.

MY TAKE
Think of it not as mould—but more akin to mushrooms.

Marketed and trademarked as Quorn, mycoprotein is low in saturated fat and is a good source of protein and fibre. But it is not as high in iron and zinc as red meat and there's no vitamin B_{12} so it's not a complete substitute for meat. It is sold in frozen form in major supermarket chains.

R

Raw Food Diets

Raw food diets consist of fresh fruit, raw vegetables, salads, raw unsalted nuts, avocado, and freshly squeezed juices. They are usually 75 per cent raw, with the addition of 25 per cent cooked legumes, fish, grains, meats and eggs.

Raw food advocates believe raw food offers the maximum level of vitamins, minerals, phytochemicals and enzymes because they are consumed in a fresh state and have not been diminished by heat from cooking. They argue food is consumed in a form closest to nature, and is a good antidote to the modern, processed and sometimes over-refined diet, lacking in nutrition.

NUTRITIONAL VALUE

Eating a diet containing lots of fruit and vegetables gives you a lot of fibre, vitamin C, B vitamins (some of which are heat sensitive) and minerals. You'll also do a lot of chewing which helps slow down your rate of eating and encourages you to listen to your stomach and eat less, which is good for weight loss. You'll also feel full on fewer kilojoules. But despite these advantages, I don't believe raw food is the answer to good nutrition.

Cooking can reduce nutrients in food, but it can also improve them. Some, such as lycopene from tomatoes, are better absorbed from the cooking process. Cooking can also inactivate anti-nutrition factors like avidin in egg whites and lectins in legumes. It also improves the digestibility of proteins and makes starch gelatinised.

Ultimately a combination of raw and cooked food makes the most nutritional sense. Any diet is improved if you aim to eat fresh fruit, leafy green salads, avocado and nuts, and cut back on processed food.

Recommended Dietary Intakes (RDIs)

See also **Adolescents and Diet; Adults and Diet; Infants and Diet; Nutrient Reference Values (NRVs); Preschool-aged Children and Diet; Primary School–aged Children and Diet; Toddlers and Diet; Appendices.**

Recommended Dietary Intakes (RDIs) are the nutrients needed (from foods not supplements) to meet the needs of healthy people of all age groups, from babies and older people to pregnant and breastfeeding women. They apply to those of average weight, height, activity and health and include a margin of safety to cover individual differences. The RDIs are revised from time to time to reflect the latest scientific research.

RDIs are used for education, planning clinical diets, formulating meal replacements and fortified foods, monitoring food supplies, checking the adequacy of rations, and labelling on foods packaging. The terminology differs from country to country—in the US it is known as Dietary References Intakes and Recommended Dietary Allowances, and in the UK it is Recommended Nutrient Intakes.

Resistant Starch

Resistant starch is a type of carbohydrate that resists digestion in the small bowel in a way that is similar to fibre, and arrives undigested in the large bowel. Once there, it is fermented by bacteria, which results in the formation of a number of volatile but beneficial fatty acids like butyrate, which is thought to promote the production of healthy cells and fight colon cancer. Resistant starch has a mild laxative effect.

Rich sources include most foods rich in carbohydrates but particularly foods like cold, cooked potatoes, unripe bananas, pasta, legumes and certain types of corn. A new variety of corn high in resistant starch (Hi-Maize) is now used to boost the fibre of breakfast cereals, bread and hamburger buns. It is undetectable and doesn't alter the colour, texture or taste of the foods.

Resveratrol

Resveratrol is a compound found on the skins of red grapes and believed to fight off grape fungal infections. It may play a role in the prevention of certain cancers, and is also thought to be one of the compounds responsible for the reduced risk of heart disease seen in drinkers of red wine.

Rice

Often called the grain of life, rice remains the main food crop for over half the world's population. It is one of the oldest cereal grains, and has been cultivated in Asia for thousands of years. In Asia, no meal would be complete without bowls of steaming rice, and it is a perfect neutral accompaniment to add to spicy foods.

Unlike other grains, rice is usually eaten as steamed grains, and only small amounts are ground into flour. It is a versatile ingredient, being manufactured into a wide range of different foodstuffs such as breakfast cereals (e.g. Rice Bubbles), rice crackers, rice cakes, rice noodles, baby food and infant cereals.

NUTRITIONAL VALUE

- ✔ Rice is high in starchy carbohydrate for energy and is a good source of protein, which is of high biological quality
- ✔ Rice has almost no fat or sugars. It's low fat content means that rice is quite low in kilojoules. Half a cup of cooked rice supplies around 350 kilojoules, which is equivalent to a thick slice of bread.
- ✔ Rice provides a number of B group vitamins and essential minerals such as potassium, phosphorus and zinc. But this will depend on whether rice is milled (white rice) or unmilled (brown rice).
- ✔ Brown rice has more nutrients than white since it retains the bran and germ where many of the vitamins and minerals are found. It has around three times as much fibre as white polished rice, with a greater content of B vitamins. It's the best choice for nutrition—you just have to have the patience to cook it, although there are a number of quick-cooking brown rice products on the supermarket shelves these days. Brown rice also provides vitamin E, plus the minerals magnesium and manganese. Brown rice contains natural oils from the bran, so it has a shorter shelf life than white rice.
- ✔ Rice contains negligible sodium, with less than 5 milligrams of sodium per 100 gram serve. It is a great food for those who need to watch their salt intake. Rice was the basis of a famous Kempner Rice Diet trialled by Dr Walter Kempner to treat high blood pressure in the 1940s before the advent of drugs for the problem.
- ✔ Rice is free of gluten, an important advantage over the other commonly consumed grains like wheat or barley. It's a great basic for meals in a gluten-free diet.
- ✔ The starch in most varieties of rice is high GI so it's rapidly absorbed and digested. However, some varieties have a low to medium GI, such as Basmati or Doongara Clever Rice, as well as other speciality rices such as some white long-grain types.
- ✔ Rice is light and easily digested—plain boiled rice is often fed to sick people or those starting to eat again after food poisoning or gastroenteritis.
- ✔ Rice is the safest of grains and produces virtually no allergic reactions, which is the main reason babies start on it as their first solid food (baby rice cereal).

White Rice and Diabetes

Several studies have suggested that white rice increases the chances of getting type 2 diabetes. This may be critical for Asian populations, who tend to eat more white rice than Western populations. The research has found that the more white rice eaten, the higher the risk of type 2 diabetes. Generally the risk increases by 10 per cent with each extra serve of white rice (which is around 160 g or 1 cup). I'd concur, as white rice is high GI and a poorer choice than brown. Swap it for brown when you can.

NUMBER CRUNCH

A quarter-cup of uncooked white rice provides 4 grams of protein, a trace of fat, a trace of sugars, 40 grams of starch, a trace of fibre and 765 kilojoules. A quarter-cup of uncooked brown rice provides 4 grams of protein, 1 gram of fat, 1 gram of sugar, 38 grams of starch, 2 grams of fibre and 780 kilojoules.

WHAT RICE IS THAT?

There are more than 40,000 varieties of rice but only 4000 of these are marketed and sold. All can be classified into five basic types:

LONG-GRAIN RICE

Long-grain rice is narrow and long in shape and cooks into separate, fluffy grains (never sticky). This type of rice is preferred for plain steamed rice and rice salads. Many Asian cooks use a fragrant long-grain rice (Jasmine rice), which is a little more costly but has a special aroma and light texture.

MEDIUM-GRAIN RICE

Medium-grain rice has grains that cling together a little more than long-grain rice, but are still distinct. Calrose rice, which has been grown in Australian for over 30 years, is a versatile medium-grain rice originally developed in California, hence the name.

SHORT-GRAIN RICE

Short-grain rice looks almost round in shape and is moist, sticky and very tender when cooked. It is ideal for risotto, soup and sweet rice dishes.

QUICK-COOK OR PARBOILED RICE

Quick-cook or parboiled rice has been soaked and steamed before milling, which shortens the cooking time and gives the grains a pale gold colour. The steaming step retains important B vitamins by driving them to the centre of the grain. So after milling, the grains have a higher concentration of vitamins than white rice. In nutritional value, it is intermediate between brown and white rice.

WILD RICE

Wild rice is the seed of an aquatic grass, related to rice. Native to North America and southern Canada, it ranges in colour from dark brown to black, with a distinctive nutty flavour. It is nutritionally similar to rice.

See also **Gluten; Grains.**

Royal Jelly

Royal jelly is a milky-white viscous secretion from the salivary glands of honeybees. It has often been promoted as a health tonic and supplement but while it contains a range of B vitamins and some antioxidants, it does not have the backing of scientific research. People prone to asthma or allergies should not take it—bee products now carry a warning on the pack.

Rye

See **Grains and Cereals.**

S

Saccharin

Saccharin was first discovered in 1879 quite by accident. Eating his lunch in the laboratory, a researcher was surprised to discover that his sandwich, which had soaked up a solution on the lab bench, tasted incredibly sweet—and the search for the chemical that created the sweetness began!

Hundreds of times sweeter than sugar, saccharin is called a 'non-nutritive' sweetener. This means it has no nutritional value—no nutrients and no kilojoules. It also has no effect on blood glucose and is not metabolised by our bodies, which is why it was popular as the earliest alternative to sugar for people on a diet or with diabetes. Its big drawback is that it leaves a bitter metallic aftertaste, which has limited its usage. It was used as the sweetener in diet soft drinks up until the 1990s when better-tasting sweeteners such as aspartame and acesulphame-K arrived on the scene.

Saccharin has been the subject of controversy almost since it was discovered in 1879. In very high doses, saccharin has caused tumours in the bladders of experimental animals but so would many other ingredients if fed in such high amounts; the equivalent consumption by humans would be somewhere around 20 cans of diet soft drink a day. The studies were always only experimental and inconclusive but left a question mark in many people's minds. Authorities in the UK, US, Australia and New Zealand now regard it as safe but it has lost ground to other sweeteners. On food labels you will see it listed as additive 954.

See also **Sweeteners.**

Salads

I love salads and eat one most days; crisp and cool in summer, or with something warm on top in winter. When I spot a salad on the menu, I'm always tempted to order it.

A salad is the perfect meal to make the most of what's fresh and in season, from tomato with basil in summer to a wintry coleslaw with cabbage and carrots. Salads are not only quick and easy to prepare, they are very adaptable—if you don't have one ingredient, just substitute with another. You can make them light to counteract a rich meal or substantial by adding protein (e.g. a can of salmon, some chicken, a hard-boiled egg, a handful of nuts) and starchy carbs for a meal in a bowl. A tossed leaf salad is a great way to make any meal, even pizza or fish and chips, more balanced. It's the perfect antidote to the average Western diet.

SUPERSTAR GREEN SALAD

Mix together a 200 g bag of baby spinach leaves with a bunch of rocket (discard the stalks). You can also throw in 100 g of lightly blanched sugar snap peas for more crunch.

For the (heart-friendly) dressing, place ¾ cup extra-virgin olive oil, the juice of one lemon (around ¼ cup), 2 or 3 teaspoons Dijon mustard, 1 or 2 cloves crushed garlic, and a little ground black pepper in a screw-top jar. Shake well to combine. Use enough dressing to moisten the salad leaves; save the rest for later.

NUTRITIONAL VALUE

There are many good reasons to eat a salad more often. It has little fat (although watch the dressing) and heaps of fibre, and helps you get those five serves of vegetables and two serves of fruit you need each day. It's also bursting with vitamins and antioxidants which are not destroyed by cooking, and is packed with potassium, magnesium and other essential minerals that can help to counteract a high salt intake.

Salad leaves contain dozens of phytochemicals—natural plant compounds that act as antioxidants to protect the body and slow the ageing process. To get the most antioxidants, select dark leafy greens or reds such as dark oak leaf, mignonette, radicchio, coral, baby spinach leaves, rocket and watercress as well as fresh herbs, particularly parsley, basil, mint and coriander.

By starting your meal with a large salad and a simple vinaigrette-style dressing, you feel fuller and so eat less of a main course, which can help you shed excess weight without going hungry. With its high fibre and water content, you can tuck into a huge plate of salad (go easy on the dressing, especially a creamy one) and yet have eaten only 200 kilojoules from 500 grams. It's what dietitians call a low kilojoule-density food, providing few kilojoules from a big volume. In contrast, chocolate has a high kilojoule density, packing a hefty 1110 kilojoules in a small snack-size 50 gram bar.

COMPARE THE DIFFERENCE

HOMEMADE DRESSING	STORE-BOUGHT DRESSING
Oil Vinegar Mustard Pepper	Water Vegetable oil Antioxidant (320) Sugar Vinegar Salt Food acid (330) Vegetable gums (407, 415, 440a) Flavour Garlic Colour (102)

SALAD DRESSINGS

A little oil with a splash of vinegar or lemon juice makes certain nutrients more bio-available, which means that you absorb a lot more of the fat-soluble vitamins (such as beta-carotene) and antioxidants (lutein, lycopene) from raw foods. Plus the dressing's acidity slows down digestion and lowers the overall GI of the meal, so you feel fuller for longer and keep your blood-glucose levels on an even keel.

Make your own dressing—it's quick, easy and best of all, you can use a quality oil and you don't get the extra salt and additives from commercial salad dressings. In a screw-top jar, measure out 3 tablespoons of extra-virgin olive oil, 1 tablespoon of lemon juice (or white or red wine vinegar), half a teaspoon of Dijon mustard plus a few grinds of black pepper. Shake well until blended, drizzle over your salad, toss and serve. If you find that bought dressings tend to make your salad go limp and watery, remember that most bought dressings are mainly water. The oil stays mixed into the water with the help of emulsifiers and gums.

Salicylates

Salicylates are a large group of natural plant chemicals found in citrus and most other fruit, many vegetables, herbs, spices, honey, tea, coffee, beer and wine. They also turn up in perfume, aromatherapy oils, toiletries and toothpaste, in minty flavours and eucalyptus oil. The painkiller aspirin is also a member of the salicylate family.

In the 1970s, US paediatrician Dr Ben Feingold proposed that hyperactive children improved when placed on a strict diet excluding foods containing salicylates (as well as artificial colours and flavours). Subsequent research has shown he was on the right track, but because he failed to eliminate all the sources of salicylates in his test diets (such as some fruit), his results were flawed.

See also **Elimination Diet.**

Salmonella *See* **Food Safety.**

Salt (Sodium Chloride)

Imagine this quick winter's lunch of a bowl of canned pumpkin soup accompanied by a round of buttered toast with melted cheese. Sounds simple and delicious, right? But this typical meal has over 2000 mg of salt; more than you need for the entire day. And that's the problem. Salt, a common kitchen ingredient, is everywhere and usually in foods that our tastebuds don't even recognise as tasting salty.

DON'T OVERDO IT

Salt is a compound called sodium chloride, of which about 40 per cent is sodium. It's the main source of sodium in the average diet and is an essential mineral. We need it to regulate our body's water balance, maintain blood volume, and control muscle and nerve function. It's also important to regulate body temperature.

	SODIUM (MILLIGRAMS)	SODIUM (MILLIMOLES*)	SALT (GRAMS)
Body's requirement	200	8.5	0.5
No high blood pressure	800	35	2
Adequate intake	460–920	20–40	1.2–2.3
Average intake	2300–4600	100–200	6–12

* Millimoles denote the number of sodium atoms present.

The problem with too much sodium is that it attracts and retains fluid inside the body and causes fluid retention. When we eat a lot of salt, there is a big increase in both sodium and fluid in the body until our hormones trigger a loss of some of the sodium by the kidneys. A new balance is set at a slightly higher fluid level in the whole body. This can lead to weight gain of up to 1 kilogram, which strains the heart and makes it pump harder to push the extra fluid through the arteries. The arteries thicken and stiffen, reducing blood flow, which then raises blood pressure. Excess sodium can also worsen kidney function in people with kidney disease, and cause calcium loss via the urine, contributing to brittle bones (osteoporosis) in later life. New research suggests that too much salt can also cause asthma to worsen.

It's a myth that the body gets rid of extra salt. The body does have good systems for managing salt levels via the kidneys, faeces and sweat. However, the amount we eat now is many, many times greater than we actually need. This excess salt is swamping our coping mechanisms so that our bodies always contain more salt than they require. Cutting back on your salt intake will make a big difference to high blood pressure and any condition where fluid retention is a feature, such as heart failure, cirrhosis of the liver and Ménière's syndrome.

And no, you don't need more salt in very hot weather if you are sweating a lot. We only lose a small amount of salt through sweat. What's important in these circumstances is to drink plenty of water to keep your body hydrated.

One level teaspoon (5 g) of salt has 2000 mg of sodium. The latest recommendation is to limit sodium to less than 920 mg a day, equivalent to half a teaspoon of salt.

DAILY REQUIREMENTS

Surprisingly we don't need much at all. Our bodies need less than 200 milligrams of sodium a day (less than 0.5 gram of salt), but the average Western diet supplies well over 2000 milligrams of sodium a day (equivalent to 6 grams or 1 teaspoon of salt).

CUTTING BACK

The big problem is not the saltshaker. It's those everyday, processed foods such as cheese, deli meats, bread, cereals, fast foods, sauces and spreads that contain a lot of salt, but don't even have an obvious salty taste. Added sugar often masks the salt, especially with some biscuits and breakfast cereals. In fact around 75 per cent of our salt intake comes from processed foods, which is why buying salt-reduced and no added salt foods will have the biggest impact on your intake.

Our tastebuds adjust very quickly to a low-salt diet. It's a question of re-educating our palates, which takes about 2 weeks. Here are some easy strategies for cutting back:

- ✔ Buy salt-reduced foods and those with no added salt whenever you can, particularly cheese, bacon, ham, salami and other deli meats, bread, cracker biscuits, takeaway food, sauces, packet meal bases and simmer sauces.
- ✔ Cut out salty-tasting foods such as anchovies, olives, pretzels, potato crisps, corn chips and pizza. They increase your desire for salty things and create a noticeable thirst, which explains why they are often served as nibbles with drinks.
- ✔ Sprinkle less salt at the table. This will not only help you re-educate your tastebuds, but it will reduce your total sodium by about 15 per cent.
- ✔ Use potassium chloride, a salt substitute, for the first few weeks if you are desperate. Like salt, it's a white crystalline powder that can be shaken over food. However, check with your doctor if you have heart or kidney problems as you may retain potassium.
- ✔ Start by using half the quantity of salt that recipes suggest (particularly older recipes), then reduce it further as you progress. Don't add salt if you are cooking with ingredients such as bacon, stock powder, soy sauce, fish sauce, hoisin sauce, olives or cheese. Use unsalted margarine, butter or oil for baking cakes and desserts.
- ✔ Add flavour with herbs, spices, curry pastes and aromatic ingredients such as lemon juice, orange rind, mustard and wine. Plenty of chilli, onions, garlic and shallots will also really boost the flavour.
- ✔ Eat more fresh food. Remember that processed foods, whether they come in packets, cans, frozen or takeaway, make up three-quarters of our daily salt intake. Fresh vegetables, fish, meat, rice and pasta cooked without salt have little sodium but contain plenty of potassium, a complementary mineral that helps to counteract the negative effects of salt.

Growing bodies

Don't add salt to your baby or child's food—their kidneys are unable to remove the heavy sodium load.

COMMON SALTY FOODS AT A GLANCE

FOOD	% SALT*
Salt	97
Stock powder or cubes	46
Asian fish sauce	19
Soy sauce	16
Soy sauce, reduced salt	9
Anchovies	14
MSG	12
Black-bean sauce	8
Yeast spread	7
Bacon	6
Pretzels	5
Cheese spread	4
Ham, salami	4
Parmesan cheese	4
Blue vein cheese	3
Sea water	3
Tomato sauce	3
Worcestershire sauce	3
Olives	2
Pickles	2

*Figures have been rounded up or down

WHAT SALT IS THAT?

TABLE SALT

Table salt is the one found in most saltshakers. It is a finely ground salt with a small, even crystal size, typically from rock salt. It usually contains an anti-caking agent such as sodium silicoaluminate or magnesium carbonate to keep it free-flowing, even in high humidity.

IODISED SALT

This form of salt looks the same as table salt but has a minute amount of iodine added, in the form of either potassium, or sodium iodate or iodide. The iodine is added to help reduce the chance of iodine deficiency, which can lead to thyroid problems such as goitre. This is the salt I prefer for cooking at home. Research shows that our iodine intake has been dropping in recent years.

SEA SALT

With its large uneven flakes or large crystals, sea salt looks 'natural' and is favoured by chefs, but it's still a form of salt (sodium chloride) and will not lower your overall salt intake to any significant extent. It's made by evaporating seawater and has 99 per cent of the sodium of ordinary salt. The other 1 per cent consists of minerals like magnesium, potassium and zinc, which are found naturally in seawater. Many claims have been made for its health qualities but none have been scientifically validated.

MY TAKE
Whether you opt for table salt, sea salt or kosher salt, there's little difference in the sodium content by weight, and they all need to be kept to a minimum. The key difference is taste, texture and iodine content. Many chefs prefer to use the coarser gourmet and sea salts. If you opt for ¼ teaspoon of a coarse-grained salt like sea salt, you'll find that less fits onto a spoon so you'll get less sodium. But that's about it when it comes to benefits.

KOSHER SALT

This salt is coarse grained and free of additives.

ROCK SALT AND RIVER SALT

These are more gourmet and it's claimed they are better for you, but they have essentially the same salt content as table salt. They appear to produce a more intense salty flavour because the salt occurs in large chunks. Some come in pink, red or grey colours due to natural minerals.

CELERY SALT, VEGETABLE SALT AND GARLIC SALT

These are also no better than regular table salt in terms of sodium content. They contain some 70 per cent salt with dried ground celery, vegetables or garlic making up the remaining 30 per cent.

COOKING SALT

Cooking salt has the same salt content as table salt, but it occurs in coarse chunks and most have no added iodine. It is sold in larger quantities and used for more industrial-sized jobs like mass-roasting potatoes on a bed of salt or getting stains out of carpet.

LIGHT SALT

This is a blend of 50 per cent potassium chloride with 50 per cent sodium chloride and allows you to halve your salt intake without giving up the taste of salt. It's the only one worth trying when you first eliminate salt.

READ THE LABEL

'SALT-REDUCED'

These generally have between 25 and 30 per cent less salt than their regular counterparts. Many light cheeses, cereals, margarines, sauces and cracker biscuits fit this category.

MAKE THE SWITCH	SODIUM (mg)	YOU SAVE (mg)
1 cup tomato soup (250 ml)	1148	
1 cup salt-reduced tomato soup (250 ml)	388	760
1 cup chicken stock (250 ml)	1300	
1 cup salt-reduced chicken stock (250 ml)	625	675
1 tablespoon soy sauce (15 ml)	993	
1 tablespoon salt-reduced soy sauce (15 ml)	536	186
1 cup baked beans (210 g)	630	
1 cup salt-reduced baked beans (210 g)	444	186
1 cup 'no added salt' baked beans (210 g)	40	590

'LOW SALT', 'LOW SODIUM'

These must not contain more than 120 milligrams of sodium per 100 grams.

'NO ADDED SALT', 'SALT FREE' OR 'UNSALTED'

These must not contain any added salt, nor any ingredient containing salt.

HIDDEN SODIUM

Sodium salts are also used as additives and in medicines, and can contribute to excessive salt intake.

INGREDIENTS OR ADDITIVES

Baking powder/baking soda—*sodium* bicarbonate
Flavour enhancer—mono*sodium* glutamate (MSG)
Preservatives—*sodium* benzoate, *sodium* nitrite, *sodium* sulphite
Emulsifier—*sodium* stearoyl lactylate
Antioxidant—*sodium* ascorbate.

MEDICINALS

Sodium bicarbonate is used in effervescent tablets to make them fizz in water. Common examples include antacids (Alka-Seltzer, Eno); soluble pain killers (Aspro Clear, Panadol Soluble); fizzy vitamins (Berocca) and urinary alkalinisers (Ural, Citravescent).

Saponins

These compounds, found in the fibre of soy beans, chickpeas, lentils, peanuts, oats, barley and spinach, are believed to lower blood cholesterol by binding and excreting bile salts and sterols.

Saturated Fats

Saturated fats are generally classified as 'bad' fats thanks to their ability to raise the harmful LDL cholesterol and set the scene for cancer. They are found in all fats and oils, but predominantly in animal fats such as dairy products (butter, ghee, cream and cheese) and the fat in meat. They are also found in palm and coconut oil, often used to fry chips and fast food. These oils have replaced beef tallow but are not nutritionally superior. Commercial shortenings and baker's fats—used to make cakes, biscuits, pastries, muesli bars and confectionery—are also usually high in saturates due to hydrogenation (hardening) of oils.

Dietary guidelines in most affluent countries recommend we reduce saturated fats to less than 10 per cent of total kilojoules. However, this is not a hard-and-fast rule as there is great variability between individual fatty acids. Stearic acid (C18), a common saturated fatty acid and one that is predominant in chocolate, does not raise cholesterol to any great extent, while the lauric acid (C12) in coconut and myristic acid in palm kernel oil and butter do raise cholesterol. In real life, it's hard to eat foods that contain just one single fatty acid so the blanket recommendation exists.

Chemically, saturated fats are a type of fat where the fatty acid chain has no double bonds. This allows the molecules to 'pack together' densely and creates a fat that is usually solid or semi-solid at room temperature, which gives a great advantage during cooking.

See also **Fats, and Fatty Acids; Trans Fats.**

Satiety

Satiety is the feeling of satisfaction or fullness after eating. It's usually the time after a meal before the return of hunger and the feeling of wanting to eat again. That means you can make it to the next full meal without having to snack, which is important if you want to lose weight.

Many things can affect your feelings of fullness and hunger: the composition of food (the ratio of kilojoules and water to the volume consumed); format (liquid versus solid, diced versus finely minced); ratio of nutrients (how much protein to fibre and fat); as well as the impact of flavour and smell. In general, foods high in protein or fibre can help you to feel fuller for longer. Protein, well known for its satiating properties, appears to slow down the rate of gastric emptying. Likewise, foods that have a low glycemic index (low GI) are slowly digested and so keep you feeling satisfied for longer. But none of these factors on their own fully explains why some foods stick with you for longer.

'FEEL-FULL' FOODS

Research has shown that when we consume foods (not beverages) that our bodies really notice we are eating, our gut and intestines send the brain the vital 'I'm full' signals. There's quite a range of 'feel-full' foods to choose from, including:

- ✔ Foods that we have to chew a lot, like lean meat, pearl barley, muesli, very grainy breads, apples and carrots
- ✔ Protein-rich foods (lean meat, fish, chickpeas and nuts) that encourage our stomach and small intestine to produce hormones that send signals to the brain telling us we're full. There's added value with these too—they make you hotter after eating, which uses up more energy
- ✔ Low-GI carbs, which can also increase the production of some 'I'm full' hormones and help keep our blood glucose steady after eating. Research from the University of Sydney has shown that eating lower-GI meals throughout the day produced significantly lower glucose and insulin concentrations, along with higher concentrations of the satiety (fullness) hormone, cholecystokinin (CCK), compared with high-GI meals
- ✔ Foods that have lots of fibre and water (high volume foods), which deliver the full feeling. This is because volume, especially 'sticky' volume like porridge, means that food really touches the gut walls and leaves the brain in no doubt that it's there. They also stick around the gut longer, clinging to the walls.

See also **Appetite and Hunger.**

Sauces and Condiments

Sauces and condiments are an easy way to add flavour to lean meats, fish, salads and stir-fries. I like to keep a range of sauces in my cupboard: a jar of mustard (Dijon or grainy) for steak or making up my own vinaigrette, a good tomato chutney for sandwiches or cold meats, horseradish for seafood or beef, a bottle of salt-reduced soy sauce for those Chinese stir-fries and steamed greens, and a bottle of Worcestershire sauce to go nicely with lamb.

NUTRITIONAL VALUE

Most sauces and condiments have few kilojoules and little fat so are generally listed as 'free foods' on diet plans, and help enliven basic meats, chicken and vegetables. They are used in such minute amounts that we can ignore any kilojoules from them. Their big drawback is that they are high in salt and contribute 8 per cent of the total salt intake of the average Australian, which is pretty sizeable considering we use them in such small quantities. Wherever you can, buy them in salt-reduced form and you'll be looking after your health. Some add a good whack of sugar too. If you've been told to reduce your salt intake, be careful to stick to a thin smear or a tiny side of your favourite, not a huge dollop.

WHAT SAUCE IS THAT?

BARBECUE SAUCE

This uses similar low-fat ingredients to tomato sauce but with more Worcestershire sauce and vinegar.

BLACK-BEAN SAUCE

Made from fermented soy beans, this sauce adds a nutty barbecued flavour and is often teamed with pork and chicken.

CHAR SIU SAUCE

This is the traditional Chinese-style barbecue sauce, which gives roast pork its characteristic red glaze.

CHILLI SAUCE

This comes in many variations, e.g. sweet, hot and with garlic flavour. Chilli sauce livens up soups, stir-fries and noodle dishes by adding heat and flavour.

COCKTAIL SAUCE

At home, you'd make this by combining tomato sauce with cream, lemon juice, Worcestershire sauce and Tabasco in a small bowl, then seasoning with salt and pepper. Commercially it's got little or no cream and is made thicker with gums and thickeners.

FISH SAUCE

Often used in Thai and Vietnamese dishes, fish sauce is made by dissolving anchovies in salt over a long period of time. It loses its pungency when cooked or mixed with other ingredients.

HOISIN SAUCE

Hoisin sauce is made from soy beans, garlic, vinegar, sugar and spices and has a sweet and spicy flavour. It can be added to a stir-fry, or used as a dipping sauce or to glaze a roast.

MAYONNAISE

Made by whisking egg yolks with lemon juice or vinegar into an emulsion, mayonnaise is all fat—about 70 per cent, but it's mainly healthy fat. Use it as a swap for oil or butter. It's low in salt and if you make it at home, you can be even more sparing with the salt.

MUSTARD

Made from ground mustard seeds, vinegar, salt, pepper and herbs, it can be smooth, grainy, mild or a nose-thumping hot English mustard. I'm a great fan of Dijon mustard and use it with all kinds of meat, on ham sandwiches and always in my salad dressing.

OYSTER SAUCE

This is a sauce made from oysters, soy sauce, salt and spices.

PLUM SAUCE

Made from salted plums, rice vinegar, chilli, sugar and spices, this is used as a serving sauce with barbecued meat.

RELISH AND CHUTNEY

These come in many different varieties. Made with anything from tomatoes, mangoes, onions, mustard seeds, dill seeds, sugar and spices, it is almost always very low in fat.

SALTY ASIAN SAUCES

Salty sauces like soy, fish or hoisin are a key feature of Asian cuisine and are used in countless ways as marinades, splashed into stir fries and soups, as a basting sauce on roasts, grills and barbecues, as a dipping sauce and a table sauce. In fact, they take the place of the table salt in Western diets. Most are low in fat and kilojoules (except satay sauce which contains coconut milk and peanuts). However, all tend to be high in salt (3–16 per cent) and should not be used as a salt substitute or by anyone on a low-salt diet. When you use these sauces, don't add salt to the recipe. Their high salt content gives them a long shelf life and means they can be stored unrefrigerated almost indefinitely.

SALSA

This is an ideal replacement for most sauces. It's typically made from fresh finely diced vegetables such as tomatoes, capsicum and onion. Salsa tastes great on omelettes, burgers, grilled steaks and fish or chicken. Usually low in sugar, it has less than 30 milligrams of sodium per tablespoon as long as you don't add any salt.

SATAY SAUCE

Containing peanuts, coconut milk, chilli and spices, satay sauce is traditionally served as a dipping sauce with chicken skewers or to top an Indonesian gado gado salad.

SOY SAUCE

This is the most popular of Asian sauces. It is a fermented sauce made from soy beans, roasted grains (usually wheat), water and salt, although better-quality brands are made solely from soy beans and aged for longer. Add to marinades, stir-fries, noodle dishes and use as a dipping sauce. *Ketjap manis* is a popular sweet soy sauce in Indonesia.

TAMARI

Gluten-free tamari is one of the authentic soy sauce recipes first introduced to Japan from China. It is a wheat-free sauce made from soy bean and has a slightly stronger flavour than regular soy sauce. It's traditionally used to flavour longer-cooking foods (soups, stews etc), but it can be used in marinades and dressings too, or as a condiment or dipping sauce. Look for reduced-salt tamari and check that wheat hasn't been added.

TARTARE SAUCE

This sauce is popular with fish dishes and is mostly made by mixing mayonnaise with pickled gherkins, capers and spices.

TOMATO SAUCE (KETCHUP)

This is made from cooked, pureed tomatoes with basil, oregano or other herbs and seasonings added. Low-salt and no added salt versions are available. However, at 25 per cent sugar, it also dumps a hefty amount of sugar over your snags and fish fingers. The concentration of tomatoes makes it a surprising source of lycopene, which may help protect against prostate cancer.

Sea Vegetables (Seaweeds)

Sea vegetables, or seaweeds as they are more commonly known, are one of nature's most biologically active resources, possessing a wealth of bioactive compounds. As a result, seaweed-derived compounds have important applications in a range of products in food, pharmaceuticals and cosmetics. In addition to bioactive components, sea vegetables are a rich source of dietary fibre (25–75 per cent dry weight), of which soluble fibre constitutes approximately half. Compounds isolated from seaweed have demonstrated various biological activities, such as antibacterial activity, antioxidant potential, anti-inflammatory properties, anticoagulant activity, antiviral activity and apoptotic activity.

The major direct use of these plants as food is in Japan, China and Korea, and in the Indian Ocean, where seaweed cultivation has become a major coastal industry. The main species grown by aquaculture in these countries are *nori* or *laver* (used in sushi), *arame*, *hijiki*, *dulse*, *kombu* (kelp) and *wakame* (the dark seaweed in miso soup). One of the main staples of the Japanese diet, seaweed accounts for some 10–25 per cent of their food intake. We all recognise the *nori* wrapped around a sushi roll or the fragments of *wakame* floating in miso soup. But it also appears in Wales in traditional laverbread and in some parts of Scotland in pudding and soup—carrageen boiled with milk to make a kind of pudding and dulse as seaweed soup. Dulse is still popular in Ireland, where it is often mixed with butter and potato and fried up as little round cakes.

NUTRITIONAL VALUE

Seaweed is high in protein (nearly 50 per cent protein content) but is very low in fat and kilojoules. It is rich in various forms of soluble fibre such as polysaccharides, fucoidan, laminarin and alginate compounds as well as lignins. It is rich in minerals, notably potassium, magnesium, phosphorus, fluoride and iodine, which is needed for thyroid function and normal metabolism. There's a little sodium but it's not clear how high this is. One sheet of *nori* has approximately 5 milligrams of sodium.

Because kelp is the saltiest-tasting of the sea vegetables, it makes a popular salt substitute, though it is actually low in sodium. Seaweed is a source of beta-carotene (converted to vitamin A) and a number of carotenoids, notably lutein. It also contains almost all the B vitamins as well as some vitamin E and C and flavonoids. However, you'd have to consume seaweed fresh to obtain the B and C vitamins. Drying or toasting seaweed—as occurs with sheets of *nori* to wrap sushi—would reduce most of these heat-sensitive vitamins. Seaweed is one of the few non-animal sources of vitamin B_{12} and it packs a decent serving; there is more vitamin B_{12} in one sheet of dried *nori* than in one egg.

USES

Seaweed has many uses in food manufacture. Chiefly it's used to extract agar (additive code 406) and carrageenan (407) or Irish moss, which are gelling substances used to set jellies, sweets, marshmallow and moulded desserts and to thicken low-fat yoghurts, salad dressings and sauces. Agar is a common substitute for normal gelatin and is called vegetarian gelatine. It is suitable for Halal foods.

Seasonal and Sustainable Eating

The wonders of food technology and a globalised distribution system mean we can eat our favourite foods year round if we want to. But I don't think this is a smart development. I relish seeing the seasonal harvest in my local fresh produce market and look forward to the first asparagus of spring, summer's juicy stone fruits, autumn's apples and pears, and winter's fennel, parsnips, oranges and mandarins.

The real health benefits to eating with the seasons is that you are naturally consuming a wider variety of foods—a key nutritional message you'll find in dietary guidelines around the world. But there are other good reasons too:

- ✔ You are eating fruits and vegetables when they are at their peak for taste and nutrition.
- ✔ You aren't paying a premium for produce that has been flown halfway around the world.
- ✔ You are supporting your local economy.
- ✔ You are making a small but important contribution to reduce the energy (and associated CO_2 emissions) needed to grow and transport the food we eat.

FOOD MILES

The concept of food miles (the distance a food has travelled from paddock to plate) is important for the environment in most, but not all, cases. It's ridiculous and wasteful when food is sent miles to be packed at a central depot and then sent back to be sold close to where it was first produced. It's equally ridiculous to freight fresh fruit by air from one country to another, simply to offer it for sale out of season. I refuse to buy, at great cost, cherries flown to Australia from the US in the middle of our winter. I prefer to wait for the Australian-grown cherries and actually look forward to the cherry season. The same goes for asparagus, mangoes and apples.

HOW YOU CAN MAKE A DIFFERENCE

- ✔ Buy what you can from farmers' markets and local growers, taking care that it is genuinely local produce.
- ✔ Eat foods in season when they're at their peak and cheapest.
- ✔ Plan a once-a-week shop using your car, and top up your perishables daily or a couple of times a week by walking. Alternatively you could find shops on your route home from work.
- ✔ Select foods with minimal packaging. Buying foods such as rice, pasta, legumes, oats and nuts in bulk saves money too.
- ✔ Reduce your food waste. Buy only what you need, plan meals in advance, check what you have already, and chill or freeze leftovers for another day.
- ✔ Compost your fruit, vegetable and grain food scraps, or use a worm farm.
- ✔ Grow your own vegetables and herbs at home. Grow herbs in pots on a balcony, or start a vegetable patch in the back garden.
- ✔ Join a community garden.
- ✔ Buy a re-usable drink bottle to carry water with you.

Shoppers are increasingly considering food miles and buying local produce from as close as possible to where it is grown. Buying food grown or caught within a radius of 100 miles (160 kilometres) can help reduce transport costs, allow fresh foods to be sold without being packaged and give small producers a better chance to compete.

However, eating locally doesn't always result in the cheapest food or have the least environmental impact—it's a complex issue with many factors that need to be taken into account. For example, coffee beans can be grown in a more environmentally friendly manner in Kenya than in most other countries due to its soil, natural sunlight and less fuel-intensive inputs. Dairy foods produced in Australia and delivered to the UK market generates fewer carbon emissions than that produced by British dairy farmers delivering to their local market thanks to more sunlight, better rainfall and open farmlands. The issue is not just distance, but the total use of energy from paddock to plate, including transport.

We have to also allow for transport costs. Freight by air is very costly in terms of carbon emissions per tonne, but sea transport is relatively efficient. The electricity generated for refrigeration adds to this impact, but then preventing food wastage could have a more positive effect on the environment overall. And it seems using your car to do the grocery shopping is more costly than all the transport used within the distribution system to get the produce to the point of sale.

FOOD WASTE

We waste so much food. Not only is it costly, but it's an environmental disaster. Think of the energy inputs it takes to grow, harvest, process, package, transport, store and cook food. Of five bags of shopping we bring home, it's estimated that we will throw out around one—that's around $5 billion worth of food in Australia each year.

FAIRTRADE

Fairtrade is an alternative marketing system designed to give disadvantaged, small-scale farmers a guaranteed price for their products. It enables growers and producers in the Third World to operate successfully in the global economy. Coffee is the movement's flagship product, followed by chocolate (cocoa) and tea. But in recent years, foods like olive oil, quinoa and Brazil nuts have entered the fairtrade market. These foods can sometimes, but not always, cost more than conventional products, but you know that no-one is being exploited. The leading certification organisations are Fairtrade, Utz Kapeh and Rainforest Alliance.

THE RAINFOREST ALLIANCE

This approach focuses on sustainability and how farms are managed. Their standards cover the full range of worker protection; the right to a safe, clean working environment; the right to be paid at least the national minimum wage; dignified housing (including potable water); access to medical care for workers and their families; and access to free education for children. Their aim is to make sure all agricultural workers are well treated. Don't confuse it with organic—it's quite different from organic standards.

Of five bags of shopping we bring home, it's estimated that we will throw out around one—that's around $5 billion worth of food in Australia each year.

Seeds

Seeds are tiny parcels of nutrition packed with good oils, fibre, protein, B vitamins and vitamin E, as well as a swag of minerals. Like nuts, they add plenty of flavour to your recipes and a little goes a long way. Seeds contain around 50 per cent oil, with little saturated fat and mostly polyunsaturates and mono-unsaturates. There's not much carbohydrate or sugar but a decent hit of fibre; sesame seeds have 12 per cent while flaxseeds are up at a high 28 per cent. You'll get plenty of potassium from seeds, a little sodium and some surprising mineral finds such as calcium, magnesium, phosphorus, copper, iron and zinc. Most seeds contain around 15 per cent protein—a similar level to wheat, yet they're gluten-free.

Seeds need to be crushed or ground to release their full nutrition package. There's research to show that the fat and minerals contained in seeds is not well absorbed; the outer seed coat does not break down easily as it's designed to protect the seed inside, which is the 'baby plant' that will grow into maturity. So whole seeds tend to pass through you undigested giving you their fibre and flavour, but not much more. So if you seek their rich content of oils, minerals and vitamins, it's best to consume them ground (like LSA) or in the form of seed butters such as tahini (sesame seed paste). Alternatively, make sure you chew and grind them between your teeth well.

MY TAKE
I store my seeds in the fridge in summer and in a cool, dark, dry cupboard in winter. This extends the life of the seeds and avoids those annoying pantry moths.

EASY WAYS TO ENJOY SEEDS

- ✔ Sprinkle over your cereal or breakfast yoghurt.
- ✔ Toss through any muesli to add a health boost.
- ✔ A tablespoon in your smoothie will boost your fibre intake.
- ✔ Add to baking such as muffins; either sprinkle on top or toss in a tablespoon for each cup of flour.
- ✔ Toast lightly in the oven or a non-stick pan and add crunch to salads and stir-fries.
- ✔ Go for soy and linseed breads.
- ✔ Make up a nutrient-packed sprinkle for fruit salad or yoghurt by grinding together 1 cup of walnut pieces with ½ cup linseeds, or buy LSA (a blend of linseed, sunflower and almond)—just make sure you buy it fresh and store it in the refrigerator, and use within two weeks.

WHAT SEED IS THAT?

CHIA

An ancient oilseed crop from Central and South America, chia are loaded with plenty of omega-3, fibre, protein and calcium. They have 18 per cent of the plant form of omega-3 called alpha-linolenic acid (ALA), which is around the same as flaxseeds, making them one of the richest sources of ALA. They're also notable for their fibre content (37 per cent), which is high in soluble fibre and some mucilages.

FLAXSEEDS (LINSEEDS)

Small, shiny, dark-brown seeds about the size of sesame seeds, flax seeds (also called linseeds) are, like chia seeds, very rich in one omega-3 called alpha-linolenic acid (ALA), a building block of the omega-3 oils found in fish. Flaxseeds are often taken for their lignans, a type of plant oestrogen that tops up female oestrogen levels, which may help minimise the unpleasant side effects of the menopause like flushing, and has anti-tumour properties. One or 2 tablespoons is all it takes to boost your intake.

> **SEEDS FOR CALCIUM**
>
> Like almonds, sesame seeds and chia have a surprisingly high content of calcium (255 mg per 100 g compared with 120 mg for milk), but how well this is absorbed is debatable. Keep two things in mind: the seeds must be ground to release their calcium, otherwise we can't break down their indigestible outer seed coat; it's also unlikely their calcium is absorbed as well as it is from milk. I take half the listed quantity as a rough guide, but no-one has tested this so far.

PEPITAS

These green pumpkin seeds really give your muesli or salad a lift. They're good to bite between your teeth and snack on.

POPPY SEEDS

Often seen as tiny black specks atop a bread roll, poppy seeds add crunch and texture to bread or can be soaked and mixed with honey, spices and walnuts for a rich filling, as in the eastern European poppy seed roll.

SESAME SEEDS

With 25 per cent protein and a high calcium content, sesame is worth including in a big way in your diet. It is a star ingredient in Middle Eastern sweets such as halva and sesame-honey cakes, as well as tahini. Tahini is sesame seed puree or paste in which the seeds are finely ground into a smooth runny paste (you can buy hulled or unhulled, which has a stronger flavour and more fibre). I find tahini is easy to use and great for adding to yoghurt, dips and satay-like sauces. Think of it as a healthy fat supplement—it's a mix of polyunsaturates and mono-unsaturates in almost equal amounts—with little carbohydrate, lots of protein, fibre and some calcium.

SUNFLOWER SEEDS

These seeds are great for munching on either raw or roasted. Raw is better, of course, as it retains more of their valuable vitamin E, but roasting allows them to remain fresh for longer storage.

SEEDS FOR OIL

Not only are seeds a very valuable food source, but they are also a valuable commercial source of oils which are all low in saturates with lots of good fats. Sesame oil is a fragrant cooking oil that's popular with Asian cuisines. Sunflower oil is high in polysaturates and vitamin E. Chia oil and flaxseed oil stand out for their omega-3 content.

Selenium *See* **Minerals.**

Serotonin

This is a neurotransmitter made in the body from the amino acid tryptophan. Changes in brain serotonin levels can influence sleep and mood. Foods that lead to an increase in brain levels of tryptophan and therefore serotonin—such as milk, malted products and carbohydrate-rich foods in general—are thought to be able to induce feelings of calmness.

Seafood

Delicate and fine-textured, shellfish is a real treat to eat and scores high points in terms of nutrition. It is generally divided into two groups: crustaceans such as prawns, lobster, crab, Balmain bugs and yabbies, which have a hard scaly outer shell; and molluscs, which inhabit shells that are bivalve (in the case of mussels, oysters, scallops, clams, pipis and cockles) or single (abalone). Also included here are the invertebrates or shell-less types (squid or octopus), as their nutrition is similar.

NUTRITIONAL VALUE

All types are similar in nutritional value to fish. They have little 'good' unsaturated fat, very little saturated fat and few kilojoules. They're packed with protein, zinc, iron and iodine as well as vitamin E. Most of the vitamins from the B group are there: thiamin, riboflavin, niacin, pantothenic acid, B_6, biotin and B_{12}. You'll also get many essential minerals such as zinc, potassium, iron, iodine, calcium, magnesium and selenium.

When it comes to getting our omega-3, we often think of oily fish like salmon, but shellfish can contribute to our intake too. At 200 milligrams in a 100-gram serve of prawns or mussels, they have the same omega-3 content as a fillet of blue-eye trevalla, John Dory, snapper and other white fish. This is around one-tenth of what's in salmon, but it's almost half your day's required intake. I suggest eating them lightly cooked or raw, to preserve the heat-sensitive B vitamins.

Shellfish was once classified as being high in cholesterol but later research found that it contains a range of cholesterol-related compounds called sterols that are not associated with heart disease. Apart from prawns, all shellfish contain low to moderate levels and can be safely included in diets to reduce blood cholesterol. Egg yolk and offal meats have four to 10 times more cholesterol than shellfish on a weight-for-weight basis.

SENSITIVITY

Shellfish are one of the foods well known as a cause of classic food allergy, causing vomiting, stomach upsets or skin rashes in sensitive people. They are always identified on food packs to alert sufferers.

SAFETY TIPS

Shellfish are extremely perishable and spoil quickly, so are well known as sources of food poisoning bacteria. Take care to store them correctly to minimise the risk of food poisoning. Make sure you buy them very fresh and keep them chilled on ice or in a refrigerator until eaten. If frozen, consume them immediately once they have thawed.

If you're catching them yourself or getting them from a friend, make sure you only catch or collect seafood when water quality is good. Do not collect shellfish after heavy rainfall, which can carry pollution.

WHAT SEAFOOD IS THAT?

OYSTERS

Oysters are light, nutritious and easy to digest. They're one of the few animal foods we can buy and eat exactly as they are—fresh and natural. Oysters in their natural state make

DID YOU KNOW?

Oysters and crab are an outstanding source of zinc. All shellfish have about half the iron of red meat, and prawns, oysters, mussels and crab are surprising sources of calcium.

the perfect appetiser for any weight-conscious person. A dozen oysters has only 555 kilojoules, the approximate equivalent of a large apple or two slices of bread.

Oysters are well known for being the richest food source of zinc, an essential mineral needed for growth and sexual maturity, healing of wounds, vision and metabolising protein and carbohydrate. They're also good for copper, a component of many enzymes that trigger chemical reactions in the body, along with a wide variety of other shellfish minerals.

Compared with fish and meats (other than liver), oysters are rich in vitamin B_{12}. A dozen oysters provides more than our total daily requirement of zinc and vitamin B_{12}.

PRAWNS

Prawns are extremely low in fat (less than 1 per cent) and kilojoules, yet they are packed with nutrition. They're tops for protein, zinc, iron and iodine as well as vitamin E. They're also good for the B vitamin niacin and for potassium (essential for muscles and nerves and for controlling blood pressure). Ditto for other seafood like oysters, squid, scallops and baby octopus.

LOBSTER, CRAB AND OTHER CRUSTACEANS

Lobster and crab have more fat than other shellfish (around 3 to 5 per cent, as opposed to less than 2 per cent for the others), and they also have higher cholesterol counts. Apart from this, they have a similar good nutritional profile as other shellfish.

MUSSELS

There's nothing more delicious than a bowl of mussels cooked in garlic, or as part of a delicious seafood stew. Like all shellfish, they're low fat and full of flavour.

SQUID AND OCTOPUS

Squid (calamari) and octopus are both low in fat and saturated fat. Opt for them barbecued rather than crumbed and fried.

See also **Fish.**

Slow Food

Slow eating is one way you can take a stand against life in the fast lane. It will make you feel less stressed, more relaxed and in tune with your body, and enjoy your food more. Research has always pointed to eating slowly helping with weight loss, but it was made prominent by the Slow Food Movement, started in Italy in 1988 by Carlo Petrini. With a snail chosen as its patron and symbol, Slow Food is everything that fast food isn't. If you read the Slow Food Manifesto, you'll see that it's not just about health—it's about a lifestyle that embraces rich varieties and traditions of local cuisines, clean farming and animal husbandry, and fair conditions of labour.

Slow eating is one way you can take a stand against life in the fast lane. It will make you feel less stressed, more relaxed and in tune with your body, and enjoy your food more.

Eating slowly is also a useful technique to help people painlessly trim their food intake. The theory is that a leisurely dining pace allows time for the body's natural fullness signals to kick in. Stomach distension and changes in several appetite-related hormones, for example, alert the body that it's time to stop eating. But these processes take time, so a rushed meal could theoretically cause overeating.

To test this theory, a recent US study gave 30 women the same pasta meal on two separate occasions. On one day, the women were told to eat the meal as fast as they comfortably could, with no pauses between bites. On the other day, they were instructed to take small bites, put their spoons down between bites and chew each mouthful between 20 and 30 times. On average, the researchers found the women ate nearly 300 fewer kilojoules when they slowed down. They also felt fuller and more satisfied after the meal. According to the researchers there are several potential reasons for the findings. Besides allowing more time for the body's fullness signals to start working, savouring a meal's flavours, textures and aromas may also help people feel more satisfied with fewer calories.

See also **Appetite and Hunger; Mindless Eating.**

Snacks

Most modern-day snacks are the downfall of a healthy diet and I believe they are one of the reasons many of us are gaining weight. Snacking itself isn't bad, it's what we snack on that makes it so unhealthy. Common snacks these days are either fatty and sugary (chocolate, muffins and biscuits), or fatty and salty (crisps, pizza, fries and savoury crackers).

Compare a healthy snack of an apple with modern snacks in the table below. You'll see how quickly they push you over your daily limit of kilojoules, saturated fat and sodium.

MOST SNACKS TODAY:

- Are loaded with fat and salt or sugar
- Fill us up but fails to contribute any of the essential nutrients we need for health such as vitamins, minerals or fibre
- Are often high GI so they are rapidly digested and absorbed and leave you feeling hungry again soon
- Are kilojoule-dense, packing a lot of kilojoules into a small volume so you overeat before your stomach feels full
- Are too generous in their portion size
- Crowd out the more natural foods like vegetables and fruit
- Are an opportunity for overeating—we all know how hard it is to stop at just one!

TO SNACK OR NOT TO SNACK?

Snacking was once frowned upon but small, healthy snacks make good sense for these three groups in particular:

SMALL CHILDREN

With their small stomach capacity, children eat better with snacks. Some 80–90 per cent of children snack between meals. If your child can't sit still for long enough to eat a full dinner, small snacks keep them topped up—just make sure they're nutritious.

FOOD	ENERGY (kJ)	SATURATED FAT (g)	SODIUM (mg)
1 medium apple	300	0	2
Chocolate bar 60 g (Mars Bar)	1145	6	114
2 glazed doughnuts	1680	8	342
2 chocolate biscuits (Tim Tams)	840	7	73
Packet of potato crisps 50 g	1150	7	450
Tub hot chips 150 g	1255	10	300
Recommended daily intake *	8700	20	920

* For a moderately active man or very active woman. Sedentary people would require less.

DIETERS

You can burn more fat and shrink your stomach size by switching to mini-meals with snacks. The theory is that your stomach gets used to feeling full after a sensible portion instead of a huge one.

PEOPLE WITH DIABETES

Spreading out the food load over small meals and snacks can keep blood-glucose levels more steady, and is less of a drain on your body than three big meals with nothing in between. Some research suggests that snacking can reduce the total (and bad) LDL cholesterol among healthy people—that is, eating six smaller meals instead of three meals daily.

HEALTHY SNACK OPTIONS

FRUIT

- ✔ Fresh fruit (bananas, mandarins and other firm fruit are best, or pack rockmelon cubes or cherries into plastic containers)
- ✔ Fruit snack-packs
- ✔ Dried apricots or sultanas (just a handful)
- ✔ Frozen orange quarters or frozen grapes
- ✔ Fresh or canned fruit (packed in water or natural juice) with yoghurt or custard.

VEGETABLES

Carrot, celery and cucumber sticks with low-fat dip (hummus, tzatiki, tuna), cottage cheese or reduced-fat cheese.

DAIRY FOODS

- ✔ Yoghurt (fruit, plain or frozen)
- ✔ A wedge or slice of cheese with rye crispbread, rice crackers or wholegrain crackers
- ✔ Cheese with celery sticks
- ✔ Small scoop of vanilla ice-cream (not premium)
- ✔ Small scoop of gelato or fruit ice
- ✔ Milkshake made with reduced-fat milk and a small amount of flavouring
- ✔ Smoothie made with reduced-fat milk, fruit and yoghurt (banana or frozen berries blend up well).

NUTS

- ✔ A handful (30–50 grams) of mixed nuts, preferably unsalted; don't open a large pack of nuts and munch mindlessly—make a portion by packing into a small tub or a bowl so you know how much is there
- ✔ Nuts and dried fruit trail mix.

BREAD AND GRAINS

- ✔ Bread or roll spread with margarine and a little honey, jam or peanut butter
- ✔ Toast (preferably wholemeal or grain) spread with peanut butter or avocado
- ✔ Toasted English muffin with reduced-fat cheese
- ✔ Raisin loaf with margarine
- ✔ Crackers or crispbread spread with peanut butter or avocado or cottage cheese
- ✔ 2–3 sushi rolls
- ✔ Date or sultana scone or pikelet with butter/margarine
- ✔ Homemade popcorn (with a drizzle of margarine or oil and a sprinkle of salt, if any)
- ✔ Cake or muffin with added fruit or grated carrot

- ✔ Toasted sandwiches made with reduced-fat cheese and tomato, baked beans, tuna or creamed corn.

CEREALS

- ✔ Bowl of wholegrain or high-fibre cereal with low-fat milk or yoghurt
- ✔ Cereal bar or cereal-nut bar.

SOUP

A mug of vegetable or lentil soup makes a warming nutritious snack. Homemade is best; however, you'll find there are a number of healthy canned or tetra-pack soups at the supermarket. Look for one with less than 250 milligrams sodium per 100 millilitres and containing at least a serve of vegetables.

If the snack has figures over one or more of these limits, it can still be OK if it is wholegrain or high-fibre, high in calcium or contains oats or nuts. Choose a snack that is not so 'light' that you're hungry again in 30 minutes but not so filling that you don't feel like eating much at the next meal. It's good to be hungry for a meal!

WHAT TO LOOK FOR IN A PACKAGED SNACK

- Less than 600 kJ
- 3 g or less of 'bad' saturated fat
- 2 g or more of fibre
- 450 mg of sodium (salt)

Soda Water

See Mineral Water.

Sodium

An essential mineral element and electrolyte vital for the regulation of the body's water balance, sodium (together with potassium) also maintains the electrical differential of the cell membrane and so controls the working of muscles and nerves. Deficiency is rare and the effects from excess intakes pose a greater health concern in modern society, contributing to fluid retention and raised blood pressure. The recommended daily intake is 420–920 milligrams or 20–40 millimoles (equivalent to 1.2–2.4 grams or one-quarter to one-half teaspoon of salt).

See also **Salt.**

Sodium Chloride

This is common table salt.

See also **Salt.**

Soft Drinks

Sweetened fizzy drinks, which are 10–12 per cent sugar, are one group of drinks you should keep to a minimum. They have come under fire as a major contributor to the obesity epidemic and are increasingly being moved out of vending machines and school canteens, while parents are urged to have only water and milk in the fridge for kids. While the occasional glass of lemonade is an OK treat at a party or when dining out, the daily consumption of cans and bottles seems to invite weight problems and dental caries.

Both regular and diet soft drinks are acidic, with a pH ranging from 2.47 to 3.35 due to the phosphoric and citric acids. Together with their sugar, it's a harmful combination for teeth through dental erosion, the chemical stripping of the natural protective layer of teeth, so the enamel begins to lose its natural minerals. Continuously sipping soft drink creates an acid bath for teeth and cola drinks also add unwanted caffeine.

Even if you don't cut them out completely, limiting them or serving smaller portions makes a difference. A US study involving school students aged 11–14 years from 23 schools found that when smaller, single-serve packs were substituted for larger-sized snacks and drinks in the school lunch program, the students' kilojoule intakes of these foods decreased by 48 per cent. Having only the smaller-sized snacks at the cafeteria meant the children consumed less overall.

DID YOU KNOW?

Theoretically, drinking just one can of sweetened drink a day over a 10-year period, with all other things being constant, can add 50 kilograms over 10 years.

A UK study of 644 primary-school children from six schools in Dorset found that rates of obesity fell when the children were encouraged to cut back on fizzy drinks over a year. The children in the study were given extra lessons by a nurse who encouraged them to cut back on fizzy drinks and the message was reinforced by teachers. After a year, they cut back by only 125 millilitres a day, the equivalent of a third of a 370 millilitre can, but the prevalence of being overweight decreased by 0.2 per cent—effectively, the children did not gain excess weight. But the weight of kids in the control group, who were not encouraged to reduce their intake rose by 7.6 per cent after a year.

Diet drinks don't contain the sugar that causes tooth decay, but they still contain phosphoric acid or citric acid, which can cause erosion in teeth. The occasional diet soft drink is convenient when out with friends and to help keep your weight down, but you don't want to be drinking these regularly. They still keep your tastebuds used to the fizzy sweetness and can stimulate your appetite.

See also **Beverages.**

Solanine

This is a toxic substance found in green and sprouted potatoes, causing gastric upset (cramps, vomiting, diarrhoea) and headaches if consumed in large amounts.

Soup and Soup Diets

Pumpkin, tomato, minestrone, leek and potato, pea and ham, or chicken and noodle—a bowl of soup is warming and nourishing on a cold winter's day. With a chunk of crusty bread it makes a complete meal in itself. And when you're unwell, nothing perks you up more. But for dieters, soup is a filling first course and hunger-buster with good research to back up its power to satisfy and help you slim down.

Over the past 10 years, Dr Barbara Rolls, Professor of Nutrition at Pennsylvania State University, has been studying how soup can help your diet efforts. She's found that dieters who eat soup as their first course in a meal consume, on average, 400 fewer kilojoules in that meal compared with those who don't start with soup. Soup is a satisfying food that can work as a high-fibre, low-kilojoule 'meal replacement'. It's filling, so you feel full before you've eaten too much. Think of it like a homemade appetite suppressant. Sounds like the perfect diet food to me, and it's a great way to get your recommended five serves of vegetables a day.

WHY SOUP WORKS

Soup is an example of a food that's low in 'kilojoule-density', which means that it doesn't pack a lot of kilojoules into its volume. Consisting largely of water and fibre, soup is big on volume but light in fat and kilojoules, even those soups finished off with cream. A mug or bowl of soup only adds 250–700 kilojoules, which is quite low. In her book *The*

Volumetrics Eating Plan, Dr Rolls says soup is the opposite of chocolate mud cake, which packs a huge 2870 kilojoules into a small 175 gram wedge—high kilojoule-density.

So why not just drink a glass of water before you tuck into dinner? Interestingly, Dr Rolls' team has tested this theory. They showed that this does decrease feelings of hunger during a meal but is not maintained after the meal. However, water incorporated into a food does. So a bowl of chicken and rice soup reduced the intake at subsequent meals more effectively than eating the ingredients (chicken and rice) with a glass of water.

MY TAKE
Ditch the silly soup diets. Follow a sensible, balanced diet but use soup as a hunger-buster between meals.

Lowest in fat and kilojoules is a clear vegetable soup, tomato soup or chicken broth. These have a tiny 300 kilojoules per mug and less than 2 grams of fat. Then varieties like pumpkin or potato and leek come next with around 600 kilojoules and 5 grams of fat, which is not much, even with a splash of cream to finish them off. Finally, the richest soups are things like pea and ham or minestrone, with their beans or starchy root vegetables, but they still contain less fat and kilojoules than potato crisps or other snack foods. Being hot and filling, it's clear why vegetable soup is so useful for diets.

VEGETABLE SOUPS AND SOUP DIETS

Remember the *KickStart Soup Diet* that was all the rage a few winters ago? You cooked up a huge pot of non-fat vegetable soup using tomato, cabbage, onion and any other vegetables and stock, and lived on nothing but that for the first week. Then you gradually introduced one 'normal' meal a day but had a bowl of the soup for the other two meals and whenever you felt hungry. The soup was the magic bullet—it was hot and filling, had virtually no fat or kilojoules, was high in fibre, and you could eat as much as you liked.

Soup diets re-appear every few years in different guises. In the 1980s there was the *Cabbage Soup Diet* supposedly followed by Arnold Schwarzenegger to tone his ripped body. You can still download this diet from the internet today. Then in 2007 everyone was doing the *Kickstart Soup Diet* thanks to publicity on a current affairs TV program. Whatever its name, the principles are always the same. You eat as much as you like (or can stomach) of the low-kilojoule, fat-free vegetable hot pot. Mind you, there were side effects. First, many dieters complained of bad flatulence and even diarrhoea if they were hard at it on the soup. Second, you quickly tire of the same mug of veggie soup day in, day out, so once it's over you can't bear to go near soup for months after.

This soup diet was far from a balanced diet. Rather, it was a last-minute desperate measure to lose those extra kilos before a wedding or to kickstart your diet efforts before you switched to a more long-term and balanced plan. Shortcomings aside, the soup diet highlighted one thing—soup is a filling and satisfying food with good research to back up its power to satisfy and help slim down.

EASY 'HUNGER-BUSTER' VEGETABLE SOUP

This is a great high-fibre filler for dieters in cold weather; heat a bowl or microwave a mug whenever you're hungry. Low in kilojoules/calories and high in veggies and fibre, this soup is a dieter's best friend.

1 tablespoon oil
1 leek, sliced (white part only), or 1 medium onion, chopped
2 garlic cloves
1 carrot, sliced
2 sticks celery, sliced
1 zucchini (courgette), sliced
¼ cabbage, shredded
440 g can diced tomato
1 litre vegetable or chicken stock (ideally make your own)
2 cups water
2 tablespoons chopped parsley

Warm the oil in a large soup pot and sauté the leek or onions and garlic over low heat for 3–5 minutes until soft. Add the vegetables, tomato, stock and water. Bring to the boil, then reduce heat and simmer for 30 minutes or until vegetables are tender. Add parsley to serve, and more hot water or stock if you prefer a thinner soup.

Variation: Replace the stock with a beef soup bone or lamb shank with the leek or onions. Brown in the oil and continue with the recipe. This makes a good salt-free soup if you need to cut out the salt.

Sorbitol

This is a sugar alcohol used to sweeten diet foods such as jam and chocolate in place of sugar. It is more slowly absorbed than sugar and has little effect on blood-glucose levels. As it supplies the same kilojoules as sugar, it is of little benefit for weight reduction, unlike no-kilojoule sweeteners such as aspartame. It can also function as a humectant. It does not cause dental decay but high doses may have a laxative effect. Its additive code is 420.

See also **Sweeteners.**

Soy Beans and Soy Foods

A cream-coloured, oval bean about the size of a common pea, the soy bean has made headlines because of its rich content of phytoestrogens, natural plant hormones known as isoflavones, which have a close chemical resemblance to our own human hormones (*phyto* means plant). Soy beans have been an integral part of the cuisines of China, Japan and Korea for nearly five centuries, where they were one of five sacred crops and earned the name 'meat of the fields' for their valuable protein content.

Today, the humble soy bean has lost its status as a 'magic bullet'. After its initial burst of publicity, the follow-up studies did not find it worked quite as well for menopausal women as hoped. But it still has influence on heart disease, cancer and bone health, making it an important bean to include in our meals.

THE WONDERS OF SOY

Soy beans are nutritional all-rounders and provide us with:

- High-quality protein—soy has twice as much protein as other beans and it's the best the plant kingdom has to offer, including the eight essential amino acids normally found in animal protein
- Lots of dietary fibre, like all beans and lentils. It's soluble fibre, the type that helps mop up cholesterol
- A number of minerals such as phosphorus, iron, calcium, zinc and magnesium
- Polyunsaturated oil—about 17 per cent of the soy bean is oil that is extracted as soy bean oil
- Plant omega-3 fatty acid alpha-linolenic acid
- Low saturated fats, no cholesterol
- Plant sterols, which can lower cholesterol.

WHAT SOY FOOD IS THAT?

MISO

Miso is a smooth, thick paste made from fermented soy beans alone or with a grain such as rice or barley and salt. It is used to flavour dishes and to make miso soup, a dark salty broth offered in Japanese restaurants.

NATTO

Made of fermented cooked whole beans, natto is more easily digested than the beans themselves. It is often served as a topping for rice, vegetables and in miso soups.

SOY AND LINSEED BREAD*

Breads such as Burgen Soy-Lin and Helga Nice Grains are good for phytoestrogens. Studies show that four slices of these breads a day reduce menopausal flush by 40 per cent.

*Good sources of plant oestrogens.

SOY BABY FORMULA*

Based on soy protein isolate, soy baby formulas have been shown to be safe, although nutritionists maintain there is no nutritional advantage in using a soy formula over a standard cow's milk–based formula. Because of their high aluminum content, soy formulas are not recommended for premature babies.

SOY BEAN OIL

Extracted from whole soy beans, it is a pale golden oil which can be used for cooking or salads. It is predominantly polyunsaturated (62 per cent) with 8 per cent omega-3 fats.

SOY DRINK* (MILK)

Soy drinks are useful for lactose intolerance, dairy allergies and vegans.

SOY FLOUR*

A gluten-free flour made from finely ground roasted soy beans, it can be substituted for one-third of the wheat flour in recipes for muffins and breads. It can be full-fat, containing all the natural oil in the soy bean, or defatted, where the oil has been removed. Defatted is thus more concentrated, making it higher in protein.

SOY GRITS*

These are coarse chunks of toasted soy, often added to breads for texture.

SOY LECITHIN

Extracted from soy bean oil, it is used as an emulsifier in oil-based foods such as margarine, mayonnaise and pastry. Soy lecithin keeps ingredients stabilised, inhibits oxidation and cystallisation. Its additive code number is 322.

SOY SAUCE AND TAMARI

This is a dark-brown condiment made from soy beans that have undergone a fermenting process. Tamari is made only from soy, while *shoyu* is a mixture of soy and wheat.

SOY YOGHURT, SOY ICE-CREAM

These are non-dairy desserts made from soy milk.

TEMPEH*

This is a fermented soy bean patty with a nutty flavour, commonly found in Indonesia. Slice thinly and grill or pan fry as a meat replacement in stir-fries, burgers and vegetarian dishes.

TEXTURED VEGETABLE PROTEIN*

Dried soy 'mince' is made from soy flour that has been defatted and compressed into granules or chunks. It's an excellent substitute for minced meat.

TOFU*

Also known as bean curd, tofu is a soft food made by curdling soy milk with a coagulant, in much the same way as cheese is produced from milk.

WHOLE SOY BEANS*

Home cooked or canned, you can add them to soups, salads, casseroles and curries.

WHAT YOU CAN DO TO INCREASE YOUR SOY INTAKE

- ✔ Add canned, drained beans to casseroles and soups.
- ✔ Make nachos with soy in place of kidney beans.
- ✔ Blend soy smoothies with soy milk (enriched with calcium) and fruit.
- ✔ Drain firm tofu and slice into strips or cubes; marinate and add to stir-fries or float on soups.
- ✔ Substitute some soy flour for ordinary flour when baking muffins and cakes.
- ✔ Switch to soy-linseed breads, soy high-fibre cereals and soy crispbreads.
- ✔ Eat more Japanese tofu dishes or miso soup (take care as they're quite salty).
- ✔ Try soy vegetarian slices or burgers.
- ✔ Use soft or silken tofu to make sauces or a creamy salad dressing.

See also **Tofu and Tempeh; Soy Milk; Emulsifiers.**

Soy Milk

Available in full-fat and low-fat versions, soy milk is similar to cow's milk in nutrients and kilojoules, but it can vary a great deal in its calcium content. Soy milk can be made in two different ways, which may influence your choice at the supermarket. It can be made from whole beans that are soaked, heated and then crushed to extract the milky juice, which is blended with water, sweeteners like malted barley or sugar, vegetable oil and salt. This method is generally lower in calcium (20–80 milligrams per glass) but rich in protein and B vitamins and regarded as more 'natural'. Soy milk can also be blended from soy protein isolate powder (which is processed from defatted soy flour and contains around 90 per cent pure protein), together with water, oil, sweeteners like sugar or maltodextrin, gums, emulsifier, vitamins, mineral salts and calcium. Generally fortified with vitamins A, B_1, B_2, B_{12} and calcium to a level similar to that in milk (250–290 milligrams per glass), this has a better flavour with a less 'beany' taste.

Soy milk would suit someone with lactose intolerance (inability to digest lactose) or a milk allergy, or for those who wish to avoid cow's milk for other reasons such as vegans and vegetarians. The best advice for vegans is to consume a soy milk that is fortified with B_{12} or else take a B_{12} supplement, particularly if you are pregnant or breastfeeding. The liver does store some B_{12}—about enough to last 3–5 years—but not enough to meet the demands of pregnancy.

See also **Milk and Milk Alternatives.**

Spices

A dusting of cinnamon, a pinch of chilli, a sprinkle of paprika—I love spices for their exotic, intense flavours that can transform the ordinary into the sublime, and for their emerging health benefits. Spices have a long history of both culinary and medicinal use, as well as acting as preserving agents for food.

Research is now revealing that they are antioxidant powerhouses and health superstars. For instance, a study published in 2010 analysed over 3100 different foods from around the world and found that culinary herbs and spices have the highest antioxidant content of all foods. The study reported that their average antioxidant activity was 300 per cent higher than that of berries (often at the top of many antioxidant lists), 2300 per cent greater than that of other fruit and 3600 per cent higher than that of vegetables.

Another study that analysed spices for polyphenols (a class of more than 4000 antioxidants) confirmed this top ranking, way ahead of the well-researched red wine, tea and cocoa. Cloves, star anise, turmeric (curry powder), ginger, cumin, cinnamon and

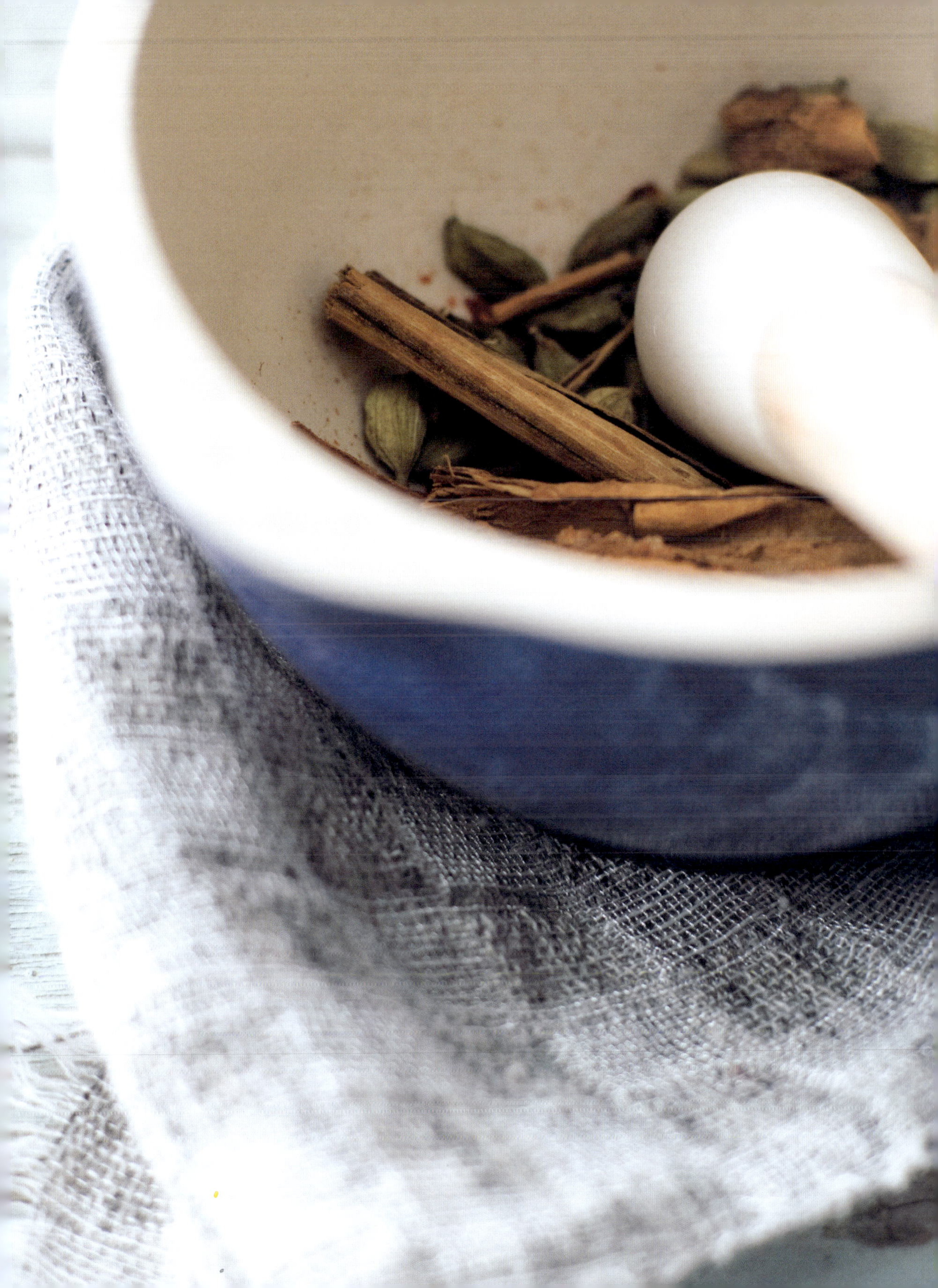

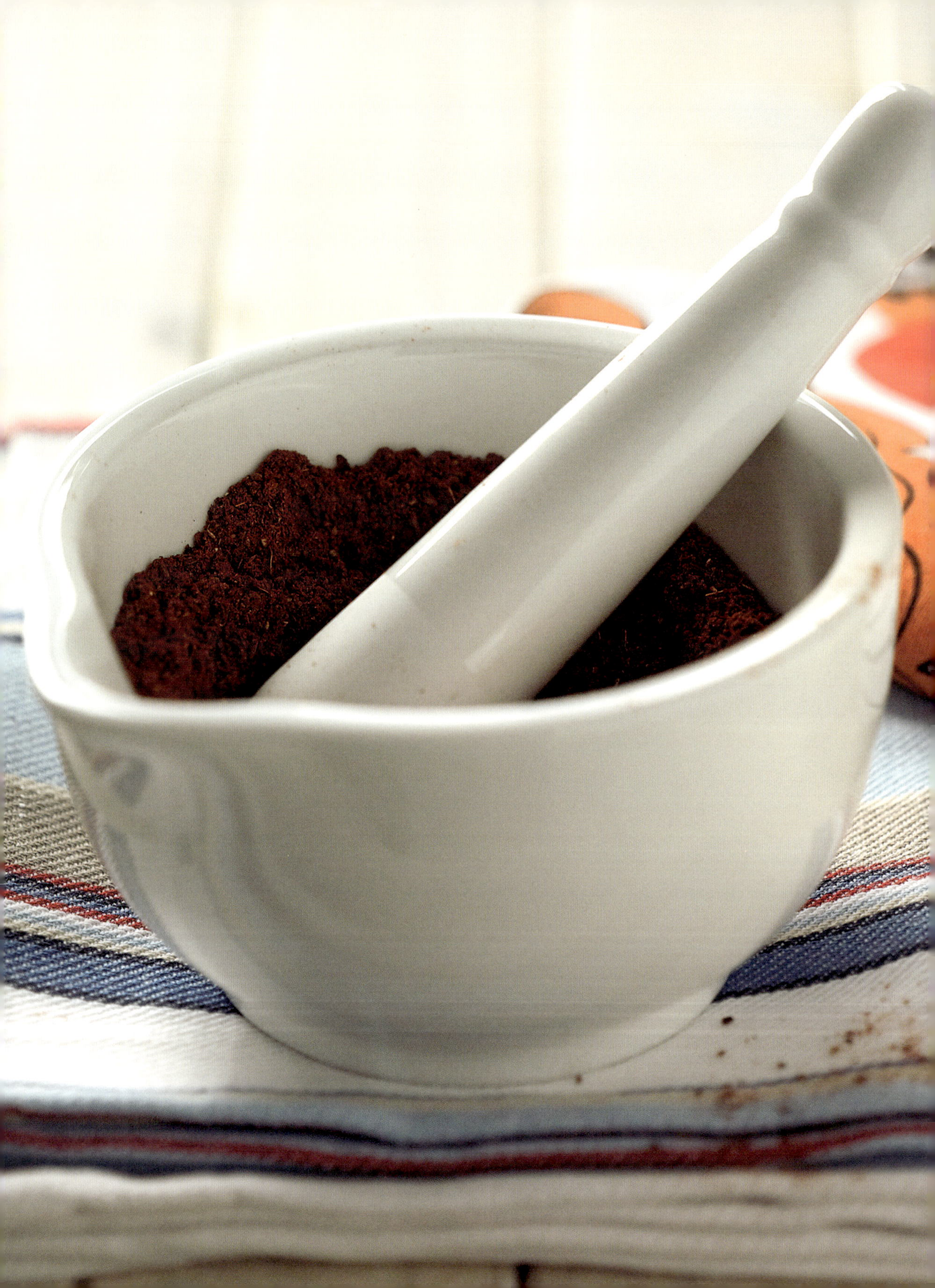

allspice have the highest levels among the spices. On the herb side, peppermint, oregano, sage, thyme, rosemary, basil, lemon verbena, parsley and marjoram are high scorers (but they all have some).

Research is now revealing that spices are antioxidant powerhouses and health superstars.

HOW THEY WORK

With their powerful antioxidant punch, spices help neutralise free radicals and slow inflammation that can set the scene for diseases such as cancer, heart and liver disease, and it can slow the ageing process. For virtually no kilojoules and little expense, spices appear to work to support our immune system, aid digestion, manage nausea, support bone and joint health, and relieve pain. Some, like cinnamon, have been studied for their ability to control blood-sugar levels. This can decrease the risk of diabetes and blood vessel damage. Scientists also believe that spices act synergistically, so they enhance the health properties of other foods and can multiply the antioxidant value of a meal.

Finally, spices make it easy for you to cut back on salt and fat. Their intense flavour lets you get away with less salt in marinades, dressings, stir-fries and curries. I estimate you can halve the amount of salt you 'need' without noticing it in hot, spicy dishes. The same goes for added fat. All good reasons to spend time building a good selection of spices in your kitchen and use them liberally.

See also **Chilli; Ginger.**

Spinach *See* **Vegetables**

Spirulina

Spirulina is a blue-green plankton promoted as a rich source of protein and vitamins A and B. Distributors claim that it is the highest known source of vitamin B_{12}, having twice the amount of B_{12} found in liver. Spirulina is also recommended as an energy booster and appetite suppressant. Some pamphlets say that spirulina supplies chlorophyll, which purifies the blood and balances your metabolism.

With all these marvellous promises, it's not surprising that spirulina is selling well. However, a study carried out by the University of California raises serious doubts about its supposed value. The majority of B_{12} in spirulina was found to be B_{12} analogues—vitamin look-alikes with a similar chemical structure but with no vitamin activity. The report concluded that it has no special nutritional advantages and its safety has not been established.

See also **Sea Vegetables.**

Spreads and Toppings

What's the healthiest thing to spread on your toast, bread or cracker biscuits? It's a common question, especially from parents, and there's not one, easy answer. The most practical answer depends on your health profile and what you're looking for. If you and your family are in good health, your overall diet is healthy (not a lot of takeaways or fatty snacks) and you want as natural a diet as you can, then butter is fine in moderation. But if you have high cholesterol or diabetes, then margarine is a wiser choice. And it spreads thinly so keeps your fat intake down.

Margarine and butter have the same fat content and the same kilojoule count. One teaspoon of either, which is roughly the amount that you spread on a slice of bread, gives you 4 grams of fat and 152 kilojoules. Whichever you go for, look for one that's

	BUTTER	LIGHT BUTTER SPREADS (DAIRY BLENDS)	CANOLA OIL SPREAD (MARGARINE)	OLIVE OIL SPREAD (MARGARINE)	STEROL SPREADS (SUCH AS LOGICOL AND PRO-ACTIV)
Saturated fat (%)	53	33	20	19	11–17
Made from	Cream	Butter usually blended with canola or sunflower oil, or butter that has had some of the harder saturated fatty acids removed, or butter that's been whipped (aerated)	Canola oil that's been blended with a lightly hardened vegetable fat	Olive oil that's been blended with canola and lightly hardened vegetable fat	Vegetable oil with added plant sterols (natural compounds extracted from soy or other plants)
Pros	Less 'processed' than margarine, it's a good source of fat-soluble vitamins A and D and it also has a great flavour.	Softer than regular butter, they spread more easily straight from the fridge but are still firm.	It has a pleasant taste and spreads easily, and is a good source of beta-carotene (vitamin A), vitamins D and E.	It has a pleasant taste, spreads easily and is a good source of beta-carotene (vitamin A) and vitamin D.	The sterols block cholesterol absorption, forcing your body to 'use up' more from its internal pool, lowering your blood cholesterol level.
Cons	It's hard to spread thinly so you often end up eating more.	They're not recommended by the Heart Foundation if you have high cholesterol.	Some people don't like the taste and mouth feel.	There's not as much olive oil as you'd think—only around 20 per cent. It contains 70 per cent total fat, so limit it if you're trying to lose weight.	You have to eat 2–3 teaspoons (25 grams) daily for the cholesterol-lowering effect to work. It may interfere with the absorption of fat-soluble vitamins, so you need to eat lots of yellow and green vegetables to make up for it.
MY TAKE	*Butter is natural (just as they say in the advertising), being made from dairy fat and salt. It has been around ever since humans started herding cows, and tastes divine. If you love the taste of butter but need to watch your cholesterol, save it for those times when you can really taste it, such as with freshly baked bread or to sauté leeks or mushrooms. For baking, use salt-free butter.*	*If you enjoy butter, this is a good compromise. Reduced-salt versions have 50 per cent less salt and still taste good.*	*Don't use for cooking; oils are better because they don't spit at high temperatures.*	*Don't use an olive oil spread for cooking; stick to olive oil which won't spit.*	*They have about half the total fat of regular margarine, which is useful, as most people with high cholesterol need to lose weight.*

salt-reduced (1 per cent salt) or salt-free and use it sparingly. We don't need much of either. Here's a guide (opposite) to the different choices ranked by their saturated fat content.

DID YOU KNOW?

Most margarines today must be called 'spreads' as they contain only 60 or 70 per cent fat. Technically only a product with 80 per cent fat can be called margarine so it is an exact match for butter.

HEALTHY SPREADS

As neither butter nor margarine are ideal spreads, I prefer to not use them and instead opt for one of these spreads on my bread or toast.

AVOCADO

It is rich in mono-unsaturated fat—the same heart-friendly fat in olive oil and macadamias—with little of the 'bad' saturated fat. With 22 per cent total fat, it is much lower than butter, margarine and most light variants. Natural and healthy!

COTTAGE CHEESE

A skim milk curd, cottage cheese is a great option for kids with its mild taste and interesting, soft consistency. Pile onto crusty bread or crackers and go for the low-fat option—you'll be loving it with about 2 per cent fat!

HUMMUS

Made from tahini (sesame seed paste), chickpeas, lemon, garlic and salt, hummus has 15–20 per cent fat. Being low in saturated fat, it is another tasty and healthy option as a spread or dip.

LIGHT CREAM CHEESE

At 14 per cent fat, light cream cheese offers you a spreadable option with around one-third less fat than the full-fat version.

OLIVE OIL

A Mediterranean favourite, olive oil is 70 per cent mono-unsaturated fat with little saturated fat. It contributes to the long life that the Mediterranean foodies are renowned for! Drizzled on toast or dunked with bread, it adds a gutsy flavour—perfect with your morning eggs and tomato.

RICOTTA CHEESE

Italian for 'twice-cooked', ricotta is like cottage cheese but smoother in texture, with no added salt. It is a by-product of cheese made from the leftover whey of other cheeses, or it can be made directly with cow's milk whey. Not only spreadable, ricotta can be used in baking, sweet or savoury, and in pasta dishes like lasagne.

TOPPINGS FOR BREAD

VEGEMITE

No kilojoules or fat, plenty of B vitamins but lots of salt. If you smear this Aussie icon on a slice of bread (around 3 grams), you get 105 milligrams of sodium, which is a little less than what you'd get from the bread itself, even though bread doesn't taste overly salty. But most people who like this salty, black yeast spread like it thick or even lick it off the knife. So a thick spread (10 grams) gives you triple what's in the bread and 17 per cent of the recommended day's intake. So spread thin and you're OK.

PEANUT BUTTER (PASTE)

This is protein for vegetarians, good fats and fibre, but it may come with more sugar or salt than you bargained for. Whether you like it smooth or crunchy, peanut butter is a convenient healthy spread. Ideally buy the 100 per cent all-peanut type even though it tends to be hard to spread and the oil rises to the top and has to be drained off. The upside is a great peanut flavour and no added salt—it's the one for the purists. Most supermarket brands give you 85 per cent peanuts blended with oil to keep the consistency spreadable, as well as some sugar and salt. Just don't spread butter/margarine before your peanut butter; there's enough fat there as it is.

> **DID YOU KNOW?**
>
> These days virtually all the margarines in Australia are free of trans fats, a situation different from the US and UK. The only exceptions are cheaper or generic margarines, which you would recognise as hard (stick) margarines. Avoid these and go for the softer types and you can be fairly sure you're not buying trans fats.

JAM

Jam has 60–70 per cent sugars derived from both the added sugar and fruit sugars. It has no fat, a bit of fruit fibre, a smidge of potassium and that's about it. There's vitamin C in most fruit but not in jam as the heat of jam-making destroys it. It satisfies a sweet tooth without fat (unlike chocolate or cake) and encourages the consumption of wholemeal bread.

HONEY

At 75 per cent sugar and no fat, honey is similar to jam. It contains little in the way of B vitamins or minerals so think of it as an extra that can enliven your slice of grainy toast or cereal on cold mornings.

NUTELLA

This is another 'treat' spread, so don't get sucked in by their advertising. It's nowhere near a health food—at 55 per cent sugar and 30 per cent fat, it is more akin to chocolate than hazelnuts or cocoa. I'd rank it between peanut butter and jam.

See also **Honey.**

Sterols (Phytosterols or Plant Sterols)

These are naturally occurring compounds related to cholesterol but which have the ability to lower cholesterol levels by inhibiting the absorption of dietary and biliary cholesterol from the gut. They are found in small amounts in most plant foods such as nuts, seeds, wholegrains and legumes, with the highest levels found in vegetable oils. The predominant ones are sitosterol, campesterol and stegmasterol. Commercially, sterols are isolated as a by-product of the processing of soy beans or wood pulp and are added to spreads, yoghurts and cheeses as a functional ingredient under the claim 'Helps lower cholesterol absorption'.

Adding 2–3 grams of sterols a day reduces LDL cholesterol by 10–15 per cent, while having no effect on the good HDL or triglycerides. This quantity translates to around 1–1.5 tablespoons of special sterol-enriched spread a day (e.g. Logicol or Pro-activ), about the amount you'd spread on three or four slices of bread. You can also buy enriched milk and yoghurt (Heart Active).

Stearic Acid

This is a saturated fatty acid that does not raise blood cholesterol. Major food sources are the visible selvage of fat around meat, chocolate and commercial fats used for deep frying and baking, many of which are derived from beef tallow (beef fat).

Starch

This is the storage carbohydrate of plant foods like cereal grains, potatoes and other starchy tubers, legumes and fruit like bananas. Chemically, starch is a polysaccharide made up of thousands of glucose molecules. Raw starch occurs in the form of partially crystalline granules, which have different structures, altering their ability to absorb water and therefore their rate of digestion in the human digestive tract. Digestible starch is broken down to glucose and yields 17 kilojoules per gram.

See also **Carbohydrates.**

Stevia

Stevia is a sweetener derived from the leaves of *Stevia rebaudiana*, a plant common in Paraguay where, for hundreds of years, it has been valued for its sweetening properties and called 'honey leaf'. To my palate there is a slight liquorice aftertaste, which I dislike but others don't mind. To me, it doesn't have the same aftertaste as sugar but is way better in taste than the older sweeteners such as saccharin or even aspartame.

See also **Sweeteners.**

Stock

Stock, whether chicken, beef, fish or vegetable, is a great flavour booster for anyone watching their weight. It has a tiny 1 per cent fat, few kilojoules (only 325 kilojoules for a cup), and significant amounts of potassium and other minerals extracted from all those bones and vegetables. Stock makes soups, risottos, noodle dishes and gravy interesting and flavoursome. Think savoury and *umami*.

Stock is easy to make at home if you have time. You just throw everything into a large stock-pot, simmer and forget about it. Every cookbook has a recipe but my standard method is to gently heat bones along with onion, celery tops, turnip, a carrot and some mixed herbs. Add enough water to cover and simmer for an hour or so. For a darker stock, brown chicken or beef bones in the oven first.

The cartilage and connective tissue in the bones are the key to a rich flavour. They have collagen, which is converted into gelatin and thickens the liquid, perfect for clear beef broth, French onion soup or coq au vin. Another bonus is that all those lovely vegetable off-cuts—including onion skins—can be used. Cool and freeze your finished stock for later. Use containers for 2 cups or 1 litre or whatever is the right amount for your soup recipes.

Bought stocks are convenient but they can be high in salt, although manufacturers have lowered the salt they add in recent years. Shop for 'salt reduced' versions or check the label and choose one with a sodium content of less than 400 milligrams per 100 grams.

See also **Glutamates and *Umami*, Natural.**

Sucralose

Sucralose is a sweetener (trade name Splenda) made from sugar that has 600 times the sweetness of sugar but none of its kilojoules. Its great advantage over other sweeteners is that it doesn't break down with heat so it can be used in cooking and baking (additive code 955). It's made by a process that changes the chemical structure of sugar whereby three of the hydroxyl ends in a sucrose molecule are replaced with chloride. So it's made from sugar but it's far from natural. It has a good safety record and pleasant taste.

Aside from the sucralose, which is present in tiny quantities, the Splenda sweeteners (granules, tablets or sachets) you'll find in the supermarket contain a variety of filler ingredients. These can be in the form of the starch maltodextrin, dextrose or lactose, a common filler added to bulk out many tablets. When Splenda is used to sweeten diet soft drinks, there is no need for accompanying starches as there is with the other forms above.

See also **Sweeteners.**

Sucrose

See also **Sugar.**

This is a double sugar composed of glucose and fructose.

Sugar

Once condemned as 'pure, white and deadly', sugar is receiving more moderate press today. While it does play a role in causing tooth decay, it does not directly cause problems such as heart disease, diabetes, cancer and hypoglycaemia; rather, it is an indirect factor in that it can lead to being overweight.

In moderation, sugar is unlikely to cause harm and adds to the enjoyment of food. A teaspoon of sugar in a cup of tea or a wedge of cake would hardly destroy the nutritional value of an otherwise healthy diet. Adding a little sweetness makes high-fibre, low-fat foods more palatable—think how much more enjoyable a spread of honey or jam is on wholemeal bread or some brown sugar over porridge. Dietary guidelines suggest that Australians and New Zealanders should eat only moderate amounts of sugar and foods containing added sugar. You don't need to avoid sugar completely for good health, but it's sensible to cut back on foods that are correspondingly low in nutrition such as soft drinks, pastries and sweets.

Foods such as flavoured yoghurts or breakfast cereals have a much better nutrient profile, and they give you important nutrients along with the sugar they contain. Sugar appears on the ingredient list of many foods, but only in very small quantities, where it functions as a flavour balancer (e.g. pasta sauce) or yeast food (e.g. bread). These sources of sugar are negligible and do not pose any health concern.

NUTRITIONAL VALUE

Sugar is sugar, whether white, brown, raw or in syrup form. They are all very similar in nutrition and kilojoule count and are all sources of sucrose, as well as some glucose and fructose, but very little in the way of vitamins, minerals or other beneficial nutrients.

- One level teaspoon (4 grams) of all sugars has 68 kilojoules.
- One level tablespoon (30 grams) of honey or any of the sugar syrups has 360 kilojoules.

All sugar in Australia and New Zealand comes from sugar cane, which is milled and refined to extract the sugar. Sugar cane is crushed in the mill and the resulting juice is purified and then boiled to produce a thick syrup. From this syrup, raw sugar crystals are formed, leaving a dark, sticky liquid called molasses behind.

Although usually taken to mean white table sugar or sucrose, there are several sugars of nutritional importance—fructose (fruit sugar), glucose, lactose (milk sugar) and maltose. Fructose ranks as the sweetest, followed by sucrose, glucose, maltose and lactose. All supply 17 kilojoules per gram, regardless of their sweetness.

TOTAL SUGARS

Food labels only tell you the total quantity of sugars present, which includes:

- Added sugar
- Naturally occurring sugars from fruit (fructose) and milk (lactose).

There is no way to tell what proportion of this is added and how much is natural. It's particularly confusing for foods such as flavoured yoghurts, cereals with dried fruit or canned fruit in syrup, which contain both types of sugar.

A bowl of Sultana Bran has around 10 grams of total sugars. Of this, 6 grams comes from the sultanas, which are high in fruit sugars, and only 4 grams comes from the sugar added to make the bran flakes. Foods that are pure sugar, like soft drink, cordial or jubes, contain only cane sugar. When checking where sugar appears on the list of ingredients, note that the closer it is to the top, the more sugar has been added. And look for sugar under different names like honey, glucose (dextrose), fructose, maltose or fruit juice concentrate.

HOW MUCH SUGAR SHOULD YOU CONSUME?

Recommended sugar levels differ according to how many kilojoules you burn off during the day. Generally speaking, around 10–12 per cent of your kilojoules can come from added sugar—a modest amount that does not cause health problems. For example, a sedentary woman who eats an 8000 kilojoule diet could happily consume 800 kilojoules or 45 grams of sugar (from both the sugar she adds to food and that found in sweetened foods). This translates to 10 level teaspoons of sugar a day. The table (right) shows how that added sugar adds up.

	SERVE SIZE	SUGAR (g)	SUGAR (tsp)
Breakfast cereal	1 bowl	10	2
Muesli slice	1 slice	17	4
Tea with sugar	2 cups	8	2
Ice-cream	1 scoop	10	2.5
TOTAL		45	10

The more active you are, the more you can eat. An active 16-year-old boy who burns off 12,600 kilojoules a day would be able to tuck into some 20 teaspoons a day. Most of us consume much more than this—adults eat on average 66 grams a day of added sugar, while teenagers consume the most at around 80–140 grams.

FOUR SIMPLE WAYS TO KEEP YOUR SUGAR INTAKE MODERATE

- Cut back on soft drink, cordial and juices. Remember, a can of soft drink gives you around 10 teaspoons of sugar! When you do buy cans of soft drink, dilute them down with ice or water. For kids, offer plain water or milk.
- Save sweet foods like lollies, chocolate, cakes and fancy ice creams for a special occasion. Don't always reward your kids with a lolly or chocolate.
- Between meals, snack on a piece of fresh fruit *or* nuts *or* yoghurt *or* cheese and crackers instead of sweet biscuits, chocolate or cake.
- Cut back on the sugar you sprinkle over cereal and use to sweeten your coffee or tea. If you cut back gradually, you'll find you won't notice the drop in your sugar intake.

WHAT SUGAR IS THAT?

WHITE SUGAR

This is one of the world's purest foods. It is 99.9 per cent sucrose, refined from sugar cane with all impurities such as mineral ash completely removed. Caster sugar has the same composition as granulated sugar, but the crystals are smaller so it dissolves quickly. Icing sugar is white sugar ground to a fine powder. All three sugars have a moderate GI of 65.

BROWN SUGAR

Brown sugar contains 95 per cent sucrose and 5 per cent molasses, which adds a toffee flavour and moistness, but no nutritional benefits over white sugar. The same applies to muscovado, demerara and black sugars, often preferred for baking.

RAW SUGAR AND COFFEE SUGAR CRYSTALS

These are made from cane juice and are golden in colour. They are virtually identical to white sugar, and at 99 per cent sucrose, they have a few minerals but not enough to give a health advantage over white sugar.

MOLASSES

A dark, sticky liquid, this is the syrup left behind after the raw sugar crystallises during sugar milling. It's a mixture of 36–38 per cent sucrose, 10–13 per cent glucose and fructose, and 24–30 per cent water. It also has some minerals and traces of B vitamins. Blackstrap molasses has been promoted as a 'healthy food' but the quantities of B vitamins present are very small.

GOLDEN SYRUP

A concentrated sugar syrup with a distinctive flavour and golden colour, golden syrup is favoured for hearty desserts such as steamed pudding.

TREACLE

Treacle is a viscous, dark-brown liquid that has a stronger flavour and aroma than golden syrup. Like golden syrup, it is produced by partly breaking down sugar into its glucose and fructose components. This process stops crystals from forming and thus creates a stable liquid product.

MAPLE SYRUP

This is the concentrated sap from the sugar maple tree and consists primarily of sugars—anywhere from 90–100 per cent sucrose and 0–10 per cent glucose or fructose. There are also traces of organic acids, vitamins and some mineral material dissolved in maple syrup, with manganese, potassium, iron and calcium being the most prevalent minerals. It's similar in food value to golden syrup or molasses.

HONEY

Honey has fewer kilojoules than sugar as it contains around 20 per cent water and only 75 per cent sugars, of which roughly half is glucose and half fructose. It also contains small amounts of plant acids, waxes, gums, pigments and volatile oils which have antioxidant properties. Honey contains B vitamins and minerals but the quantities are tiny and not significant nutritionally. You would have to consume enormous amounts of honey to obtain a decent intake.

See also Honey.

FRUCTOSE

Fructose contains the same kilojoules as sugar but, being slightly sweeter, can be used in smaller quantities to achieve the same degree of sweetness. Now marketed as a sugar replacement, it has a low GI of 19. Fructose is metabolised differently from sugar and doesn't trigger the hormones that regulate appetite and intake.

HIGH-FRUCTOSE CORN SYRUP

A sweetener derived from corn or maize starch, this syrup is popular in the US where it's used to sweeten soft drinks and doughnuts. It is a mix of 50 per cent sucrose and 50 per cent glucose. Over the past 30 years, it has gradually replaced sugar in the US food supply and researchers suspect it may somehow contribute to obesity. It also seems to trigger the body to overproduce triglycerides.

TRUE OR FALSE?

SUGAR GIVES YOU ENERGY

True and false. Sugar is a carbohydrate and, like all carbohydrates, is a source of energy (measured in kilojoules or calories). But it is a common myth that sugar 'picks you up' and boosts your vitality when you're feeling tired or run down. Studies of the ways different foods are absorbed into the bloodstream (their glycemic index or GI) show that sugar has only a moderate effect on blood-glucose levels and is not as quickly absorbed as glucose itself or white bread. Many starchy foods such as potatoes and Rice Bubbles are better foods for quick energy boosts than sugar.

SUGAR MAKES YOU FAT

False. Sugar alone cannot be held responsible for excess weight; too much food and too little exercise are the real culprits. Sugar has less than half the kilojoules of pure fat. Two teaspoons of sugar supply 130 kilojoules, which is equivalent to only half a slice of bread. Nonetheless, sugar is a refined food and easy to over-consume, a major reason for its restriction in weight-loss diets. Because sugar often keeps company with fat, watch out for sweet high fat foods such as chocolate, puddings, muffins, pastries and biscuits.

SUGAR IS A USELESS FOOD

False. Apart from its sweet taste, sugar has indispensable functions in cooking. It acts as a preserving agent by inhibiting the growth of moulds in jams and chutneys. It helps activate the yeast in bread and retains moisture in cakes and biscuits. Sugar brings out the flavour of fruit products, tomato dishes and sauces. It also helps create a smooth, creamy texture in ice-cream and adds 'mouth feel' to soft drinks and toppings.

SUGAR ROTS YOUR TEETH

True and false. Sugar does contribute to dental caries (cavities), but so do all fermentable carbohydrates, including those in biscuits, savoury crackers, bread, muffins and dried fruit. Any sugar or cooked starch that the bacteria in your mouth can break down into acid (which gradually eats away at tooth enamel) is a potential danger food for teeth. It's worse if it comes in a chewy, sticky form that clings to teeth long after we've finished eating. You can minimise the damage by brushing teeth after meals and by allowing saliva, which can repair some of this acid damage, to do its job. This means less frequent snacks—it is better to eat lollies or potato crisps all at one time than to nibble or suck on them all day. Chewing sugar-free gum also helps, by stimulating the flow of saliva.

KILOJOULES FROM SUGAR ARE EMPTY KILOJOULES

True. Apart from its carbohydrate, sugar contains no essential vitamins, minerals or fibre. If it is eaten in large amounts and at the expense of more nutritious foods, then an unbalanced diet can result.

SUGAR GIVES YOU DIABETES

False. Diabetes is frequently believed to be the direct result of eating too much sugar. This misconception is understandable, since the dietary treatment for many years was to avoid sugar and it is easy to confuse terms such as blood sugar (glucose) with sugar in food (sucrose). Excess weight and a sedentary lifestyle have been identified as the two major causes of type 2 diabetes, not how much sugar is eaten.

Once diabetes is diagnosed, proper control of diet is essential to prevent sudden surges of blood glucose, so large quantities of sweets or sweetened drinks on an empty stomach should be avoided. Studies have shown, however, that sugar taken with a meal (e.g. dessert or ice-cream) does not lead to high levels of blood sugar as had commonly been supposed. Foods vary in the rise of blood glucose that they produce and people with diabetes now have a greater latitude with sugar and are allowed it as an exchange for starchy foods. A little sugar also improves the palatability of low-fat, high-fibre diets, so they are more likely to be followed.

SUGAR CAUSES HYPOGLYCAEMIA

False. Sugar has been condemned as the cause of hypoglycaemia or low blood sugar. Many writers have claimed that hypoglycaemia is responsible for much of the depression, anxiety and mood swings people experience today. Sugar, they claim, overloads the pancreas, forcing it to overproduce insulin. The insulin clears the blood of glucose and, despite having just eaten, the body tissues become starved of energy. In an attempt to correct the lack of glucose, the body instinctively puts out signals for sweet foods, which only starts the sugar craving cycle again.

True hypoglycaemia is a rare condition. A valid diagnosis requires that blood glucose drops below normal and is accompanied by shakiness, an inability to think clearly, fainting attacks and sweating. It is especially important that symptoms are immediately relieved by eating something sweet (or by injecting glucose into the bloodstream). Sugar in moderation is rarely the cause of hypoglycaemia. The only exception is when it is taken as a large drink with alcohol on an empty stomach.

SUGAR MAKES KIDS HYPERACTIVE

False. Hyperactivity, one of the key symptoms of attention deficit hyperactivity disorder (ADHD), has often been linked to sugar, but without solid evidence. A number of studies of ADHD children have used artificially sweetened foods as dummy controls to assess children's behaviour with and without sugar. The most recent and thorough study was carried out in Tennessee, USA, which found that even large amounts of sugar produced no significant alteration in behaviour or cognitive performance of children. Even though the researchers selected children whose parents described them as 'sugar sensitive', the parents couldn't tell when their children were on the high-sugar diet or on one of the two diets incorporating sweeteners (saccharin or aspartame).

Because kids often become unruly after parties where sugary foods are consumed, many parents blame the high load of sugar. But there's more evidence to condemn some of the other substances commonly present with sugar, such as:

- caffeine in cola soft drinks and chocolate
- artificial colours in cordial, soft drink, lollies, ice-blocks and cheese snack foods
- preservatives in frankfurts, party pies, dips and pizzas.

All these compounds, but not sugar, are removed in a standard elimination diet used to test whether food is a trigger for behaviour problems.

HIDDEN SUGAR

Only about 25 per cent of the total sugar we ingest is sugar that we consciously add to foods—in tea, coffee or in home baking. The remaining 75 per cent comes from the everyday packaged and pre-prepared food we consume, such as biscuits, cakes, yoghurt, ice-cream, fruit juice drinks and breakfast cereals, as well as the more obvious soft drinks, cordial, chocolate and lollies.

This is a dramatic reversal of the situation early last century. Up until the 1950s, most sugar was used at home to prepare jams, biscuits, cakes, bottled fruit, sweets and puddings as well as for table use to sweeten tea, coffee and cereals. Today, with the growth of convenient ready-made foods and the decline in home cooking, sugar usage at home has dropped dramatically. Despite this, our total intake has changed relatively little.

While it does play a role in causing tooth decay, sugar does not directly cause problems such as heart disease, diabetes, cancer and hypoglycaemia.

Superfoods

Hardly a month goes by without us reading about a new 'superfood' or 'magic ingredient' that can prevent cancer, lower our cholesterol, boost the immune system or keep us looking young. A dietitian may encourage you to eat a piece of fruit but the choice you reach for can bring vastly differing nutrients. Put simply, an orange is not equivalent to an apple.

- An orange has 10 times more vitamin C and beta-carotene, 4 times more thiamin and a huge 40 times more folate (a B vitamin that prevents birth defects) than an apple.
- Broccoli and its relatives cauliflower, cabbage, kale and Brussels sprouts are nutritionally superior to beans, zucchini or other green veggies.
- Nutritionally, liver towers over red meats including kangaroo and venison.
- Garlic lords it over leeks, onions, shallots and chives, even though they are all cousins.
- Dark chocolate is the one with the catechin antioxidants (the more bitter, the better); milk chocolate has only around one-third and white chocolate—forget it!

Sometimes the headlines are premature; sometimes they don't tell you the huge quantities you need to eat to see a clinical effect—such is the case with cranberry juice. While there is some research to show it can keep urinary tract infections at bay, you need to drink at least 300 millilitres (a large glass) every day to see any benefit.

To be free of hot flushes during those menopausal years means a real commitment to soy; around 1 litre of soy beverage a day was what was consumed in the studies to get enough of those mighty phytoestrogens. Garlic, king of the superfoods, has been shown to lower cholesterol in many, but not all studies, but the volunteers were taking in at least four cloves a day, or the equivalent in garlic extract or powder.

DEFINING A SUPERFOOD

Despite the hype, it's clear that foods are not created equal. Although there is no formal definition on what exactly is a superfood, here's what I look for in deciding whether a food is 'super' or not. It should have one or more of these eight qualities:

- ✔ Be rich in vitamins, minerals, omega-3 fat or fibre compared with its kilojoule/calorie count (have a high nutrient density)
- ✔ Have 25 per cent or more of the recommended intake of 2 or more nutrients in a serve *or* be outstandingly rich in one nutrient, having 50 per cent or more of its recommended intake for the day
- ✔ Contain significant quantities of what could be regarded as health-promoting and/or protective substances, such as phytonutrients or other substances not usually found in foods in its class (in addition to the normal nutrients)

- ✔ Be minimally processed without being enriched
- ✔ Provide essential nutrients without overloading the body with salt, saturated fat, trans fat, sugar or other compounds linked to poor health
- ✔ Have research linking it to a potential reduced risk of illness or poor health
- ✔ Be easily available and affordable
- ✔ Have medicinal or healing qualities that have been acknowledged by traditional medicine and induce effects beyond nutrition—think of the folklore behind garlic or ginger.

In a nutshell, a superfood should be nutrient-rich and natural, won't overload you and should be easy to incorporate into your daily diet.

SUPERFOODS FROM EACH FOOD GROUP

VEGETABLES

All vegetables are a nutritionist's delight, but the superstars that turn up time and time again are spinach, members of the cruciferous family (cabbage, broccoli, Brussels sprouts), dark-green lettuces (mignonette, rocket, baby spinach leaves), avocados, beetroot and orange sweet potato (kumara). These foods give you the highest quantities of vitamin C, folate, fibre and minerals without overloading your system. Also included in this group is fresh garlic, thanks to its ability to fend off bacteria and viruses, reduce cholesterol levels and thin the blood.

GRAINS AND GRAIN FOODS

Concentrated sprinkles such as wheat germ and lecithin rank highly for B vitamins and minerals. They are an easy nutritional supplement for your breakfast. Brans have concentrated fibre and make a handy addition to top up fibre intake and prevent constipation; examples include wheat bran, rice bran, oat bran and psyllium.

DAIRY FOODS

Hardly surprisingly, it's low-fat yoghurt (and milk) that gives you the most bang for your nutritional buck.

MEAT, CHICKEN AND FISH

When it comes to animal protein foods, top of the class are pink or red salmon, lean beef steak, pork loin and eggs. Liver and kidney are concentrated in things like iron and vitamin A, but have long suffered in popularity with their strong flavour.

NUTS AND SEEDS

Almonds, walnuts, hazelnuts and peanuts rank the highest for nuts. Flaxseed and chia tick the most boxes for the seeds.

LEGUMES

It's soy that shines over the other beans and peas.

FRUITS

While all fruit is nutritious and variety is important, two main types are outstanding. Go for the berries, especially blueberries (but also strawberries, raspberries, blackberries and cranberries) and any of the citrus fruit (grapefruit, oranges, mandarins). Kiwi fruit come close as a contender.

HERBS AND SPICES

Of all the foods, spices and dried herbs are the most concentrated in phytonutrients. Those that pack the most powerful punch are cloves, cinnamon, turmeric, oregano, sage, rosemary, thyme, marjoram, sage, mint, saffron and ginger. Chilli also makes this list. Just remember you need to use culinary herbs and spices in generous quantities—not just as a garnish—and consume them regularly.

Supplements *See* Nutritional Supplements.

Sweeteners and Sugar Substitutes

Sugar substitutes can be a useful aid for dieters wishing to satisfy a sweet tooth without adding kilojoules. In addition, they do not cause dental caries, so are kind to teeth between meals. How helpful they are in keeping weight off probably depends on the individual. Some research suggests that slimmers make up the kilojoule deficit at later meals, thus negating the savings from a sugar-free food. Substituting a sweetener in your cappuccino and then tucking into a Danish pastry is not a winning, sensible trade-off! You can cut back on your intake by using a sweetener. The table shows what you'll save:

Opt for three pieces of sugar-free gum	SAVE 45 KILOJOULES
Skip the teaspoon of sugar in your cappuccino	SAVE 100 KILOJOULES
Swap your soft drink for a diet drink	SAVE 645 KILOJOULES

WHAT SWEETENER IS THAT?

ACESULPHAME K (ADDITIVE CODE 950)

Acesulphame remains stable after heating, making it suitable for sweetening baked foods such as sweets and biscuits, flavoured milks and sugar-free yoghurts. Like aspartame, it's an 'intense' sweetener as a little goes a long way—they are around 300 times sweeter than sugar.

ASPARTAME (ADDITIVE CODE 951)

Sold under the names Nutrasweet or Equal, aspartame is made from two amino acids (components of protein), which give a pleasant sweet taste. It is the most widely used sweetener today, and turns up as the sweetener in many diet drinks, sugar-free chewing gum and diet yoghurts, as well as a tabletop sweetener. It carries a warning for sufferers of phenylketonuria (PKU), a rare illness diagnosed in infancy, since one of its amino acids is phenylalanine which has to be avoided in PKU. Rumours of a possible link with brain cancer surfaced years ago, but aspartame has been given the all-clear by US and Australian food authorities.

CYCLAMATE (ADDITIVE CODE 952)

Cyclamate has a better flavour than saccharin, but has been banned in many countries due to early reports that very high doses of it caused bladder cancer in rats. Later studies showed it caused no harm in the small amounts consumed, but its reputation was sullied. It is often combined with saccharin to achieve a nicer sweetness without the aftertaste. You'll still find this combination in many diet cordials.

ISOMALT (ADDITIVE CODE 953)

Also made from sugar but with half the kilojoules, isomalt is often combined with intense sweeteners like aspartame or acesulfame K. Stable to heat, it's ideal for making confectionery like hard lollies, lozenges and chocolate. It too carries a laxative warning.

SACCHARIN (ADDITIVE CODE 954)

Saccharin is 300 times sweeter than sugar and has no kilojoules, which is why it was seen as such a godsend in years gone by. Now saccharin has fallen out of favour due to its bitter metallic aftertaste (which today's newer sweeteners don't have) and its cancer scare in rats in the 1970s, which saw it banned in the US but not in Australia.

SORBITOL (ADDITIVE CODE 420), MANNITOL (421), XYLITOL (967), ERYTHRITOL (968)

Collectively known as sugar alcohols, these four have the same kilojoules as sugar but they are absorbed more slowly, so don't disturb blood-sugar levels as much. Because of this, they were once promoted for diabetes and they're OK if your weight is healthy.

Unfortunately, most people with diabetes need to shed weight, so these sugar alcohols have no advantage over sugar—there's no kilojoule saving, unlike with aspartame or stevia. These are often combined with another intense sweetener like aspartame to give sweetness and body to diet foods such as jam, chocolate, chewing gum, mints and pastilles. If you eat a lot of them, they can cause wind or diarrhoea, which explains the laxative warning you'll read on the label.

STEVIA (ADDITIVE CODE 960)

This is a natural sweetener with a slight liquorice taste derived from the leaves of a plant native to Paraguay. The crude stevia leaf is 30 times sweeter than sugar but supplies virtually no kilojoules/calories. Steviol glycosides, extracted from the leaves and refined as a white powder, are now sold as tabletop sweeteners and in low-sugar iced teas (Purevia, Natvia, SteviaSweet). Stevia powder is 200–300 times sweeter than table sugar.

SUCRALOSE (ADDITIVE CODE 955)

Made by modifying the sugar molecule so it's indigestible, sucralose has a sugar-like taste. Unlike other sweeteners it is sold as a spoon-for-spoon sweetener, which is handy for cooking and baking, as well as in tablet form. Its brand name is Splenda.

SAFETY ISSUES

All sweeteners have passed stringent testing to ensure they are safe, both here and overseas. Rumours about the safety of aspartame have been circulating on the internet for several years. These are groundless—aspartame is one of the most studied additives with an established safety record.

Studies of heavy long-term users of sweeteners, such as older people with diabetes who have 'grown up' with no-sugar diabetic diets for years, report no higher frequency of brain or kidney cancers. But having said that, I don't want anyone having too much of any chemical sweetener, no matter how good its safety at the time. New research can overturn things we hold for certain and a sweetener does keep your tastebuds locked into that sweet taste, which you should aim to lose.

As with most things in nutrition, it's all about the quantity. If you have one diet soft drink every day or second day that's fine, as is popping a sweetener into your daily tea or coffee. But guzzling a litre of diet drink a day isn't a long-term strategy I'd recommend.

Syndrome X *See* Metabolic Syndrome.

TUV

Taurine

This is a sulphur-based amino acid formed in the body from methionine and cysteine. It is considered conditionally essential in infants because of its crucial role in prenatal and postnatal development of the nervous system. Taurine is obtained from the diet and is found in seafood, poultry, beef, pork and dairy.

Theanine

Theanine (technically L-theanine) is an amino acid found in tea. Research conducted in the UK suggests theanine is responsible for promoting that feeling of relaxation while maintaining an alert state of mind after you drink tea. This reinforces earlier research by Japanese scientists—the Japanese are big tea drinkers, especially green tea. Theanine may also curb the over-stimulating effects of caffeine to enhance concentration and diminish mental fatigue.

DID YOU KNOW?

One standard cup of black tea has 14–18 mg of theanine and green tea has 10–20 mg.

Early research appears to show that just 50 milligrams of L-theanine—found in two to three cups of tea—stimulates brain activity known as alpha waves, which is commonly present when you are very relaxed. High alpha brain-wave activity occurs in people during meditation and yoga practice, helping to promote a relaxed yet clear and focused mind.

Theanine is also sold as a 'feel-good' supplement in doses of 100 milligrams. In Japan, drinks and chewing gum are also sometimes fortified with theanine, and claim to induce relaxation. It causes no adverse reactions.

See also **Tea.**

Teeth and Diet

Despite great improvements in dental health over the last 20 years, dental caries are still estimated to be the most common and most costly health problem for most Western countries, including Australia. A healthy diet combined with fluoride and good brushing and flossing habits are the keys to keeping teeth strong and decay-free. Use these tips to keep teeth free of caries.

Chew sugar-free gum

Chewing gum between meals can help fight tooth decay. Chewing (it can be anything really—even a piece of rubber) stimulates the flow of saliva, which bathes the teeth and moves any leftover food away from the teeth and gums.

WATCH OUT FOR FOODS WITH FERMENTABLE CARBOHYDRATES

Bacteria that live in our mouth can ferment some carbohydrates and produce acids, which erode away strong tooth enamel. Fermentable carbohydrates can be found in all foods that contain cooked starches or sugars (sweets and lollies, fruit juice, soft drinks, sports drinks and cordial, sweet and savoury biscuits, cakes, buns and pastries, soft bread, potato crisps, pretzels and dried fruit). Restrict these foods or brush teeth after having them.

LIMIT HIGH-ACID FOODS

Soft drinks, energy drinks, sports drinks and fruit juices are high in acidity and this can erode the tough enamel that coats the tooth surface.

SNACK LESS OFTEN

Each time we eat or drink, our saliva works to repair damage to tooth enamel caused by acid build-up (remineralisation). This process takes two or three hours, so those who graze or constantly snack don't do their teeth any favours.

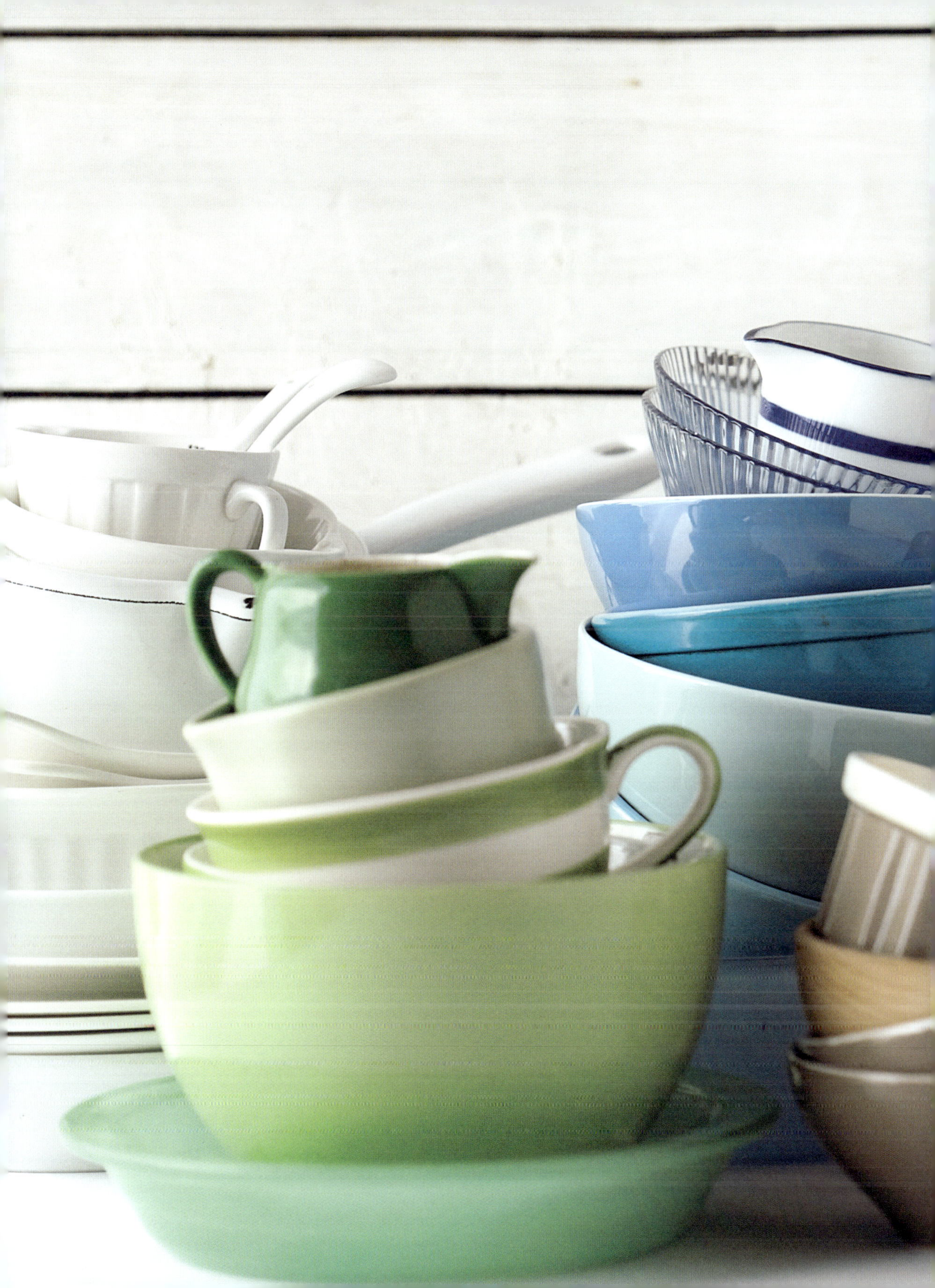

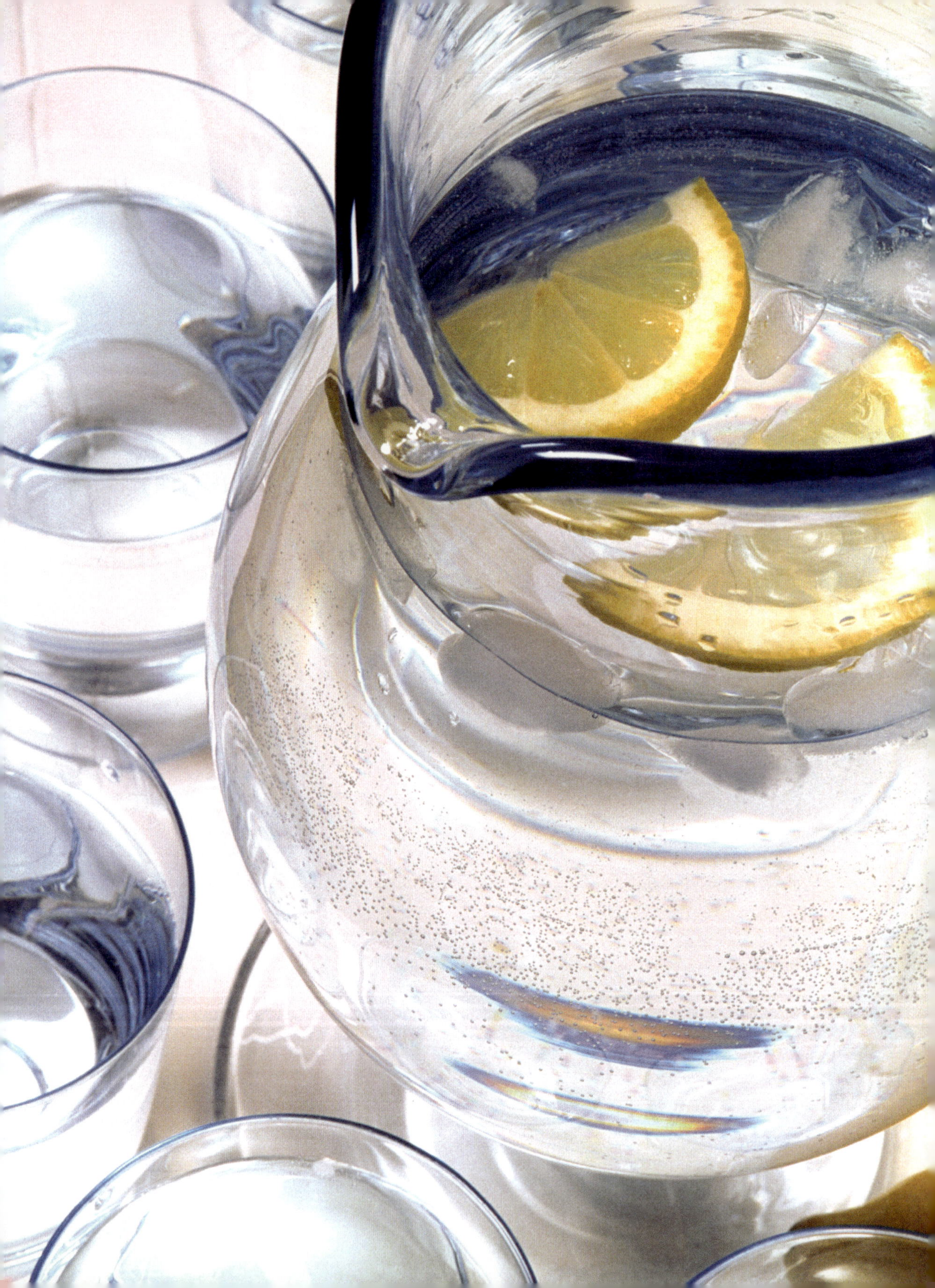

Tea

Black or white, strong or weak, with or without sugar, tea is the world's favourite hot drink. I love tea and drink it every day. I find a cup of tea refreshes and revives me, without the adrenalin rush you get from coffee.

The Chinese have been drinking tea for thousands of years. It spread to Japan around 805 AD and to other parts of Asia, but did not reach Europe until 1610, when the Dutch East India Company imported samples to Holland.

Recent studies support what these ancient people knew—there's definitely something in tea that acts as a pick-me-up. It's a rare combination of the amino acid theanine, which stimulates brain activity that enhances relaxation, and low levels of caffeine.

DID YOU KNOW?

The belief that tea contains the same amount of caffeine as coffee is incorrect. A standard-size cup of black tea has less than half the amount of caffeine (about 10–50 mg) of a cup of instant coffee (60–100 mg). Green and black tea leaves have a similar level of caffeine; however, because fewer tea leaves are used to brew green tea, a cup of green tea tends to be lower in caffeine than black tea.

NUTRITIONAL VALUE

When drunk as an infusion, tea is not especially rich in minerals, vitamins or fibre, but it can be a significant source of fluoride in the diet, especially in areas where the water supplies are not fluoridated. However, it's the healthy dose of polyphenols called flavonoids—as antioxidants, vasodilators and blood thinners with their potent properties, that sets this beverage apart. While both black and green teas are a rich source of flavonoids, green tea contains EGCG (epigallocatechin gallate) while black teas are rich in theaflavins and thearubigens.

Best of all, if you take it black with no milk or sugar, tea has no kilojoules.

NUMBER CRUNCH

A cup of black Ceylon tea supplies a trace of protein, a trace of fat, a trace of sugars, a trace of starch, a trace of dietary fibre, 5 kilojoules and 140–300 milligrams of total flavonoids, depending on the brew time and tea origin.

TEA'S MANY HEALTH BENEFITS

TEA AND HEART HEALTH

Dozens of studies have examined the link between tea and heart disease and found that people who drink it regularly (three or more cups a day) have a significantly lower risk of heart troubles than those who don't. It seems that tea catechins help maintain heart health by decreasing inflammation, lowering the tendency for clotting (an early factor in heart attacks) and by keeping the arteries more elastic so your blood flows freely. The addition of milk or lemon makes no difference.

TEA AND IMMUNITY

A number of studies (predominantly in vitro or animal) have demonstrated tea to have anti-microbial and anti-inflammatory effects. For example, studies have demonstrated that tea can inhibit the growth of the 'bad' Helicobactor bacteria and reduce inflammation in the body. A Chinese study of green tea consumption in patients undergoing their first endoscopy found that the more tea they consumed the less likely they were to have the bad bacteria in their stomach.

HEALTHY HYDRATION

The popular belief that tea is dehydrating due to its caffeine content is a myth. Tea is a hydrating liquid and counts towards our recommended daily intake of 2–3 litres of fluid a day. Earlier studies discounted the contribution of fluid from drinks that contain caffeine, including tea and coffee, on the basis that the caffeine (a diuretic) would cancel out the fluid consumption. However, recent research has shown that at low intakes, and for people who regularly consume caffeine, this is not a problem.

DID YOU KNOW?

These same 'good' flavonoids can potentially inhibit iron absorption from the body. It's true. High intakes of tea can bind with certain forms of iron (mainly non-haem iron found in vegetables) and prevent its absorption. For this to occur, tea has to be consumed at the same time as the food—if not, then there is no effect. Anyone who is low in iron or at risk of low iron (pregnant women, young children and adolescents), should drink tea separately from meal times. Allow at least 1 hour to pass after eating a meal before consuming tea.

ASSISTING WEIGHT LOSS

Best of all, if you take it black with no milk or sugar, tea has no kilojoules. Early research suggests that tea may speed up the body's metabolic rate (which is good for weight control), and possibly burn abdominal fat at a faster rate.

DIABETES AND TEA

There's also good news for people with diabetes. A small clinical study from King's College in London suggests that black tea may stimulate an insulin response and blunt blood-glucose spikes, keeping the body's blood-glucose levels relatively steady throughout the day.

RICH IN POLYPHENOLS

Both green tea and regular (black) tea are a good source of phytochemicals known collectively as flavonoids or polyphenols. These are shown to be more potent than the well-studied beta-carotene or vitamin E. Green tea has a number of simpler catechins, while in black tea some catechins are converted into more complex ones known as theaflavin and thearubigens. One of these catechins, Epigallocatechin gallate (EGCG) is known to inhibit the growth of tumours in animals.

Study into the polyphenols in tea also suggests that tea consumption may protect smokers from oxidative damage, and could potentially reduce cancer risk or other diseases caused by free radicals associated with sun damage.

There is some concern that milk affects the absorption of the antioxidants in tea. At this point, research shows this is not the case. There is some interaction between tea's flavonoids and the casein proteins of milk, but the small quantity of milk added to tea does not appear large enough to overcome the benefits from tea.

WHAT TEA IS THAT?

All tea comes from the bush Camellia sinensis. The difference lies in the way teas are processed (traditionally known as fermented), after picking.

BLACK TEA

The leaves are left to undergo oxidation, which changes their colour from green to red-brown and converts the simple catechins to longer, more complex molecules called theaflavins and thearubigens. It has a stronger flavour and accounts for 78 per cent of all tea consumed.

GREEN TEA

Green tea leaves are heated soon after harvesting, so that they wither. They are then rolled and dried. This stops the oxidation or fermentation activity, and retains most of the simple tea polyphenols known as catechins. It accounts for 20 per cent of all tea consumed.

HERBAL INFUSIONS (TISANES)

These are not strictly tea in the true sense, but infusions of fruits, herbs, flowers and spices. Some are rich in vitamins or plant extracts, but none have the solid bank of research behind them that true teas do. However, they add variety to tea choices, and make a pleasant caffeine-free hot drink before bed.

ICED TEA

Available in citrus, mango, peach and other fruity flavours, iced tea contains around half the sugar of soft drinks and fruit juices. Without carbonation, it makes a refreshing drink for hot days. Made from a dried tea extract, there's much less actual tea present and therefore less of the health benefits of hot tea.

OOLONG TEA

Oolong tea is halfway between green and black. It's drunk without milk or sugar, like green tea.

WHITE TEA

Rare and expensive, white tea is produced from the bud and first few leaves only. It has a sweet subtle flavour.

TEA VARIETIES

Specialty teas can either be made from teas from a specific area which gives its name to that blend (e.g. Assam, Darjeeling or Ceylon), or they can be a blend of different tea leaves to produce a tea with a characteristic aroma and flavour (e.g. English Breakfast, Earl Grey or Russian Caravan). Chinese and Japanese teas have their own traditional names.

MY TAKE

Here's how I make the perfect cup of tea:

- ✔ *Start with fresh, cold tap water to provide plenty of dissolved oxygen*
- ✔ *Boil it completely*
- ✔ *Warm the teapot with hot water*
- ✔ *Add one teaspoon of loose tea or one teabag per person to the teapot*
- ✔ *Infuse your tea for 3–5 minutes—any longer and it begins to stew*
- ✔ *Add your milk first if pouring from a pot; add it last if jiggling a tea bag in a cup.*

Tocopherols

These comprise four of the eight naturally occurring compounds that make up the family of fat-soluble vitamins known as vitamin E. One synthetic form also exists. They act as antioxidants and are found in wheat germ, oils, margarine, nuts and seeds.

See also Vitamins.

Tocotrienols

These comprise four of the eight naturally occurring compounds that make up the family of fat-soluble vitamins known as vitamin E. They are found in palm oil, barley and oats.

See also Vitamins.

Tomatoes *See* Vegetables.

Thickeners

These are compounds that thicken foods such as sauces, soups, toppings and custard, or give them a smooth, uniform texture. Similar in function to cornflour or arrowroot used at home, they include a number of lightly modified starches (additive numbers 1400–1405) and more extensively modified starches like acetylated distarch adipate (additive code 1422). If you need to avoid wheat or gluten, check the ingredient list—it must list wheat as a major allergen. Today most manufacturers use thickeners derived from potato or maize to make life easier for those with allergies.

See also Additives.

Toddlers and Diet

12 months to 3 years.

At this early stage of life, it's critical that toddlers see parents eating, preparing and enjoying healthy food including vegetables. If parents can be good role models for healthy eating habits, it's the best start for kids and creates food preferences that will last a lifetime.

Recommended daily intake
3 year old—ranges from 5300 kJ for a sedentary, inactive girl to 6900 kJ for a sporty, active boy.

For fussy eaters, encourage them to taste just one mouthful of the food they don't like. Once tasted, let them leave the rest of that food on their plate. Continue to serve them this food, following the same pattern of one mouthful, and then leaving the rest. Studies have shown that a number of repeated tastings of a disliked food over time changes the child's taste preferences and acceptance of the food. In other words, children have to see and taste a new food at least five or six times before it looks 'normal' to them.

Allergies often surface at this age stage. Introduce one new food at a time, every second day or so, according to your child's readiness, so that any reactions can be easily identified. Consult your GP if you suspect your child has an allergy of some kind. The most common type of test to investigate allergies is a skin prick test.

Tofu

Tofu has been a staple of Asian diets for thousands of years, and it is now moving into the mainstream in the Western world. It is made from soy beans—the basis of a variety of protein-rich products and meat substitutes that also includes textured vegetable protein (TVP), nutmeat, vegetarian sausages and soy burgers.

Also known as bean curd, tofu is a soft cheese-like food made by curdling soy milk with a coagulant in much the same way as cheese is produced from milk. In fact, it's often referred to as the 'cheese of Asia'. It's bland in taste and needs to be teamed with other stronger-flavoured ingredients to create an appetising dish.

NUTRITIONAL VALUE

Tofu is rich in high-quality protein and is a good source of B vitamins, potassium, zinc and other minerals. It is also low in kilojoules and saturated fat. Like other foods high in soy protein, it is also rich in isoflavones, which have been shown to reduce the risk of osteoporosis and reduce the risk of heart disease by reducing bad cholesterol and helping to maintain good cholesterol levels.

The coagulant is traditionally nigari, which is magnesium chloride, a white powder produced from sea water (additive code 511), but other coagulating agents may also be used and this is important as it determines whether tofu is a good source of calcium or not. If calcium chloride or sulphate is used, the tofu is a good source of calcium—around 300 milligrams per 100 gram serve, which is the same as a glass of milk. If magnesium chloride is used, the tofu will be low in calcium—less than 50 milligrams.

Tofu comes in two forms. Soft tofu (silken or Japanese-style) can be used as a replacement for cream, sour cream and cream cheese, and in creamy desserts and cheesecake. Firm tofu (Chinese-style) can be sliced or diced and added to kebabs, stir-fries and salads.

EASY WAYS TO GET MORE TOFU

FIRM TOFU

- ✔ Marinate tofu slices in soy sauce and mirin, and add to vegetable stir-fries.
- ✔ Marinate tofu in soy sauce or teriyaki marinade and grill or barbecue.
- ✔ Mix mashed tofu with chopped onion and fresh chopped herbs and shape into patties, then roll in breadcrumbs and pan-fry.
- ✔ Thread tofu chunks onto skewers with capsicum, zucchini and cherry tomatoes.
- ✔ Use tofu to replace meat in dishes such as burrito fillings, curries and soups.
- ✔ For Asian stir-fry dishes, use firm tofu or tempeh with red capsicum strips, carrot strips and snow peas with garlic, ginger, chilli and soy sauce.

SOFT OR SILKEN TOFU

- ✔ Mix half sour cream and half soft tofu for a reduced-fat topping for a baked potato.
- ✔ Blend it into cream cheese for use in a baked cheesecake.
- ✔ Blend half tofu and half sour cream and add your favourite herbs and spices for a vegetable dip.
- ✔ Blend silken tofu with banana and peaches (or banana and strawberry) and a touch of honey to make a protein-rich smoothie.
- ✔ Replace all or part of the cream in a creamy soup or sauce with silken tofu.
- ✔ Scramble tofu instead of eggs and serve on toast for breakfast.

DID YOU KNOW?

Tempeh (pronounced *tem-pay*) is a patty made from fermented soy beans. Common in Indonesia, it has a firm texture and a nutty flavour. Grill or pan-fry slices as a meat replacement in burgers, or add it chopped to stir-fries and vegetarian dishes.

NUMBER CRUNCH

Half a cup (around 125 grams) of firm tofu contains 570 kilojoules, 14 grams of protein (important for vegetarians), 9 grams of fat, only 1 gram of saturated fat, a generous 8 grams of fibre and 3.5 milligrams of iron. In contrast, the same amount of soft or silken tofu will deliver half the number of kilojoules and only 2 grams of fat. As well as being lower in kilojoules and fat, soft tofu usually contains minimal amounts of calcium, a quarter of the fibre and two-thirds the amount of iron found in firm tofu. Both varieties of tofu contain the same level of isoflavones, on a par with soy milk. Manganese, iron and vitamin E are also found in tofu.

See also **Soy Beans.**

Trace Elements

These are mineral elements that are required by the body in only small amounts for health and growth. The best researched are copper, chromium, cobalt, fluorine, iodine, manganese, molybdenum, selenium and zinc.

Trans Fats

Trans fats (or trans fatty acids or TFAs) are a group of fatty acids chemically classified as unsaturated, but the molecules have been 'rearranged' or 'straightened' so they act like saturated fatty acids in the body. This alters the way it behaves in food, and in your body. There are two types of trans fats.

1. **Naturally occurring:** These are made by bacteria in the stomach of cattle, sheep, goats and deer, and so occur naturally in the meat, milk, butter and other foods derived from these animals. They make up only a minor proportion of the fat we eat.
2. **Industrial:** This is the type of trans fats nutritionists are concerned about. They are formed through the hydrogenation of liquid vegetable oils, which converts liquid oils into semi-solid fats. They turn up in solid cooking margarines and hydrogenated commercial fats, but trans fat–free margarines and spreads are available now.

MY TAKE

While trans fats are not the problem here that they are in the US, we do need to worry about the amount of saturated fats we consume. Don't choose foods based on trans fats alone—try to choose products with the lowest total of saturated plus trans fat possible.

Food manufacturers find these hydrogenated fats useful as they have a higher melting point than non–trans fats. This means they are more solid and so make for crispier biscuits and crunchier chips, nuggets and corn chips. They are also more stable and less likely to go rancid, so they have a longer shelf life. These are all handy things when you want your product to keep longer and taste better.

The problem with trans fats is that they increase your total cholesterol, raising the bad (LDL) cholesterol levels and lower the good (HDL) levels, causing a deficiency of essential fatty acids. This significantly increases your risk of heart disease, type 2 diabetes and possibly infertility.

SHOPPER'S GUIDE

Foods likely to be high in trans fats include:

- Deep-fried fast foods such as fries, chips, wedges and nuggets—they are cooked in partially hydrogenated oils unless stated otherwise
- Potato crisps, corn chips and other salty snack foods
- Baked goods like meat pies, sausage rolls, apple pies and croissants
- Doughnuts
- Solid cooking margarines
- Biscuits and cookies
- Muffins and cakes
- Instant fried noodles
- Microwave popcorn
- Non-dairy coffee whitener
- Frozen foods including fish fingers, crumbed chicken and spring rolls.

READ THE LABEL

It's not compulsory for manufacturers to list the amount of trans fats in foods, unlike the requirement to list total fat and saturated fat in the nutrition information panel. It is only labels with claims such as 'no cholesterol', 'low in saturated fat' or 'free of trans fats' that include figures for trans fats. If you see 'hydrogenated fat' or 'partially hydrogenated fat' (where the hardening process is not complete) on a list of ingredients, it means the product contains trans fat, but it does not tell you how much.

DON'T COMPARE AUSTRALIA WITH THE US

The intake of trans fat in Australia in relatively low compared with the US, so it pays to be wary when you're reading material from overseas—often the hype about trans fats simply doesn't apply here. This is largely because we have not had to rely on hydrogenated soy bean oil like the US (until recently, around half the soy bean oil in the US was hydrogenated for processors and fast-food operators).

DID YOU KNOW?

In the US the average American consumes 2–3 per cent of their daily kilojoules from trans fats, compared with 0.6 per cent for an Australian.

We have mainly used palm oil for frying and processing, which is already a semi-solid fat with good shelf life, so doesn't need to be hydrogenated. While this has no trans fats, it is high in saturates, so it's not kind to your heart. In the 1990s, the two major margarine manufacturers (Flora and Meadow Lea) made all their spreads virtually trans fat–free, dropping them from around 12 per cent down to less than 1 per cent. This early move dropped the intake of trans fat here significantly.

U

Ubiquinol

Also known as co-enzyme Q, this is a substance found in most foods, particularly fish, red meat and oils, which can be synthesised in the body. It is needed for oxygen production by cells and is essential for mitochondria, which converts fuel into energy. It works in synergy with vitamin E to keep bad (LDL) cholesterol from being oxidised, and is often promoted as a supplement for heart health.

Ulcers and Diet

There is no special diet to treat a gastric or duodenal ulcer. Bland, milky or low fibre diets are no longer prescribed. However, spicy or rich foods, alcohol, strong tea and coffee, and vegetables like onion, garlic, cucumber or cabbage may aggravate the ulcer and cause discomfort. Personal trial and error is the only way to find out. Small frequent meals are recommended. Most ulcers are due to overgrowth of a type of bacteria (*Helicobacter pylori*) and can be treated successfully with antibiotics.

Ulcerative Colitis *See* Crohn's disease.

Underweight

While most people in the Western world are battling the bulge, others struggle to gain or maintain their weight. These may include people born naturally thin, young males or those recovering from chemotherapy or other illness, or surgery. Another group is older people who have to eat a soft diet, or dementia sufferers.

Growing bodies

Many young males want to put on weight, especially around the upper torso (chest, shoulders and arms). To achieve a bulkier look, you need to combine a healthy diet that is rich in kilojoules with a graduated weight-training program at a gym or with a trainer. You may need to drop your level of aerobic exercise too, so that you're not burning off muscle as soon as you create it. This means less running or cycling and more weights for the upper body—ask your gym instructor or coach to plan a program for you.

IT'S IN THE GENES

If you come from a family with a lean build or a slight body shape, your genetic predisposition will probably override whatever you eat and how much (or little) exercise you do. As you age, a slim build can become an asset, rather than a liability, as it means you are less likely to suffer from heart disease, type 2 diabetes, gallstones and other illnesses that effect people who are overweight.

HOW TO GAIN WEIGHT

The secret to eating for weight gain is to eat regularly and include foods that are dense in kilojoules and nutrients. These foods generally include more fat than is recommended for the general overweight population. Try these tips in your day-to-day diet.

- ✔ Eat little and often, especially if your appetite is small or you fill up quickly.
- ✔ Ensure you eat a protein food such as red meat, chicken or fish in at least one meal each day.
- ✔ Eat kilojoule-dense foods like avocado, peanut butter, extra margarine on vegetables and pasta, dressing on salads and sour cream or cheese on potatoes.
- ✔ Enrich soups and porridge with cream or milk rather than water.
- ✔ Avoid using diet or fat-free products.
- ✔ Snack on foods like nuts, dried fruit, sandwiches, cheese and crackers, yoghurt and flavoured milk or smoothies.
- ✔ If you enjoy fruit, combine it with custard, yoghurt or ice-cream for a higher kilojoule boost.
- ✔ Use protein-enriched milk in drinks, on cereal and in cooking.
- ✔ Aim for drinks with kilojoules like full-fat milk, fruit juice and cappuccinos.
- ✔ Try adding a supplement such as Sustagen or Ensure to your drinks.
- ✔ Do things to boost your appetite, like taking a brisk walk before mealtime.
- ✔ Enjoy a pre-dinner drink—think of it as a medicinal; it does add kilojoules.
- ✔ If you smoke, stop—it blunts your tastebuds and decreases your appetite.
- ✔ Try to eat out more often.

WEIGHT GAIN AND CHOLESTEROL

If you are worried about cholesterol when increasing your fat intake, choose lean meat, poultry and fish, and use fats that are either polyunsaturated or mono-unsaturated. These won't raise your blood cholesterol or increase the risk of heart disease.

V

Vegetables

Eating plenty of vegetables is one of the best things you can do for your health. They are packed with the vitamins, minerals, fibre and antioxidants we need for health, growth and energy—and all for very few kilojoules.

The key nutrients we get from vegetables are vitamin C, folate, beta-carotene (converted to vitamin A), potassium, fibre, carbohydrate and water. There are also plenty of minor substances such as trace elements, enzymes, anti-cancer compounds and phytochemicals.

MY TAKE

Don't say 'no' to potatoes just because most have a high GI. They are fat-free (when you don't fry them), nutrient rich and filling. Look for the lower-GI varieties like Carisma, developed here in Australia, which from a nutritional, and taste perspective stand head and shoulders over the rest.

ROOT VEGETABLES

These vegetables store food in their swollen roots. As a group it includes the starchy staples like potatoes, as well as leeks and green onions (members of the onion family), although the part we eat is actually a bundle of leaf sheaths.

- Beetroot
- Carrot
- Celeriac
- Jerusalem artichoke
- Onion and leek
- Parsnip
- Radish
- Swede/rutabaga
- Turnip

STARCHY STAPLES

- Potato
- Sweet potato
- Taro
- Yam

NUTRITIONAL VALUE

Root vegetables are a good source of fibre (especially when you don't peel them) and micronutrients including beta-carotene (plentiful in yellow and orange-coloured vegetables), B vitamins, vitamin C and potassium. They tend to be vegetables that fill you up. Their high fibre and water content means they are bulky, and help to satisfy your appetite. They aren't fattening by themselves. It's how you cook them and what you pour over them that adds the kilojoules.

Carrots and parsnips have low GI values; beetroot is moderate and swedes have a high GI. But they have much smaller amounts of carbohydrate than the starchy staples and a typical serving size won't give your blood-glucose levels an excessive boost, even the ones with higher GI values. When it comes to the carbohydrate-rich, starchy staples, however, you need to think of them as the vegetable kingdom's equivalent to rice or pasta. Their place is the 'carb quarter' of the dinner plate (and within the inner rim too, and not piled up like a pyramid). This is because their GI is very relevant when it comes to managing blood-glucose levels.

Growing bodies

The number of serves children need a day depends on their age, appetite and physical activity levels, but those older than 9 or 10 should also be aiming for five. Adequate folate intake from vegetables is also essential to growing a healthy baby.

VEGETABLE FRUITS AND SEEDS

Included are all fruits and members of the legume family where the seed is enclosed within a pod and either the seed (lima and butter beans) or the seed and pod (French and runner beans) are eaten.

- Beans and peas
- Capsicum (pepper)
- Cucumber
- Eggplant (aubergine)
- Okra
- Pumpkin
- Tomato
- Zucchini

NUTRITIONAL VALUE

> In Australia, 11 per cent of all cancers are thought to be related to people not eating enough fruit and vegetables.

This is a varied group as you can see, but they are all packed with micronutrients and, like all vegetables, make a valuable contribution to your diet. Their high fibre and water content means they are bulky and satisfy your appetite without adding a lot of kilojoules—providing you don't fry them! I love to serve green beans and peas with a meal but if I had to pick a favourite, it would be tomatoes, which are high in lycopene, vitamin C and fibre and great for sandwiches, salads and soups, or simply slow roasted to top a piece of toast for breakfast.

I have devoted a special section to the dried form of peas, beans and lentils, as these are very nutritious foods that provide us with a good dose of B vitamins, protein and fibre.

See **Legumes.**

LEAF VEGETABLES

These are all the familiar leafy greens, along with brassicas such as broccoli and cauliflower, where the immature flower heads are eaten, and celery and rhubarb, which we eat for their succulent plant stems.

- Asian greens
- Asparagus
- Broccoli and cauliflower
- Cabbage and Brussels sprouts
- Celery
- Globe artichoke
- Lettuce
- Radicchio and endive
- Rocket
- Spinach, silverbeet and other beet leaves
- Sprouts
- Watercress

> **EAT BY THE RAINBOW**
>
> It's important to eat a variety of different coloured vegetables each day including:
>
> - Dark-green vegetables (spinach and broccoli)
> - Orange or yellow vegetables (pumpkin and carrots)
> - Cruciferous (broccoli, cauliflower and cabbage)
> - Root vegetables (potatoes, kumara, turnips, taro, yams and corn)
> - Salad vegetables (lettuce, fresh green herbs like rocket and basil, capsicum, tomato and cucumber).

NUTRITIONAL VALUE

Enjoy all these vegetables in season. When you hear nutritionists talk about 'piling your plate with veggies' or 'free veggies'—the ones below are the ones they mean. In my book these are the superstars!

- ✔ Spinach, silverbeet and Asian greens are packed with vitamin C, folate, antioxidants and fibre, for almost no kilojoules.
- ✔ Dark-green lettuces (mignonette, rocket and baby spinach leaves) are a nutrient-rich addition to any meal, big on volume but small on kilojoules.
- ✔ Cruciferous (cabbage, cauliflower, broccoli, Brussels sprouts, kale and rape) contain cancer-fighting sulphur compounds, lots of fibre, beta-carotene, a host of minerals, a little iron and calcium.

HOW MUCH

Research shows that we are much healthier if we eat at least five serves of vegetables and salad a day. This helps prevent heart disease, some types of cancer (in Australia

11 per cent of all cancers are thought to be related to people not eating enough fruit and vegetables), excess weight and constipation. Five serves a day can also reduce blood pressure and blood cholesterol. Most of us currently only get about two or three serves a day. One serve is:

- ½ cup diced, cooked vegetable such as carrots or broccoli
- 1 cup salad leaves or raw sliced vegetables
- 1 medium potato
- ½ medium kumara or sweet potato.

RAW VS COOKED

I believe a balance of cooked and raw veggies is the key to good health, and salad at lunch and cooked vegetables at dinner is one way to do this.

Cooking vegetables makes certain nutrients more biologically available to the body—for example, beta-carotene and the antioxidant lycopene are absorbed better from cooked carrots or tomatoes than from raw. What are lost are the heat-sensitive vitamins including vitamin C and two key B vitamins (thiamin or B_1, and folate). The minerals (like potassium and magnesium) and fibre are unaffected by cooking.

Uncooked fresh vegetables therefore give us a higher intake of those heat-sensitive vitamins. I often recommend a salad a day for this reason.

PRESERVING NUTRIENTS

- Don't overcook vegetables. Serve them tender, so when you pierce them with a knife they're only just soft inside.
- The healthiest cooking methods are steaming, microwaving with little or no water, and stir-frying.
- The shorter the cooking time and the less water there is to leach out nutrients, the better.
- Add a splash of olive oil to vegetables after cooking; this enhances the absorption of fat-soluble vitamins (beta-carotene) and antioxidants such as carotenoids.
- Don't hold vegetables warm for more than 5 minutes; this destroys more (but not all) of the nutrients.

FROZEN VS FRESH

Frozen vegetables can be as nutritious as fresh—as long as you cook them quickly in as little water as possible according to the directions on the packet. Frozen vegetables are already half cooked, so they only need to be heated.

Freezing (at –18°C for no more than 6 months) is the most nutritious and efficient way to preserve food. It is better than canning as frozen vegetables retain a lot more of the heat-sensitive nutrients (particularly vitamin C, thiamin and folate). There is also little additional salt, which is a big drawback with canned vegetables.

Vegetable Gums

These are compounds that thicken and gel foods like ice cream, desserts, dressings, sauces, toppings and mayonnaise. Alginates (additive codes 400–405), agar (406) and carrageenan (407) are extracted from seaweeds, while pectin (440), guar gum (412) and xanthan gum (415) come from plants. Other gelling agents are produced from cellulose, like carboxymethyl cellulose (466).

Growing bodies

If you want your kids to eat up their vegetables, then make sure you set a good example as a parent. Also try these easy, tempting ideas.

- ✔ Pack raw vegetable sticks into lunch boxes.
- ✔ Serve vegetable soup or hot corn on the cob on cold afternoons after school.
- ✔ Grate vegetables into Bolognese sauce, rissoles, homemade hamburger patties, stews, muffins and cakes.
- ✔ Use leftover vegetables for bubble and squeak.
- ✔ Serve sliced vegetables with salsa or low-fat dip.
- ✔ Grow a vegetable garden if you have the space; if not, grow baby tomatoes, lettuces, baby spinach or herbs in pots on a sunny window sill or balcony.

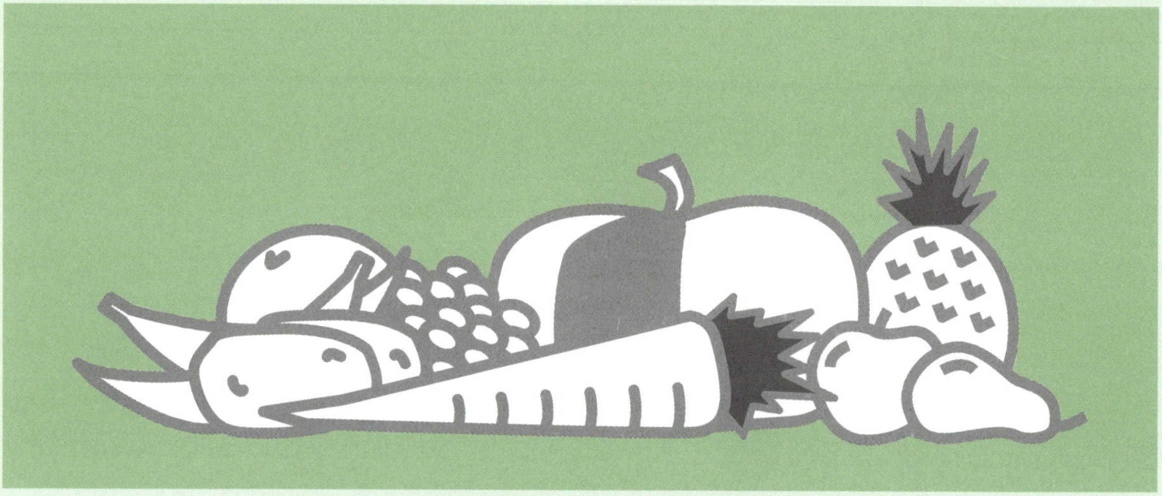

Vegetarian and Vegan Diets

Vegetarianism has long been practised by many communities, who have enjoyed excellent health into old age. George Bernard Shaw, Socrates, Plato and Aristotle were all vegetarians. It is built into the philosophy of several religious faiths like Seventh Day Adventists, Buddhists and Hare Krishnas. Many people today are vegetarian for a range of reasons. These include concern about the world environment or the practices around farming animals for consumption, or because they seek optimum health. While only 2–3 per cent of the population are completely vegetarian, many more are eating meatless meals (think of Meatless Monday dinners and the Weekday Vegetarian campaign) and restaurants now offer a wider range of meat-free choices.

DIFFERENT TYPES OF PLANT-BASED DIETS

VEGANS

Vegans are total vegetarians, avoiding all foods of animal origin, including honey and gelatin. They live on products of the plant kingdom, relying on grains, vegetables, pulses, nuts and fruits. They also avoid leather, wool, cosmetics, soap and shampoo products derived from animal ingredients or tested on animals.

LACTO VEGETARIANS

Lacto vegetarians eat dairy, but avoid all other foods derived from animals.

LACTO-OVO VEGETARIANS

Lacto-ovo vegetarians consume dairy foods and eggs as well as plant foods. This diet is recommended for children and pregnant or breastfeeding women.

SEMI-VEGETARIANS OR PESCO-VEGETARIANS

People on this diet eat dairy foods and eggs, plus the occasional meal with fish or chicken (white meats). The key is the quantity of vegetables and legumes they consume. Many early studies reported positive findings on vegetarians but in reality they were eating more of this type of diet—which is nutritionally closer to the ideal.

FRUITARIANS

Those on this diet subsist on only fruit and nuts. It is considered too limited, and may lead to nutrient deficiencies.

THE HEALTH BENEFITS OF VEGETARIAN DIETS

Once viewed as fringe or extremist, vegetarianism is now accepted as having proven health benefits. Compared with the general omnivore population, research shows that on average vegetarians:

- ✔ Have lower levels of bad (LD) cholesterol
- ✔ Are less likely to suffer heart disease
- ✔ Are less likely to suffer cancer, notably of the bowel, breast and lung
- ✔ Have lower blood pressure
- ✔ Weigh less
- ✔ Have a lower risk of type 2 diabetes.

This positive health profile is attributed to two diet factors—less saturated fat from meat and dairy products and more fibre and phytochemicals from nuts, grains, pulses, fruits and vegetables. In addition, the indications are that vegetarians tend to smoke less and drink less alcohol and caffeine, all of which helps to keep them in top health.

THE POTENTIAL PITFALLS OF VEGETARIAN AND VEGAN DIETS

There are some nutrients likely to be in short supply when following a vegetarian diet.

VITAMIN B_{12}

Strict vegan diets lack vitamin B_{12}, which is found only in animal foods. Although needed in minute quantities, it is essential for healthy red blood cells, DNA genetic material and nerve tissues. Insufficient supply can bring on pernicious anaemia and degeneration of the nervous system. However, because vitamin B_{12} is stored in the liver, it takes 3 to 5 years for a healthy vegetarian to develop a deficiency. Though rare, deficiency has been reported in elderly vegetarians and in the babies of vegan mothers, where it caused impaired mental functioning. The demands of pregnancy and breastfeeding soon deplete the mother's B_{12} stores, and leave her breast milk without sufficient supply. Pregnant and breastfeeding vegetarian women should therefore make sure that any soy drink they buy is fortified with B_{12} or take a supplement (2 milligrams a day is recommended; supplements contain between 2 and 100 milligrams).

Sources: yoghurt, milk, cheese, eggs and fortified soy drink. Once considered reliable sources, seaweed and fermented foods like tempeh are now not recommended since tests revealed that any B_{12} they contain is in the form of inactive B_{12} analogues.

IRON

Anaemia is caused by iron deficiency and is one of the most common nutrition problems for vegetarians, especially women. Lack of iron can also prevent children achieving their full brain potential. The iron found in plants is also not as easy for the body to absorb as that found in meat. Due to the presence of phytates and oxalates in plant foods, less than 5 per cent of their iron is absorbed, compared with 20 per cent or more of the iron in red meat.

Sources: fortified breakfast cereals, dark-green vegetables, beans, lentils, meat substitutes like tofu or soy steaks, dried fruit and cocoa powder. Vegetarian meals are typically high in vitamin C, which greatly boosts the absorption of non-haem (plant) iron.

Growing bodies

Nutritionists recommend that children in vegetarian families eat eggs and dairy products to ensure they are getting adequate sources of protein, vitamin B_{12}, calcium, iron and zinc. For the first 6 months of life, breast milk can provide all the nutrients a baby needs, provided the mother is well nourished. The infant can then be weaned onto yoghurt, baby cereals, mashed avocado, soft tofu, pureed vegetables, fruit juices and soft-cooked eggs. Difficulties arise when a toddler starts eating general family food with its bulky vegetables, filling beans and wholegrains. These all have plenty of fibre, which may be an advantage for an adult but not for a rapidly growing child who needs lots of kilojoules but has a small stomach with limited capacity.

CALCIUM

Calcium is critical for growing children and pregnant women. Deficiency causes stunted growth and malformed bones and teeth. Vegetarians who consume milk, yoghurt or cheese are fine, but many avoid these dairy products and need non-dairy calcium.

Sources: fortified soy drink (about 100 milligrams per 100 millilitres), green leafy vegetables, tahini (sesame seed paste), almonds, Brazil nuts, hazelnuts, tofu and dried figs.

ZINC

Zinc is vital for the function of many enzymes in the body and for a strong immune system. The richest sources are animal foods such as meat, fish, oysters and chicken. Zinc from these foods is better absorbed than from plant foods.

Sources: wholemeal and grain breads, bran and wholegrain breakfast cereals, legumes and nuts.

Vegetarian Toddlers

Small meals and lots of snacks is the key. Concentrated foods like cheese, avocado, eggs, honey, dried fruit or oil are handy for adding kilojoules without bulk. Nuts and seeds should be chopped or ground to break up their fibrous hulls and improve digestion. Milk or soy drink should be full-cream, not low-fat.

OMEGA-3 OILS

Vegans consuming no animal foods at all may miss out on essential omega-3 oils from fish and lean meat.

Sources: linseeds (flaxseeds), flaxseed oil, canola oil, omega-3 enriched products (eggs are the best), walnuts, pecans, soy products, green vegetables and herbs.

SUGGESTED DAILY AMOUNTS

Each day you need to eat the following serves, to ensure a nutritionally balanced vegetarian diet:

- ✔ Grains (rice, pasta, couscous, burghul, bread, noodles, breakfast cereal and oats)—6 serves.
- ✔ Vegetables, salads and sprouts (some raw, some cooked)—5 serves
- ✔ Fruit and juices—2 serves
- ✔ Protein sources (60 grams cooked or canned legumes, beans and peas or 125 grams tofu or tempeh)—2 serves; *or*
  Nuts or nutmeat (30 grams of almonds, walnuts, pecans, macadamias, hazelnuts or peanuts)—2 serves; *or*
  Eggs—2 serves; *or*
  Cheese (40 grams)—1 serve; *or*
  Yoghurt (200 grams)—1 serve; *or*
  Any combination of the above.
- ✔ Calcium sources (300 millilitres milk for adults; 600 millilitres for children and pregnant and breastfeeding women)—1 serve; *or*
  Cheese (40 grams)—1 serve; *or*
  Cottage cheese (60 grams)—1 serve; *or*
  Buttermilk (300 millilitres)—1 serve; *or*
  Yoghurt (200 grams)—1 serve.
- ✔ Unsaturated oil (20 grams of any of mono- or polyunsaturated oil, mono-unsaturated margarine, tahini, peanut butter, mayonnaise, salad dressing, seeds, avocado, wheat germ or olives)—1 serve.

Vinegar

Vinegar has been used since ancient times. The word comes from the French word *vinaigre*, meaning 'sour wine'. Vinegar is the fermentation of alcohol converted into the key ingredient, acetic acid. Natural vinegar also contains small amounts of tartaric acid, citric acid and other food acids. Vinegar can be made from almost anything that contains sugar or starch, including fruits, grains or roots.

Vinegar is often used in pickling and to make vinaigrettes and other salad dressings. It is also used in mustard, sauces, mayonnaise and chutneys (often as a substitute for lemon juice).

WHAT VINEGAR IS THAT?

BALSAMIC VINEGAR

This is an aromatic, aged vinegar traditionally crafted in the Modena and Reggio Emilia provinces of Italy, from the concentrated juice of white grapes. It is very dark brown in colour with a rich, sweet and complex flavour. True balsamic vinegar (which has a Protected Designation of Origin) is aged for 12 to 25 years. Balsamic vinegars that have been aged for up to 100 years are available, though they are usually very expensive. The commercial balsamic sold in supermarkets is typically made with concentrated grape juice mixed with a strong vinegar that is laced with caramel and sugar.

CIDER VINEGAR

Cider vinegar is made from cider or apples and has a brownish-yellow colour. It is often sold unfiltered and unpasteurised with the mother of vinegar present, as a natural product. Because of its acidity, apple cider vinegar may be very harsh, and can even burn the throat. It is very popular, partly because of the hype about its possible weight loss properties. Often promoted as a 'slimming aid' by the health-food industry, cider vinegar has no magical properties. It is sometimes marketed in combination with kelp, vitamin B_6 and lecithin as a diet supplement, but none of these have been scientifically proven to speed up weight loss.

DID YOU KNOW?

Adding a tablespoon of vinegar to a meal (in your salad dressing, for example) has long been known to lower the body's blood-glucose response to the meal by up to 30 per cent. The theory is that adding vinegar to a meal slows down the rate at which food empties from the stomach and enters the small intestine for digestion, therefore slowing the absorption of glucose into the blood.

As far as we know it works for all types of vinegar. The acidity from the acetic acid and resultant low pH is thought to slow stomach emptying and balsamic, wine or raspberry vinegar all work in the same way. You get the same effect from any acidic food like lemon juice or acidic fruits (grapefruit, kiwi fruit) or pickled vegetables (pickled gherkins, pickled onions).

A recent paper reported that the vinegar effect is more pronounced after a high-GI meal and not the low-GI meals nutritionists suggest for good health. So if you're already choosing legumes, grainy breads and pasta you may not notice as much of an effect. But if you choose high-GI foods (e.g. potatoes) you may notice an effect.

FRUIT VINEGARS

These are made from fruit wines such as apple, raspberry or quince. The flavours of the original fruits usually remain in the final product.

MALT VINEGAR

Malt vinegar is made by malting the barley, which causes the starch in the grain to turn to maltose. An ale is then brewed from the maltose and allowed to turn into vinegar, which is then aged. It is typically light brown in colour.

RICE VINEGAR

Rice vinegar is the most popular in the cuisines of South-East Asia. It is available in white (actually light yellow), red and black varieties. The Japanese prefer a light rice vinegar for the preparation of sushi rice and salad dressings. Red rice vinegar is traditionally coloured with red yeast rice. Black rice vinegar (made with black glutinous rice) is most popular in China.

WHITE DISTILLED VINEGAR

One of the most versatile and economical vinegars, it's very sour and mostly used for cleaning and disinfecting, rather than consumption. In fact, it's a great eco-friendly alternative to chemical cleaners, good for cleaning teapots, coffee makers and windows.

WINE VINEGAR

Wine vinegar is made from red or white wine and is the most commonly used vinegar in Mediterranean countries and central Europe. As with wine, there is a considerable range in quality. Better-quality wine vinegars are matured in wood for up to 2 years and exhibit a complex, mellow flavour. Wine vinegar tends to have a lower acidity than that of white or cider vinegars.

Vitamins

Vitamins are a group of organic compounds needed in minute quantities (less than 1 per cent of our food is composed of vitamins). There are 13 known vitamins essential for health and growth, and nine of them are grouped together as the B group or B-complex vitamins. These are thiamin (vitamin B_1), riboflavin (B_2), niacin, pyridoxine (B_6), cyanocobalamin (B_{12}), folate, biotin, pantothenic acid and a recent addition, choline. Not all carry the number designation as some were discovered and numbered, then later found to be other compounds—not vitamins. Vitamins are usually classified as fat-soluble or water-soluble.

FAT-SOLUBLE VITAMINS

A, D, E and K vitamins are stored in the body, so excess of these vitamins can cause unpleasant side effects. They occur in association with food fats and are fairly stable during cooking and processing.

WATER-SOLUBLE VITAMINS

B group and C vitamins dissolve in body fluids and excess intakes of most of them are excreted in the urine. They are distributed in many foods including vegetables, grains, meat and milk, and are often sensitive to heat.

NUTRITIONAL VALUE

Vitamins regulate the body's metabolism by speeding up chemical reactions (they are often enzymes or co-enzymes), acting as antioxidants or forming an integral part of the structure of proteins, hormones and blood. Think of them as spark plugs for your body's engine.

With a few exceptions, the body cannot produce them so they must be supplied by food. Vitamins are needed in minute amounts for health and growth and to prevent deficiency diseases such as scurvy (lack of vitamin C), beriberi (vitamin B_1), pellagra (vitamin B_2) or rickets (vitamin D).

Following is an individual overview of each vitamin; also see the tables on pages 335–38 for recommended intakes.

VITAMIN A

Occurs as retinol and beta-carotene, which is converted into retinol in the body. It is needed for:

- ✔ Eyesight—protects against night blindness
- ✔ Normal growth in children
- ✔ Healthy skin and mucous membranes
- ✔ Resistance to infection
- ✔ It is also currently being studied for its role as an antioxidant in cancer prevention.

THIAMIN (VITAMIN B_1)

It was the discovery of thiamin in the early 1900s that led to our understanding of the existence and importance of vitamins. Clinical deficiency of thiamin is known as beriberi. The major cause of thiamin deficiency in developed countries like Australia is heavy alcohol intake. To combat this, many countries have added thiamin to staple foods such as flour and bread. In Australia, flour was first enriched with added thiamin in 1989. Although thiamin supplements are recommended in alcoholism, there is no scientific evidence to support an effect for this B vitamin on hangovers as a result of binge drinking. Thiamin supplements have also been shown in some studies to improve mood and mental function. Thiamin:

- ✔ Metabolises carbohydrate in the body
- ✔ Releases energy into the body from food
- ✔ Aids normal appetite and digestion
- ✔ Ensures proper function of the heart and nervous system.

RIBOFLAVIN (VITAMIN B_2)

Riboflavin is highly sensitive to light, which is why milk is best stored in non-clear containers or away from light. The bright yellow-green colour of urine that occurs when taking vitamin supplements is due to riboflavin because the excess is excreted in the urine. It is difficult to suffer from excess riboflavin because the human body can't absorb it in large quantities. Riboflavin helps the body:

- ✔ Maintain healthy skin and eyes
- ✔ Release energy from food
- ✔ Metabolise carbohydrate, protein and fat.

NIACIN (VITAMIN B_3)

Niacin is the common name for the two compounds nicotinic acid and nicotinamide (or niacinamide). A deficiency of this vitamin causes a disease known as pellagra. It was first seen in populations that used corn as their staple food. The form of niacin found in corn is not well absorbed. Niacin (as nicotinic acid) is used for the treatment of high LDL cholesterol and triglycerides. Niacin can also be formed in the body from the amino acid tryptophan. Niacin:

- ✔ Releases energy from food
- ✔ Metabolises carbohydrate, protein and fat
- ✔ Is essential for growth.

PANTOTHENIC ACID (FORMERLY KNOWN AS VITAMIN B_5)

Although rats fed a diet deficient in pantothenic acid ended up with grey hair, no role for this vitamin has been found in determining the colour of human hair. Deficiency is rare in humans—it's only ever been seen in severely malnourished prisoners of war. Pantothenic acid is one of the constituents claimed to be responsible for the benefits of royal jelly (which contains bee pollen and may trigger life-threatening allergic reactions in susceptible people). Pantothenic acid aids in the:

- ✔ Metabolism of carbohydrate, fat and protein for energy
- ✔ Formation of red blood cells, helping prevent anaemia.

PYRIDOXINE (VITAMIN B_6)

Vitamin B_6 exists in three forms: pyridoxine, pyridoxal and pyridoxamine. High doses can damage nerve endings producing symptoms that include tingling in the hands and feet. Vitamin B_6 supplements should not be used when taking medication for epilepsy or Parkinson's disease as they reduce the effectiveness of these drugs. Vitamin B_6:

- ✔ Metabolises protein
- ✔ Forms red blood cells and prevents anemia.

CYANOCOBALAMIN (VITAMIN B_{12})

Vitamin B_{12} is found only in foods of animal origin such as eggs, milk, meat and fish, so it is important that vegans and others who eat little of these foods get the recommended amount. Pregnant women following vegan diets should take vitamin B_{12} supplements because adequate vitamin B_{12} is crucial to the development of the baby's nervous system. It is also important in the:

- ✔ Formation of red blood cells
- ✔ Prevention of pernicious anaemia
- ✔ Formation of nerve cells and DNA genetic material
- ✔ Metabolism of carbohydrates and fat.

DID YOU KNOW?

It is a widely held belief that vitamin B_{12} can be obtained from tempeh, miso and spirulina but this is not true. Vitamin B_{12} in a form that can be absorbed by humans is only found in foods of animal origin.

BIOTIN

Another of the B group vitamins, biotin was once called Vitamin H. Biotin:

- ✔ Metabolises fat and protein
- ✔ Aids growth
- ✔ Nourishes nerve cells.

FOLATE (FOLIC ACID)

Extra folate is now recommended for women before conception to prevent neural tube defects such as spina bifida in babies. Fortification of some foods (breakfast cereal, flour and juices) is now common in Australia, the US and the UK to assist women in increasing their intake of folate. It is important to assist in the:

- ✔ Formation of enzymes and red blood cells
- ✔ Prevention of anaemia
- ✔ Metabolism of DNA
- ✔ Prevention of neural tube defects (spina bifida and anencephaly).

ASCORBIC ACID (VITAMIN C)

A powerful antioxidant, vitamin C's main job appears to be to regenerate vitamin E and inhibit the formation of carcinogenic nitrosamines in the stomach. Smokers have an increased requirement for vitamin C and low intakes of vitamin C from food have been associated with an increased risk for many forms of cancer including the stomach, mouth, oesophagus, pancreas and cervix. A deficiency of vitamin C results in scurvy, a disease whose symptoms include swollen and bleeding gums, and bruising. Studies into its impact on colds and flu have been conflicting. These days research supports only a reduction in the length and severity of colds—not avoiding it completely. It is also currently being studied for its role as an antioxidant. Vitamin C helps to:

- ✔ Keep gums, teeth and bones healthy
- ✔ Speed wound healing and help resist infection
- ✔ Form collagen, a cementing material in blood vessels, bones and teeth
- ✔ Assist in the absorption of non-haem iron from vegetables and grains.

CHOLECALCIFEROL (VITAMIN D)

Vitamin D is a hormone-like compound made by the skin through exposure to sunlight, and found in only a small number of foods. A deficiency of vitamin D results in softening of the bones known as rickets in children and osteomalacia in adults. Vitamin D is often used as part of the treatment for osteoporosis in post-menopausal women and it's usually combined with calcium as a supplement for this older age group, who are prone to brittle bones. It is also being researched for its role in preventing cancers and boosting our immune system. Vitamin D helps to:

- ✔ Build strong bones and teeth
- ✔ Prevent rickets, a bone disease in children which results in stunted growth and bowed legs
- ✔ Boost the absorption of calcium and phosphorus
- ✔ Contribute to normal cell division, growth and development.

TOCOPHEROLS (VITAMIN E)

Vitamin E is a group of eight substances known as tocopherols and tocotrienols, of which alpha-tocopherol is the most potent. It is being researched for its role in the prevention of cancer and heart disorders—clinical studies using supplements have not been positive to date, but further study is underway. Vitamin E:

- ✔ Acts as an antioxidant to protect polyunsaturated fats and vitamin A
- ✔ Maintains the stability of the fats found in cell membranes.

PHYLLOQUINONE (VITAMIN K)

Vitamin K is made by the bacteria in the intestine and is also available from foods. Because newborn babies don't have bacteria established they receive an injection of vitamin K immediately after birth to prevent bleeding. Anyone taking anticoagulants or blood thinners such as Warfarin is generally advised to maintain a steady intake of vitamin K because it is involved in blood clotting. Greatly varying intakes can interfere with the function of medication. Vitamin K helps your blood to clot.

Growing bodies

All newborn babies receive an injection of vitamin K soon after birth. Babies do not get enough vitamin K from their mothers during pregnancy. Without vitamin K, they are at risk of developing a rare blood disorder.

CHOLINE

Choline has only recently received vitamin status, with the US first recommending levels of intake in 1998. Typical diets contain twice the amount of choline currently

OTHER VITAMINS

- Vitamin B_{15}—The name coined for pangamic acid. Many unfounded claims have been made about it, including an ability to cure diabetes, heart disease and cancer, and to strengthen the body's immune system against infections and pollution. Pangamic acid is a derivative of glucuronic acid, but there is no evidence that it is an essential vitamin, or that it can alleviate disease.
- Vitamin F—An obsolete name for essential fatty acids.
- Vitamin H—An obsolete name for biotin.
- Vitamin P—From permeabilitas vitamin, it is a name once given to a group of plant flavonoids that were reported to affect the strength of blood vessels. It is no longer used.
- Vitamin PP or PP factor—A former name for the B vitamin niacin, it refers to the vitamin's ability to act as a pellagra preventive.

MY TAKE

If you do take supplements, think of them only as a 'top-up' to your daily diet. Supplements aren't magic bullets. They won't supply everything we get from good food, nor can they counteract a bad diet with too much fat or salt.

recommended, so supplements are rarely needed. Excessive intake may cause low blood pressure and a fishy body odour in some people. Choline is:

- ✔ A component of cell membranes and the neurotransmitter acetylcholine
- ✔ Important in fat and bile metabolism.

FOOD VERSUS SUPPLEMENTS

Ideally, it is best to obtain all your vitamins from food rather than pills. Food provides vitamins in the most biologically available form, in the right amounts and combined with other complementary nutrients. Except under special circumstances, there is low risk of vitamin overdose from food.

Vitamins work best together. Too much of one can disturb the balance of others. Vitamin C increases the absorption of iron; vitamin E acts together with selenium and vitamin C as antioxidants; folate supplements can mask the symptoms of B_{12} deficiency.

Food also naturally contains a variety of compounds that we don't know a lot about yet, such as the many phytochemicals. These are not yet in supplement form and can only be derived from food.

In recent years, however, attitudes to supplements have changed, as numerous studies have emerged suggesting that supplements, especially the antioxidant supplements, are associated with better health outcomes. That said, supplements cannot provide you with all 27 essential vitamins and minerals you need. While there are certain groups who can definitely benefit from a supplement (such as smokers, fussy eaters or the elderly), be wary of the over-enthusiastic promises made by vitamin sellers. Often the scientific evidence is not reliable, consisting of anecdotes from 'satisfied' patients or the people treating them. One example is an often-quoted examination of studies into vitamin C and the common cold showed that it could slightly shorten the duration of colds, but not prevent them entirely.

VITAMIN OVERDOSE

For some vitamins, there's the possibility of overdose. Here are some examples:

- Excess vitamin A is toxic and causes loss of appetite, nausea and a dry itchy skin—one to watch during pregnancy.
- Excess beta-carotene can turn the skin and whites of the eyes an orange-yellow (which slowly disappears once the excess stops).

WHEN YOU MAY NEED EXTRA VITAMINS

Before conception	A high intake of folate can protect against birth defects.
During pregnancy	Extra iron, folate and calcium are needed, as well as omega-3 fatty acids.
When breastfeeding	Extra calcium and omega-3 fatty acids are needed.
Vegans	May run short on vitamin B_{12}, iron, zinc, calcium and omega-3 fatty acids.
Smokers (and passive smokers)	Smokers have around double the vitamin C requirement and may need more zinc, folate, beta-carotene and other antioxidants.
Heavy drinkers	Excessive alcohol depletes B group vitamins such as thiamin and folate as well as zinc, potassium and vitamin E.
Those with malabsorption problems such as coeliac disease and irritable bowel syndrome	Extra iron, calcium, zinc and vitamin C may be needed.
Athletes	Various vitamins and minerals are needed but generally the antioxidant vitamins C and E as well as iron.
People aged over 60 and who are housebound	Absorption of nutrients declines in later years but requirements for vitamins B_6, B_{12}, calcium and vitamin D are increased.
Those on an elimination diet for allergy or food intolerance	The removal of whole food groups such as grains and/or dairy also eliminates related vitamins and minerals.
During illness and after surgery or burns	More vitamin C and protein are required for tissue synthesis.
Restricted weight-loss diet	Very low-kilojoule intakes cannot provide sufficient vitamins and minerals—a multivitamin and mineral supplement is recommended.
People with certain types of anaemia	Iron supplements may be needed, as well as B_{12} for pernicious anemia.

- Excess vitamin D causes calcium to be deposited in soft tissues, as well as vomiting and diarrhoea.
- Excess niacin causes flushing and interferes with liver function. This is checked for when patients are given high doses of niacin doses for lowering cholesterol.
- Overdose of vitamin B_6 produces a loss of sensation in the body's extremities (due to damage to the sensory nerves).

VITAMIN SUPPLEMENTS AND CHILDREN

As a rule, I don't think it's a good idea to give children vitamin pills. If they're eating a reasonably balanced diet, they should get all the vitamins and minerals they need from foods, so supplementation isn't necessary. If you believe your child needs a supplement, it's best to talk to your doctor, early-childhood nurse or a paediatric dietitian about the right type and the correct dosage. Don't believe the persuasive marketing of naturopaths, health-food shops and even well-meaning pharmacists.

PROS

✔ If a child has been sick or has had an operation and been unable to eat, then extra vitamins, minerals or protein can help for the short term until they're eating fully.

Q

I've heard the soils are depleted so I need to take supplements to get all the vitamins and minerals I need.

A

This is a myth. If the soils were depleted, the produce would be stunted and wouldn't grow properly or yield commercially viable amounts. A 2004 survey carried out by FSANZ compared the minerals in 44 common fruits and vegetables. It found no significant changes over the years between 1981 and 1985, and 2000 and 2001. They suggested that different stages of ripeness or different cultivars could have accounted for any variations. Also, while organic farming is kinder to the environment, there is no significant nutritional difference between crops grown under organic and non-organic conditions.

- ✔ Kids on any type of restricted diet can be vulnerable and need a little nutritional help at times. This can include fussy eaters who refuse to eat whole groups of foods such as meat or vegetables, and those with allergies (like dairy intolerances) who miss out on particular nutrients (like calcium).
- ✔ Kids on elimination diets or gluten-free diets (don't do this without proper advice) need a supplement. This will be advised by a health professional when you embark on the diet.
- ✔ Teens who have decided to eat vegetarian can miss out on iron and zinc without meat. Teens on fad diets, such as no-carb diets for weight loss, can miss out on getting what they should like fibre, B vitamins and vitamin C.

CONS

- ✖ Children can find tablets difficult at the best of times. You may find it a battle to get them to take any supplement regularly. Syrups and liquid tonics for children overcome the problem but then you have to check for colours, added sugar or sweetener, and preservatives.
- ✖ Multivitamins taken as a chewable tablets can cause dental erosion from the acidic nature of their vitamin C.
- ✖ It's easy to get the dose wrong—children of different ages can be different sizes and pills are based on body weight, not on age.
- ✖ Avoid large doses of supplements. There are side effects from too much of some nutrients, particularly iron and vitamins A and D.
- ✖ Keeping toddlers away from medicines is always a problem. Accidentally swallowing iron supplements is the most common cause of poisoning in young children, who mistake them for lollies. Excess iron can be fatal for a small child. Keep all supplements well out of reach of children.
- ✖ Don't think that a pill can be a substitute for nutrition. There's no way that taking a pill can replace all the nutrients available in vegetables and fruit. Parents still need to ensure their children are eating a balanced diet.
- ✖ Some of the food your child is eating may already be fortified or enriched with vitamins and minerals. Most breakfast cereals have four B vitamins and iron, most bread has extra iodine and thiamin (vitamin B_1) while orange juice is sometimes sold with added calcium.
- ✖ Many so-called 'complete' multivitamins do not have all of the recommended amounts of vitamins and minerals that your child needs each day. For example, most don't have enough calcium because it's impossible to fit 1 gram into a 'one a day'.

See also **Nutritional Supplements.**

RECOMMENDED DIETARY INTAKES OF VITAMINS

RETINOL/VITAMIN A			
RECOMMENDED DAILY INTAKE (MCG RETINOL EQUIVALENTS)		SAFE UPPER LIMIT FOR SUPPLEMENTS	SOURCES
Adult women	700 or 2300 IU	3000 mg or 10,000 IU—it is stored in the body, primarily in the liver, and toxicity can occur with high doses of retinol, but not carotenoids. Excess doses in pregnancy can cause birth defects and should be avoided.	Retinol is found in liver, oily fish (fish liver oils such as cod liver oil are a very rich source), butter, table margarine, cream, full-cream milk, egg yolk and cheese. Vitamin A is a fat-soluble vitamin, so relies on a little dietary fat for its absorption.
Adult men	900 or 3000 IU		
Children 1–3 years	300		
Children 4–8 years	400		
Children 9–13 years	600		
Girls 14–18 years	700		
Boys 14–18 years	900		

BETA-CAROTENE (CONVERTED TO VITAMIN A)			
RECOMMENDED DAILY INTAKE (mg)		SAFE UPPER LIMIT FOR SUPPLEMENTS	SOURCES
No Australian or US figures available	5–6 suggested	25 mg—turns the skin and whites of the eyes an orange-yellow (which slowly disappears once you cease taking excess). May also produce hair loss, nausea or blurred vision.	Beta-carotene can be gained from orange and green fruit and vegetables including carrots, carrot juice, spinach, silverbeet, parsley, basil, apricots, mango, rock melon, pumpkin, pawpaw and chilli.

THIAMIN/VITAMIN B_1			
RECOMMENDED DAILY INTAKE (mg)		SAFE UPPER LIMIT FOR SUPPLEMENTS	SOURCES
Adult women	1.1	None established but 50–100 mg a day is considered the maximum.	Thiamin is found in yeast extract, wheat germ, bran, nuts, fortified breakfast cereals, liver, kidney, lean pork, peas, wholemeal flour, wholemeal bread and sesame seeds.
Adult men	1.2		
Children 1–3 years	0.5		
Children 4–8 years	0.6		
Children 9–13 years	0.9		
Girls 14–18 years	1.1		
Boys 14–18 years	1.2		

Figures given in the tables in the following pages for each vitamin are either Recommended Dietary Intake (RDI) or, if not yet set, the Adequate Intake (AI) set by the National Health and Medical Research Council of Australia.

RIBOFLAVIN/VITAMIN B_2			
RECOMMENDED DAILY INTAKE (mg)		SAFE UPPER LIMIT FOR SUPPLEMENTS	SOURCES
Adult women 19–70 years	1.1	Not established, but 200 mg a day is considered the maximum.	Riboflavin is derived from milk, cheese, yoghurt, yeast extract (Vegemite), meat extract (Marmite), liver, eggs, almonds, mushrooms, wholemeal flour, wholemeal bread, fortified breakfast cereals and green vegetables.
Adult women > 70 years	1.3		
Adult men 19–70 years	1.3		
Adult men >70 years	1.6		
Children 1–3 years	0.5		
Children 4–8 years	0.6		
Children 9–13 years	0.9		
Girls 14–18 years	1.1		
Boys 14–18 years	1.3		

NIACIN/VITAMIN B_3			
RECOMMENDED DAILY INTAKE (mg)		SAFE UPPER LIMIT FOR SUPPLEMENTS	SOURCES
Adult women	14	35 mg—can cause a mild flushing reaction at doses over 1000 mg a day.	Niacin is found in lean meat, liver, yeast, bran, peanuts, tuna, salmon, kidney, legumes, fortified breakfast cereals, eggs, vegetables and milk.
Adult men	16		
Children 1–3 years	6		
Children 4–8 years	8		
Children 9–13 years	12		
Girls 14–18 years	14		
Boys 14–18 years	16		

PANTOTHENIC ACID			
RECOMMENDED DAILY INTAKE (mg)		SAFE UPPER LIMIT FOR SUPPLEMENTS	SOURCES
Adult women	4	Not established but 1000 mg a day is considered the maximum.	The best sources are lean meat, liver, poultry, fish, yeast, yeast extract, soybeans, nuts, whole grains (brown rice, wholemeal breads, barley) and vegetables.
Adult men	6		
Children 1–3 years	3.5 (AI)		
Children 4–8 years	4 (AI)		
Girls 9–13 years	4 (AI)		
Boys 9–13 years	5 (AI)		
Girls 14–18 years	4 (AI)		
Boys 14–18 years	6 (AI)		

PYRIDOXINE/VITAMIN B_6			
RECOMMENDED DAILY INTAKE (mg)		**SAFE UPPER LIMIT FOR SUPPLEMENTS**	**SOURCES**
Adult women 19–50 years	1.3	50 mg—more than 200 mg a day can lead to neuritis, a painful numbness or tingling in the hands and feet due to damage to the nerves.	Vitamin B_6 is derived from lean meat, liver, poultry, fish, yeast, soy beans, nuts, wholegrains (brown rice, wholemeal breads, barley) and vegetables.
Adult women > 50 years	1.5		
Adult men 19–50 years	1.3		
Adult men > 50 years	1.7		
Children 1–3 years	0.5		
Children 4–8 years	0.6		
Children 9–13 years	1.0		
Girls 14–18 years	1.2		
Boys 14–18 years	1.3		

CYANOCOBALAMIN/VITAMIN B_{12}			
RECOMMENDED DAILY INTAKE (mcg)		**SAFE UPPER LIMIT FOR SUPPLEMENTS**	**SOURCES**
Adults	2.4	Non-toxic even in large doses.	It is only found in animal foods such as liver, kidney, lean meat, oysters, fish, seafood, eggs and milk. Vegetarians should drink fortified soy milk and eat cultivated mushrooms.
Children 1–3 years	0.9		
Children 4–8 years	1.2		
Children 9–13 years	1.8		
Children 14–18 years	2.4		

BIOTIN			
ADEQUATE DAILY INTAKE (mcg)		**SAFE UPPER LIMIT FOR SUPPLEMENTS**	**SOURCES**
Adult women	25 (AI)	Not established, but 2500 micrograms (mcg) a day is considered the maximum.	The best sources are in egg yolk, liver, kidney, heart, oats, wholegrains and legumes. Biotin is also made by bacteria in the intestine.
Adult men	30 (AI)		
Children 1–3 years	8 (AI)		
Children 4–8 years	12 (AI)		
Children 9–13 years	20 (AI)		
Girls 14–18 years	25 (AI)		
Boys 14–18 years	30 (AI)		

FOLATE			
RECOMMENDED DAILY INTAKE (mcg)		**SAFE UPPER LIMIT FOR SUPPLEMENTS**	**SOURCES**
Adults	400	1000 micrograms (mcg).	Folate is derived from yeast extract (Vegemite), Marmite, fortified breakfast cereals, fortified juices, leafy vegetables, wholegrains, peas, nuts, avocado and organ meats (liver, kidney and heart).
Children 1–3 years	150		
Children 4–8 years	200		
Children 9–13 years	300		
Children 14–18 years	400		

ASCORBIC ACID/VITAMIN C			
RECOMMENDED DAILY INTAKE (mg)		**SAFE UPPER LIMIT FOR SUPPLEMENTS**	**SOURCES**
Adults	45	1000 mg, although many people take more than this during the winter via vitamin C supplements. Vitamin C is not toxic, but doses greater than 2000 mg a day can cause upset stomach and diarrhoea. It also increases the risk of iron overload.	Vitamin C is found in a wide range of fruit and vegetables, the richest being citrus fruit and juices, berries, guava, mango, capsicum, pawpaw, parsley, broccoli, pineapple, spinach and cabbage.
Children 1–3 years	35		
Children 4–8 years	35		
Children 9–13 years	40		
Children 14–18 years	40		

CHOLECALCIFEROL/VITAMIN D			
RECOMMENDED DAILY INTAKE (mcg)		**SAFE UPPER LIMIT FOR SUPPLEMENTS**	**SOURCES**
Adults 19–50 years	5 (200 IU)	80 mcg or 3200 IU if you're taking supplements (for those unable to get exposure to sunlight). Vitamin D is fat soluble so is stored by the body and is toxic at low levels. If you take supplements—including combination calcium supplements for bones or cod liver oil—check how much vitamin D you're taking in. More than 80 mcg a day can lead to nausea, bone pain, liver damage, muscle weakness and lethargy. Too much vitamin D causes calcium to be deposited in soft tissues like the liver and kidneys.	The best food sources are in cod-liver oil as a liquid or as capsules (not fish oil), oily fish such as salmon, trout, sardines, mackerel (fresh or canned), egg yolks, foods fortified with vitamin D (such as table margarine and specialty milks like Anlene), rice milk, soy milk, butter and cheese. Vitamin D is also derived from sunshine—you'd think we get plenty in a country like Australia, but there's increasing recognition that significant numbers of the population do not get enough Vitamin D, especially in winter. Generally you'll get enough if you can expose your hands, face and arms to sunlight for 10–20 minutes every second day. But it will need to be longer if you have dark skin, are over 60 or living at a low latitude.
Adults 51–70 years	10 (400 IU)		
Adults > 70 years	15 (600 IU)		
Children 1–3 years	5 (200 IU) (AI)		
Children 4–8 years	5 (200 IU) (AI)		
Children 9–13 years	5 (200 IU) (AI)		
Children 14–18 years	5 (200 IU) (AI)		

IU means International Units. These units are a measure of the biological activity of a vitamin. They were used before vitamins were available in pure form. 1000 micrograms (μg or mcg) = 1 milligram (mg).

TOCOPHEROLS/VITAMIN E

RECOMMENDED DAILY INTAKE (mg)		SAFE UPPER LIMIT FOR SUPPLEMENTS	SOURCES
Adult women	7 (10 IU)	300 mg or 450 IU as d-alpha tocopherol.	The best food sources are wheat germ, vegetable oils, nuts, unsaturated margarine, eggs, seeds, wholegrains, fish, fruit and vegetables.
Adult men	10 (15 IU)		
Children 1–3 years	5 (AI)		
Children 4–8 years	6 (AI)		
Girls 9–13 years	8 (AI)		
Boys 9–13 years	9 (AI)		
Girls 14–18 years	8 (AI)		
Boys 14–18 years	10 (AI)		

PHYLLOQUINONE/VITAMIN K

RECOMMENDED DAILY INTAKE (mcg)		SAFE UPPER LIMIT FOR SUPPLEMENTS	SOURCES
Adult women	60	Not established but it appears safe even at quite high intakes.	It is found in green leafy vegetables (spinach, silverbeet, Asian greens, watercress and dark lettuces), broccoli, cauliflower, liver, eggs, cheese, wholemeal flour and wholemeal bread. It is also made by bacteria in the intestine.
Adult men	70		
Children 1–3 years	25		
Children 4–8 years	35		
Children 9–13 years	45		
Children 14–18 years	55		

CHOLINE

RECOMMENDED DAILY INTAKE (mg)		SAFE UPPER LIMIT FOR SUPPLEMENTS	SOURCES
Adult women	425	3500 mg.	The best sources of choline are lecithin, egg yolks, wheatgerm, liver, meat, brewer's yeast, legumes (particularly soy beans), wholegrains (particularly maize), nuts and green leafy vegetables.
Adult men	550		
Children 1–3 years	200 (AI)		
Children 4–8 years	250 (AI)		
Children 9–13 years	375 (AI)		
Girls 14–18 years	400 (AI)		
Boys 14–18 years	550 (AI)		

WX YZ

Waist Circumference

Waist circumference is a simple measurement that tells you whether you're carrying too much of the dangerous abdominal fat. People who carry fat mainly around the stomach and have abdominal obesity (an apple shape) have a higher risk of diabetes, high blood pressure and heart disease. People with most of their fat around hips and thighs (pear shape) have less risk of these problems. The pear shape is typical of a woman's fat pattern and is known to be harder to shift than the fat around the middle—of which the beer gut is a good example.

The safe upper limit for a healthy waist size varies for different ethnicities. Run a tape measure around your waist at the narrowest part (usually at the navel) and check your measurement against the following figures. These are the upper limits for people over 19 years old.

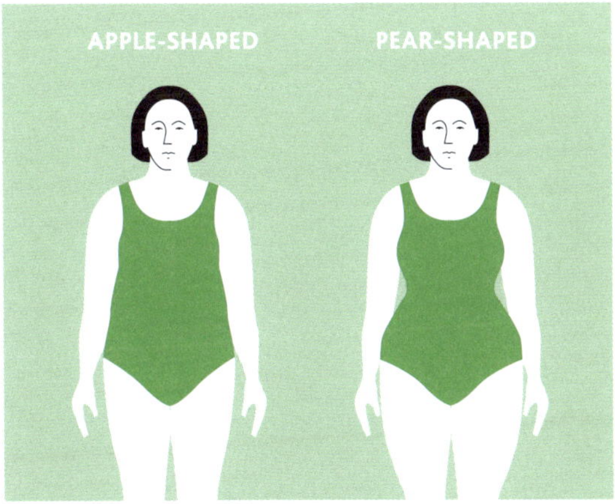

	MEN	WOMEN
European background	up to 94 cm	up to 80 cm
Asian background	up to 90 cm	up to 80 cm
Australian Aboriginal background	up to 90 cm	up to 80 cm
Pacific and Torres Strait Islander background	up to 102 cm	up to 88 cm

See also Weight Loss.

Waste, Food

Wilted herbs, milk past its use-by date, stale bread, and last weekend's leftovers—who isn't guilty of throwing uneaten food away? According to an online survey carried out by The Australia Institute in 2009, Australians discard around $5 billion worth of fruit and vegetables, meat and fish, pasta and rice and dairy products each year. The cost of waste per household is AUD$616 in Australia and AUD$458 in New Zealand.

We need to think of food scraps as a resource, not a waste. By recycling them into compost at home or via a food waste recycling facility, your food scraps become something valuable that can be used by landscapers and farmers.

WHAT TO COMPOST

- ✔ Fruit waste and vegetable peelings
- ✔ Leftovers and table scraps
- ✔ Coffee grounds, filters, tea leaves and tea bags
- ✔ Food-soiled paper, including pizza boxes
- ✔ Paper towels and napkins.

DID YOU KNOW?

Edible, unwanted food, including restaurant leftovers, is often 'rescued' these days to feed the hungry by organisations such as Foodbank and OzHarvest.

RECYCLING TIPS

- ✔ Have separate kitchen bins for bottles and cans, paper and cardboard and green waste.
- ✔ Buy a re-usable drink bottle to carry water with you. If you don't like the taste of your tap water, invest in an inexpensive filter jug to remove impurities and off-tastes.

See also Seasonal and Sustainable Eating.

Water

Water is critical to our health and our very existence. It moistens our breath, keeps our internal body temperature constant, transports nutrients and wastes, keeps the kidneys working, facilitates chewing and prevents constipation.

Signs you are dehydrated include headache, tiredness, a dry mouth and constipation. If the dehydration gets worse, you'll find yourself unable to think clearly and may experience muscle cramps. Lack of fluid also affects the skin, which loses its plumpness, and our kidneys.

WHAT WATER IS THAT?	
Tap water	Tastes OK in most places in Australia. Check whether fluoride is present—tank rainwater won't contain fluoride; bore water may.
Filtered tap water	Pleasant taste—a filter removes taints and that strong chlorine smell. Charcoal filters are inexpensive and retain fluoride. Reverse osmosis filters under the sink remove both fluoride and harmful bacteria like cryptosporidium.
Bottled water	Clean neutral taste. Lacks fluoride so don't allow your children to drink this all the time.
Still mineral water	Pleasant taste. Certain spring waters contain low concentrations of sodium carbonate and bicarbonate, sodium chloride (common salt) and salts of calcium, magnesium, iron and sometimes hydrogen sulphide—varies depending on the source.
Sparkling mineral water	Fizzy so more thirst-quenching than still water. Some are naturally aerated with carbon dioxide and may be slightly alkaline or salty. They are generally low in sodium.
Flavoured mineral water	Sounds healthy, but has only a little less sugar content than soft drink—think of it as another sweetened drink with kilojoules to count.

EIGHT GLASSES A DAY

About 2.5 litres of water are lost from the body each day. In hot climates and during exercise or illness, as much as 9 litres can be removed via the kidneys, bowel movements, perspiration and expired air. Office workers in dehumidified, air-conditioned environments also require extra water. Over half our daily water intake comes from food (even 'dry' foods like bread contain 30–40 per cent water) and the remainder comes from beverages.

Drinking at least 8 glasses (2 litres) of fluid per day is generally recommended. If it's plain tap water, that's good. Water has no kilojoules and no extra sugar or sodium. An inexpensive water filter jug removes any taints, without taking out the fluoride, which is good for your teeth—it really does make water taste better. I serve it chilled with a slice of lime or lemon.

THE BOTTLE CONTROVERSY

Most of the tap water in Australia and New Zealand is potable—suitable for drinking. However, much of it doesn't taste that great, which is why people won't drink it. Bottled water may taste better, but it has a huge environmental impact. Massive resources are used to produce billions of plastic bottles each year, which then end up as litter, in waterways or in landfills. There's no genuine need for this when tap water is safe and plentiful. I am a big fan of the trend to carry water with you—I find keeping a bottle in the car or at work encourages people to drink more—but we should use our own personal refillable bottle wherever possible. I started using one when I learned that 60 per cent of plastic bottles are *not* recycled and so end up in landfill as waste. Rinse, drain well and fill. It's easy and will save you money too.

DRINK MORE, EAT LESS

A drink of water before a meal can be a simple, inexpensive and effective weight control strategy. I used to think the reason was simply kilojoule subtraction—replace soft drink, juice or alcohol with water and you save kilojoules (it can be a considerable—one 600 millilitre 'buddy' Coke packs 1080 kilojoules). But research shows that drinking water distends your stomach, reduces sensations of hunger and leaves you feeling fuller, all desirable feelings when you're on a diet. US researchers have reported that kilojoule intake among habitual water drinkers is approximately 9 per cent less (81 kilojoules a day) than those who do not drink water.

See also Hydration.

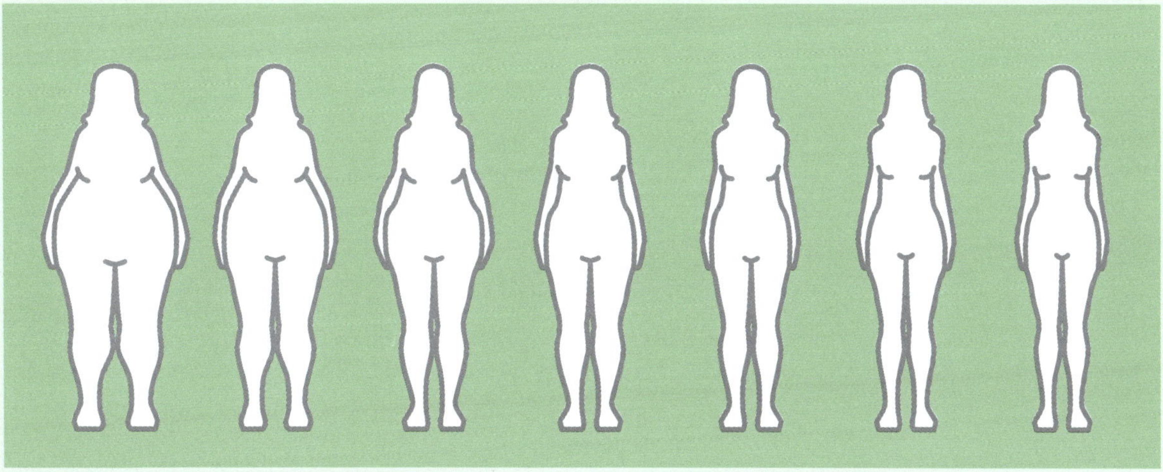

Weight Loss

Of all the topics I write about in nutrition, dieting and weight loss are always the most popular. In our sedentary world with less and less opportunity for physical activity, overeating is the norm. It's easy to put on weight and difficult to take it off and keep it off. I'm not immune to our obesogenic environment (a relatively new word that refers to the modern conditions which make it easy for us to put on weight), so I understand the hurdles and pitfalls.

People often ask me how to lose weight. In reply, I could simply say 'eat less and move more'. Long term, that's the truth in a nutshell but it's not helpful, nor does it address the daily questions of what to eat, how to eat and how to fit in exercise when you're busy. I believe there are 3 key areas that need to be addressed to lose weight, and keep it off—daily eating habits, thoughts and emotions, and physical activity.

DEVELOP HEALTHY EATING HABITS

NEVER SKIP MEALS, PARTICULARLY BREAKFAST

Breakfast kickstarts your body's metabolism and prevents you from becoming ravenously hungry before lunch. Take the time to sit down to fruit and cereal (900 kJ) before you start your day, and you'll be less likely to reach for fattening snacks like a muffin (1800 kJ) or pastry (1460 kJ) at morning tea. If you can't face food first thing in the morning, have a sandwich or smoothie mid-morning.

BE CAREFUL WITH FAT AND FRIED FOODS

Cutting back on fat, especially saturated fat, is still the easiest way to eat fewer kilojoules. Gram for gram, fat supplies more kilojoules than carbohydrate or protein and tends to be stored more efficiently. Fat is also difficult to oxidise and burn off. Refined carbs often occur in combination with fat—think of potato chips and doughnuts.

DRINK ALCOHOL IN MODERATION

Alcohol is a concentrated form of kilojoules. Just one small glass of dry wine or a nip of spirits has 300 kJ. Many people also eat more following a couple of drinks. Try to drink no more than a couple of drinks once or twice a week.

DOWNSIZE YOUR PORTIONS

You don't need to eat everything on your plate or have second helpings. Get used to leaving the table feeling comfortable, not stuffed full. When you eat out, go for two entrées instead of an entrée plus a main, or try a main plus a salad.

SPREAD YOUR FOOD OVER THE DAY

Four or five mini-meals a day can help increase you body's metabolic rate, so you burn fat faster. Regular, small meals also stop extreme hunger and bingeing.

DON'T EAT BIG LATE AT NIGHT

Evenings are inactive times for most people so whatever you eat is more likely to be converted to fat. Aim to eat your main meal at lunch or have an early dinner.

MAKE SAVINGS WHERE YOU CAN

Substitute diet or light foods whenever you can. Genuine diet products have less fat and fewer kilojoules (always check the label) and can offer good kilojoule savings, as long as you use them in the same quantities as normal items. For example, reduced-fat cheese has 25 per cent fat, one-third less than normal cheddar at 33 per cent. But if you eat twice as much as usual, there's no saving in kilojoules.

The best diet foods worth substituting are soft drinks, cordials, dips, yoghurts and dairy desserts, beer, wine and milk. The least helpful are light muffins, biscuits, muesli bars, cereals and snacks.

Whether using diet or regular versions, make a habit of spreading margarine thinly on sandwiches or toast, trimming the fat off meat, removing chicken skin, and frying in a non-stick pan brushed or sprayed with a just little oil.

COOK AT HOME

Avoid takeaway foods as much as possible—they are notoriously high in fat and are soft and easy to swallow. Plan ahead so you don't arrive home feeling tired and hungry. If you have a balanced meal waiting for you, you'll find it easier to eat well. Spraying on oil, using lean meat, being frugal with cream or sour cream, and adding plenty of vegetables or salad that fill you up are all things fast food places never do.

DON'T WEIGH YOURSELF EACH DAY

Everyone's weight has daily fluctuations, which reflect fluid balance, bowel movements, monthly periods and recent food intake. Once a week is enough.

SLOW IT DOWN

Eat slowly and chew each mouthful thoroughly. Stretch each meal out to last 20 minutes so your brain's appetite control centre has a chance to register when you are full. Put down your fork or spoon between mouthfuls.

MANAGING THOUGHTS AND EMOTIONS

THINK LONG TERM

Your excess weight won't disappear in three days (despite diet promises), but it will over three weeks. Aim for small, gradual losses and you won't trigger your body's natural famine/starvation responses, which serve to preserve your fat stores for lean times. This is why strict diets often leave you fatter than before.

KEEP A FOOD DIARY

Make a note of your eating schedule. Record the time and place where you eat and when you feel most hungry. Try and be aware of unconscious eating; for example, when cooking, clearing away leftovers or feeding children. Plan an absorbing activity for these times or rearrange your food plan to allow for a snack.

KEEP BUSY

The busier you are, the less time you'll have to be tempted to overeat. Keep away from the kitchen in your down time and do something that occupies your hands.

MANAGE CRAVINGS

When you feel a craving for a particular food, say to yourself, 'I can eat this food but I'll postpone it for 10 minutes.' When the 10 minutes is up, check how strong your craving is. You may have become involved in something else and no longer feel like eating. But if you're still dreaming of, say, chocolate, have one piece. Sit somewhere by yourself and place the chocolate on your tongue. Don't chew. Just suck it slowly for as long as you can. Enjoy it. That may be all you need to satisfy your desire.

DON'T USE FOOD TO RELIEVE ANGER OR TENSION

A piece of cake or a chocolate bar generally won't help change a situation. If you have learnt to use food as an emotional crutch, it can be unlearnt. Take up yoga or meditation to help yourself unwind without food. A walk is a good way to clear your head and the air.

ENJOY YOUR MEALS

When you're eating, devote your attention to the experience. Enjoy the aroma and savour each mouthful. Don't watch television or read while eating. This only associates the two activities mentally.

KEEP FOOD OUT OF SIGHT

It's easier to avoid eating if you are not constantly facing temptation.

SHOP AT THE RIGHT TIME

Buy groceries when you are not hungry. Don't buy foods you know are hard to resist.

GET MOVING

INCREASE YOUR METABOLIC RATE

Exercise was once believed to be of limited help for fat loss because you needed to exercise strenuously just to burn off a few kilojoules (caloric counters would previously list equivalents such as one cream bun is equal to 60 minutes of jogging). But it is now recognised that regular exercise increases the resting metabolic rate for 24–48 hours afterwards, so your body 'revs' at a higher rate, burning up more kilojoules (resting metabolism accounts for some 70 per cent of total kilojoule expenditure). Exercise also helps to regulate your appetite.

ENJOY THE HEALTH BENEFITS

Exercise helps to lower blood cholesterol, including the dangerous LDL cholesterol. It also reduces blood pressure in mildly hypertensive people, reduces blood glucose levels and improves insulin resistance.

IMPROVE MUSCLE STRENGTH AND JOINT FLEXIBILITY

This helps fight osteoarthritis and reduces the risk of bone fractures and development of osteoporosis in later life, particularly in women (it should be weight-bearing exercise).

BOOST YOUR MENTAL HEALTH

Exercise can help alleviate mild depression and stress, and improve your sense of wellbeing. It can also improve sleeping patterns.

WHAT YOU SHOULD AIM FOR WHEN YOU WANT TO LOSE WEIGHT

NON-STARCHY VEGETABLES

Eat freely. With no fat and less than 80 kilojoules per serve, non-starchy vegetables can be eaten freely. The list is long and varied and includes asparagus, bean sprouts, beans, Asian greens, broccoli, Brussels sprouts, cabbage, capsicum, cauliflower, celery, choko, cucumber, eggplant, kale, leeks, lettuce, mushrooms, radish, silverbeet, spinach, tomatoes and zucchini.

DID YOU KNOW?

You need to rev your body at a higher rate to shed body fat successfully. This can be any aerobic activity that exercises the heart and lungs and increases the oxygen needs of the body—using the large muscles of the body (thighs, trunk and shoulders) over an extended period is a particularly good form of aerobic conditioning. Walking, swimming, bicycling, skipping, jogging or gym classes are all good, and any exercise is better than none at all. If you are unfit, check with your doctor before undertaking vigorous exercise.

FRUIT

Two serves a day. Fruit is a year-round treat, and one with virtually no fat. It is an ideal way to finish any meal and makes a convenient, refreshing snack. Choose whole fruit rather than juice for maximum fibre and filling value. One serve is one piece of fresh fruit or ½ cup of canned or stewed fruit.

MEAT, FISH AND POULTRY

Two to three serves a day. Lean meat, trimmed of visible fat, can definitely be part of a low-fat diet, as can skinned chicken, fish and eggs. It is acceptable if it is grilled, barbecued, dry-baked, stir-fried with a spray of oil or cooked in the microwave. Do not fry or roast in fat. One serve equals 175 grams of lean meat or chicken (raw weight), 200 grams fish or seafood (raw weight), a 100 gram can of tuna or salmon (in spring water) or two or three eggs. For vegetarians, one serve means 1 cup of cooked or canned beans or lentils.

PASTA, GRAINS, BREAD AND STARCHY VEGETABLES

Four serves a day. These foods are low in fat and high in starchy carbs, and are filling and satisfying. Aim for versions that are slowly digested with a low GI, or are wholegrain or high in fibre. One serve means one slice of bread, one medium potato, ½ cup of mashed pumpkin or sweet potato, ½ cup of cooked rice or pasta, ¾ cup of breakfast cereal, or 1 cup of rolled oats.

MILK, YOGHURT AND ALTERNATIVES

Two to three serves a day. Go for skim milks and yoghurts and you can have twice as much as you can if eating the full-cream version. Hard yellow cheeses should be restricted or avoided. In their place, look for the reduced-fat cheese varieties now being made. One serve is 250 millilitres of reduced-fat milk, a 200 gram carton of yoghurt, a 30 gram wedge of low-fat cheese or ½ cup of cottage cheese or ricotta.

10 DIET TRAPS

Trying to slim down? Don't fall into these common traps.

- **Wanting to lose weight too fast**—sure, you can shed a few kilos in a week on a juice-only fast but the weight will come straight back on once you resume your normal eating patterns.
- **Eating big after the gym**—don't let yourself think you can tuck into a big feed just because you've done a workout. Your goal is to slightly under-eat so your body is forced to tap into fat stores.
- **Going vegetarian to save kilojoules**—cutting out meat will cut your kilojoule intake, but it also cuts out vital nutrients like iron, zinc and vitamin B_{12}, which many women in particular run short on. It also cuts out one of the most filling and satisfying foods for dieters.
- **Forgetting about kilojoules**—with all the hype about high-protein diets, it's easy to think that meat, fish, chicken or eggs can be consumed in any quantity without being converted into body fat, or that all carbs are bad for you. The bottom line is if you eat more kilojoules (of any type) than you burn off, you won't lose that excess fat.
- **Giving up after a binge**—everyone falls off the wagon at some stage! The trick is to pick yourself up and get back on track. A single pig-out isn't the problem. It's when you give up and start a week-long marathon meal that the weight piles on. In fact, some diets allow you a small daily treat to prevent that deprived feeling.
- **Skipping breakfast to save kilojoules**—eating a nutritious breakfast kickstarts your metabolism, helping you burn off fat during the day and avoid starting your day feeling tired or sluggish.
- **Pigging out on low-fat snacks**—even when a product has 30 per cent less fat, the most the total kilojoules will drop is 10–15 per cent, so, you can't eat twice as much! Many light biscuits and muesli bars are sold in smaller serve sizes (20 g for a light biscuit compared with 40 g for the regular version) so the kilojoule savings appear hefty, simply because you're eating less food.
- **Trying every new diet you read**—cabbage soup, Dukan, Atkins, Sugar Busters, detoxing, liver cleansing, and blood type diets—you've done them all. You lose some weight, but then it slowly creeps back. Why? Because you haven't changed your eating habits long term.
- **Giving up the carbs**—the Dr Atkins–style protein diets may have left you thinking carbs are responsible for obesity, and that you just have to avoid all bread, potatoes, pasta, fruit and sugary foods. The reality is carbs can't be avoided completely. If you want to cut back, choose the healthier wholegrain or high-fibre foods, and eat smaller portions of them. But as a minimum you need 120 g of carbs a day.
- **Cutting out all fat**—the explosion of '97 per cent fat-free' foods has made many dieters paranoid about fat eating. Cutting down on fat is a good strategy for cutting kilojoules, but it shouldn't be cut out completely.

FATS AND OILS

Two serves a day. Oil, nuts and avocado—these are high-fat foods, so use them sparingly. Cream and sour cream are best avoided, and mayonnaises vary greatly so look for those that are labelled 'light' or 'low-oil' when shopping. One serve is 1 teaspoon of oil, margarine or butter for cooking and spreading, 1 tablespoon (10 grams) of nuts, or half an avocado (50 grams).

FAT-FREE FILLERS

You can rely on these foods when you're feeling peckish. Their fat is so low, they have negligible kilojoules and are a healthy snack option to have at hand. These fillers include clear soup, mineral water, diet soft drinks, herbal teas, sugar-free jellies and passionfruit.

FAD DIETS

'Lose 14 kilograms in 30 days!' 'Drop a dress size in a weekend!' 'Block the absorption of fat and carbs!' 'Lose weight with our miracle juice!' 'New diet melts away flab!' I'm sure you've heard them all. Losing weight quickly and without effort is so appealing that it's hard not to be sucked in with sensational claims like those above. Forget the false promises and magic bullets. The reason there is a new fad diet each month is because the last one didn't work. Sure, you can reduce your weight while you're on the diet, but once it's finished and you go back to eating normally, you put it back on. Because they've been so deprived and real food looks so good, people generally lash out after a fad diet and overeat. They then embark on another fad diet and the downward cycle starts again.

Yoyo dieting is not only ineffective and expensive, it is also considered to be even more unhealthy than being overweight. It can place a physical strain on your heart—not to mention being disheartening! Fad diets are not nutritionally balanced. They usually leave you irritable, hungry, sleepless, and lacking energy. They can make you constipated and prone to infections. Often, they cause you to lose lean muscle, which creates a drop in your metabolic rate and in turn decreases the number of kilojoules you burn each day. This means you must eat less and less to maintain your weight loss.

MY TAKE

There are no magic foods or diets that will dissolve fat—not grapefruit, kelp or cider vinegar, nor chitosan, brindle berry or chromium picolinate. Nutritionists recommend a steady weight loss of 1 kg per week (of body fat, not fluid). It won't be dramatic, but hopefully it will be permanent. Your excess weight took months or even years to accumulate—it's not going to melt away overnight.

CHECK THE CREDENTIALS

If you hear about a new diet (and there will be one coming to a magazine or website near you!), look over it and ask yourself if the diet:

- Makes enticing claims about losing weight quickly and effortlessly
- Allows you to eat as much as you like of any one food and not put on weight
- Makes one food appear important, giving it 'miracle' properties
- Requires you to buy special diet supplements or pills or formula
- Claims to be new or revolutionary
- Only mentions food and says nothing about exercise.

If the answer to any of these questions is yes, then this is not a balanced program and it is unlikely to be based on a healthy eating plan that will lead to healthy weight loss and eating habits that will help you maintain it. Forget it!

If you feel confused about what's best for you, make an appointment with an accredited practising dietitian. To find one near you, contact the Dietitians Association of Australia on 1800 812 942 or go to www.daa.asn.au.

SPOT THE NEXT FAD BEFORE YOU OPEN YOUR WALLET

SINGLE-FOOD DIETS—WEIGHT LOSS THROUGH BOREDOM

Based on one food (like hard-boiled eggs or grapefruit) or one food group (like vegetables), these diets offer you unlimited quantities of a food, knowing that you will quickly get tired of the same thing and curtail your total kilojoule intake. They work on the principle of boredom and monotony. You end up eating very few kilojoules, so your body basically goes into starvation mode. Examples include the Kickstart Soup Diet, the Cabbage Soup Diet, the Heart Foundation 3 Day Diet (disowned by the Heart Foundation), the Grapefruit Diet, the Mayo Clinic Diet (also known as the Egg Diet), the Israeli Army Diet, the Beverley Hills Diet and the Bananas and Milk Diet.

SEMI-FASTS—WEIGHT LOSS THROUGH STARVATION

Semi-fasts allow small amounts of light foods like juices, fruit, salads, herbal teas or brown rice. They promise you will feel euphoric and cleansed afterwards. Semi-fasts are attractive as they produce rapid weight loss in only a few days. They can be a health hazard and cause dizziness, muscle cramps, nausea, bad breath, dehydration and constipation. Follow with caution. Examples include detox diets, the Lemon Detox Diet (based on syrup drink) and water diets.

HIP AND THIGH DIETS—WEIGH LESS BUT KEEP YOUR BODY SHAPE

It is impossible to lose fat from a single area. Weight is lost from all over your body—if you are pear-shaped, you may be larger or smaller, but you will always be pear-shaped. That said, most diets that target 'problem areas' combine low-kilojoule intakes with an exercise plan and are generally healthy. Examples include the Flat Belly Diet, Rosemary Conley's Hip and Thigh Diet, and the Cellulite Diet.

LIQUID DIETS AND MEAL REPLACEMENT—WEIGHT LOSS THROUGH CONVENIENCE

You replace one, two or three meals a day with a special shake (or soup, bar or biscuit) on this type of diet. The good thing is this keeps you out of the kitchen and away from food so you're not tempted to nibble or overindulge. The downside is that they can be expensive and may leave you short on vitamins or minerals that are plentiful in food (although many shakes are fortified these days). And because you're not chewing and taking time to eat as you would over a proper meal, you may not feel as satisfied as you would be from whole foods. Examples include Slim Fast, Tony Ferguson, Kickstart, Herbalife, Optifast, Biggest Loser, Celebrity Slim, Betty Baxter and the Cambridge Diet.

DID YOU KNOW?

When you exercise aerobically on a regular basis and follow a diet, you may find the scales show no weight loss at all, or sometimes even a weight gain. Don't become discouraged. Muscle is heavier than fat and, as you lose body fat, you are replacing it with heavier muscle, and increasing your muscle-to-fat ratio. Rather than registering on the scales, it will show up in your measurements. It is best not to weigh yourself more than once a week, but rely instead on the measuring tape and how your clothes fit.

VIRTUALLY ZERO-CARBOHYDRATE DIETS—WEIGHT LOSS THROUGH WATER LOSS

Diets that tell you to avoid all bread, potatoes, pasta and cereals come into fashion every few years. They claim these carbohydrate foods are the cause of obesity and that by cutting them out, you will lose your flab. Living without carbohydrate means a diet of meat, cheese, fish, eggs, mayonnaise, butter and cream, which creates a high-fat, high-cholesterol regime—not very good for the heart. You definitely shed a lot of weight on these diets, but the weight is largely water and will return when carbohydrates are eaten again. Examples include Dr Atkins' Diet Revolution (initial phase), The Scarsdale Medical Diet, the Boston Police Diet and Dr Stillman's Quick Weight-Loss Diet.

Don't be tricked by massages, rubs, vibrator belts or muscle stimulation that promise to 'break up' fat. Passive exercise is of no benefit. Nothing can break up the fat or work your muscles without effort from you.

MEAL REPLACEMENTS

Meal replacement shakes such as Tony Ferguson, Optifast VLCD, Optislim, Biggest Loser, Betty Baxter, Dr Sandra Cabot QuickLoss Meal Replacement powder,

Kickstart VLCD, Xantrax, Isowhey Complete, Musashi SLM, the Cambridge Diet and Dymatize 12 hour Meal are generally made from non-fat milk powder, with added vitamins and minerals. Some have a little fibre (psyllium or guar), so you don't get constipated and feel fuller. Some also have probiotic, omega-3 or soy protein present so they sound more impressive—think of them as milk drink combined with a vitamin pill.

MY TAKE
I think the most practical way to use these is to replace one meal a day and eat two balanced meals. Nutritionally you won't lose out, and research shows this approach has lower drop-out rates.

Meal replacements including shakes, soups and bars are recommended by dietitians to help people who are very overweight kickstart a weight-loss program. In these situations, the meal replacement phase of the program is typically 8–12 weeks and the participants then start learning how to eat a healthy long-term diet.

Meal replacement diets are also marketed direct to consumers, but I recommend checking with your doctor or dietitian before trying them. They can play a role at the start of a new eating plan or as a replacement for one meal a day, but I believe a healthy, low-kilojoule diet combined with regular exercise is the best long-term way to lose weight and keep it off.

PROS

- ✔ Single packaging makes it easy to control portion sizes.
- ✔ You know exactly how many kilojoules/calories you've consumed.
- ✔ There's no choice, so you have no opportunity to stray.
- ✔ They are quick and convenient making them easy to use at work.
- ✔ They keep you out of the kitchen (or fast-food court) and away from temptation.

CONS

- ✖ They don't teach you to make healthy 'real food' choices day to day.
- ✖ They aren't as nutritious as eating whole foods.
- ✖ They don't help you learn the kilojoule content of a normal diet.
- ✖ They can be linked to gallstones if you lose weight too fast.
- ✖ Many are sweet, encouraging a 'sweet tooth'.
- ✖ They can pall after a while—there are only so many 'chocolate or vanilla shakes' you can take.
- ✖ They can be expensive.

See also **Dietary Requirements (by age group); Energy; Exercise; Fasting; Fat-Burning Foods and Drinks; Food-combining Diets; Mindless Eating; Mood and Food; Obesity; Portion Distortion; Waist Circumference.**

WEIGHT-LOSS SUPPORT GROUPS

Clubs and groups such as Weight Watchers, Jenny Craig, Biggest Loser and Fernwood do a great job by offering a support system of regular weekly meetings or online forums led by group leaders who have successfully lost weight themselves. Like Alcoholics Anonymous and similar programs, a group of people battling the same problem can provide encouragement and peer support to keep even the most unmotivated dieter on the right track.

Such groups generally have a fairly standard diet plan with the emphasis on balanced meals that the whole family can eat, combined with exercise, behaviour modification and group support. No supplements or special foods are necessary, although larger groups do promote their own range of diet products for members. They generally have a board of scientific advisors who monitor research and adapt the basic food plan from time to time. They encourage members to lose weight at a healthy rate of between 0.5 kilograms and 1 kilogram per week.

Wheat

Wheat was first cultivated about 7000 BC in the valley of the Fertile Crescent and spread to other parts of the Middle East, then Egypt, Rome and Europe. Today, thanks to its adaptability and endless uses, it is grown on all continents and is sometimes called the 'king of grains'.

Wheat is consumed in a diverse variety of forms. Bulgur, pasta, bread, puffed wheat and biscuits might all look and taste different, but they're all derived from the same versatile grain—wheat.

The simplest and earliest way to consume wheat was probably by soaking and parching whole grains over a fire. Alternatively, wheat can be soaked and cooked in water, and eaten as a coarse porridge or gruel. Throughout history, however, wheat's main end-use has been to be ground into a meal or flour and used to bake bread, either leavened (with yeast) or unleavened (flatbread).

Unleavened breads are made by mixing flour with water to make a dough, shaping the dough and then baking it on hot stones or in an oven. Examples include the Jewish matzoh, some types of Indian chapattis, Mexican tortillas and Middle Eastern flatbreads.

Leavened bread is baked from a dough of flour, water, yeast and salt. Originally wild yeasts from the air settled on the dough and this created the first sourdough breads. Modern breads are made with cultivated strains of yeast to produce the familiar risen baguettes, rolls, cobs, roggenbrots and today's sliced square loaves from the supermarket.

After milling, wheat grains are separated into the three parts—the starchy inner endosperm which goes to become white flour, the fibrous outer bran layers and the oil-rich embryo called wheat germ. Wheat products include bran, wheat germ, bulgur, couscous, rolled wheat, kibble and semolina (the basis of pasta), cereals, bread and baked goods like biscuits, cakes and pastry.

NUTRITIONAL VALUE

Wheat, in the form of grains or flour, shares many similar nutritional features with the other cereal grains:

- ✔ Wheat has been valued for its starchy carbohydrate, which makes up over 70 per cent of its composition, and which gives bread, noodles, macaroni or bulgur their filling power. Generally the starch in wheat is high GI so it's rapidly absorbed.
- ✔ Wheat is low in fat, with less than 2 per cent fat.
- ✔ Wheat contributes a fair quantity of protein, especially from bread wheats and durum wheats, which are used to make pasta. Protein ranges from 7 to 15 per cent, but figures as high as 20 per cent have been reported.
- ✔ Wheat contributes a good dose of fibre, particularly from bran-based food like bran cereals, wholemeal breads and whole-wheat cereals.
- ✔ Wheat is a major source of B vitamins, notably thiamin and niacin (needed to release energy from carbohydrate) and folate (nerve function)
- ✔ Wheat foods supply a range of minerals including phosphorus, potassium, iron, magnesium and selenium, but this depends on the mineral content of the soil in which it's grown.
- ✔ Research has uncovered lignans in whole-wheat, compounds that can influence oestrogen levels in women.

See also Bran; Bread; Grains and Cereals; Gluten.

Wheat Intolerance

Bloating, wind, diarrhoea and tummy pain—many people avoid wheat, complaining it upsets their digestive system. An intolerance to wheat is not necessarily coeliac disease, and until a few years ago, I would have dismissed them as faddists. But new Australian research has found evidence for the first time that gluten may trigger gut symptoms and fatigue in individuals who do not have coeliac disease. In addition, wheat is high in fructans—fructose-based carbohydrates that can upset anyone with irritable bowel. People with a wheat intolerance need to avoid large quantities of bread, pasta, cereals and crackers. Rye and spelt breads seem to be better tolerated, as are oats. Small amounts of wheat like thickeners, are usually not a problem.

It's important not to self-diagnose. Avoiding wheat unnecessarily can leave you short on fibre, B vitamins and carbohydrates—not to mention making eating out a hassle! It can be difficult to tell the difference between the symptoms of allergy and intolerance. Food intolerance reactions are usually related to the amount of the food consumed. They may not occur until a certain threshold of the food is eaten. Keeping a food and symptoms diary, following an elimination diet for two weeks, skin prick tests and blood (RAST) tests can all help. Make an appointment with a gastroenterologist or a dietitian, and speak to an expert.

See also **Food Allergy and Intolerance.**

Whey

Whey is one of the two main proteins in milk. It is the liquid by-product left over when milk is turned into cheese. It contains water, lactose, minerals (a little calcium), active peptides, proteins and fat. It is used to produce ricotta.

Whey goes through a process called micro-filtration, which separates the lactose and fat from the protein. The end result can be whey concentrate or whey isolate, the two major forms. Concentrates have the highest amount of fat and lactose and are about 75 per cent protein. Isolates are similar to concentrates but with the fat and lactose removed. They are usually 90 per cent or more protein, providing a greater amount per serve. They also cost more than the concentrates. Both forms have a mild, slightly milky taste.

Whey protein can be further 'digested' into whey hydrolysates, which taste very bitter. This makes them more easily absorbed, and also the most expensive. They are used to make infant formula and protein supplements for medical use.

Whey protein is commonly sold as a dietary supplement (think of the protein powders loved by body builders), and is added to protein bars and some drinks. It is digested very rapidly, and used after workouts to help increase the levels of amino acids (small units of protein) in the blood. These are then taken up by the muscles to help with faster muscle repair, decreased recovery time and increased muscle mass. Protein supplements should never be used as the sole source of protein.

Whole Foods

Whole foods are foods that are unprocessed or processed as little as possible. They are foods that are close to their natural state and don't typically contain added sugar, salt or fats. They are usually high in fibre and low GI. Eating foods that are in their natural state provides the essential nutrients that are often lost in the processing of foods. Examples include unrefined grains (brown rice, spelt and buckwheat), legumes, fresh fruit, fresh vegetables and non-homogenised full-fat dairy foods. The term is often confused with organic food, but whole foods are not necessarily organic, nor are organic foods necessarily whole foods.

What's missing is important. Oranges are a whole food, but orange juice (even home-squeezed) isn't because the fibre has been removed and with it goes the natural brake to over-consumption. When you eat whole foods with their natural high-fibre structure intact, there's more chewing involved so you take longer to eat them. As they fill the stomach and the intestines, your eating is slowed and your stomach gets full, giving you the signal to stop eating. This doesn't happen with juice.

Wholegrains

Wholegrain is the new black. These foods have enjoyed a boost in popularity in the last few years, with numerous studies showing wholegrain versions of grain foods are the best choice for health and wellbeing.

Wholegrain used to be limited to intact, unmilled grains like brown rice. Very few products qualified under the old definition, but now wholegrain can include any grains that have been dehulled, ground, milled, cracked or flaked, as long as the three original components—the outer bran layer, nutritious inner germ and the starchy endosperm—are recombined in their original proportions. This more inclusive definition means a large number of cereals, breads, snack foods, porridges and soups now qualify—both satisfying and confusing the health-conscious shopper.

NUTRITIONAL VALUE

There is a lot of evidence supporting the many benefits of eating plenty of wholegrain foods:

- ✔ Wholegrain cereals reduce the risk of certain types of cancer, heart disease, stroke and type 2 diabetes.
- ✔ A higher fibre intake, especially from whole cereal grains, is linked to a lower risk of cancer of the large bowel, breast, stomach and mouth.
- ✔ Wholegrains help with weight loss because fibre makes you feel full longer.
- ✔ They improve bowel health and regularity.
- ✔ Rye adds lignans to the diet, which work in a similar way to soy's phytoestrogens to help with the menopause.
- ✔ Oats and barley are good for beta-glucans, a type of gelling fibre that can lower cholesterol.

MAKE THE SWAP

You don't have to eat everything wholegrain, just aim to swap half of all the grain foods you eat for wholegrain. For women, this usually means two or three

NOT ALL WHOLEGRAINS ARE LOW GI

Some people use wholegrain and low GI as though they are interchangeable terms. That's not the case at all. Wholegrain foods can be high or low GI, and it's essential to know what is and what's not, to manage your blood-glucose levels. In fact many processed wholegrain foods, such as wholemeal bread, have a high GI. When wheat fibre has been finely divided, as it is in wholemeal bread, it does little for constipation or blood-glucose levels. But if your favourite wholegrain food has a high or moderate GI, combine it with a low-GI ingredient like legumes to reduce the glycemic load of the meal or snack.

serves a day. This could be a bowl of wholegrain cereal and two slices of bread in your sandwich at lunch. Wholemeal pasta and brown rice are also alternative options. For men, this usually means 3–6 serves a day, depending on how much physical exercise they do.

WHOLEGRAIN VS WHOLEMEAL

Wholegrain foods contain the 3 parts of the grain—the bran, germ and endosperm. Wholemeal foods are important for fibre and nutrients, but they have been processed to a finer texture and we digest them faster. That's why wholemeal foods often have a GI about the same as their white counterparts. Wholemeal is wholegrain, but it's not the case the other way around.

Wild Rice *See* Grains and Cereals.

Wind *See* Flatulence.

Wine *See* Alcohol.

X

Xylitol

See also Sweeteners.

Xylitol is a sugar alcohol used to sweeten diet foods. Its additive code is 967.

Y

Yeast

Yeasts are single-cell organisms related to fungi-like moulds. Over 500 different species of yeast exist but only a few are important in food production. Bread, beer and sparkling wines all rely on yeast and there are special food yeasts and extracts of yeast used to flavour food.

NUTRITIONAL VALUE

Yeast contains fibre, and little or no fat or sugars. As they grow, yeasts also produce proteins and B vitamins. Dried yeast, whether brewer's, baker's or torula food yeast, is the richest known source of seven B vitamins—it's like a multi-B vitamin supplement—but the vitamins are not necessarily in the same ratio as required by humans. One tablespoon of dried baker's yeast supplies 35–65 per cent of our needs for thiamin, riboflavin and niacin, but as little as 20 per cent of biotin and up to 400 per cent of folic acid. It also supplies plenty of potassium, phosphorus, zinc and the trace elements chromium and selenium. It is such a rich source that decades ago it was taken to treat diseases caused by B vitamin deficiencies, like pellagra and beriberi. Many healthy food advocates prefer yeast tablets or flakes as a natural food-derived supplement over ordinary B vitamin tablets, which are likely to be synthetic, and I concur. Generally yeast supplements are derived from brewer's yeast, which is the leftover yeast that remains from the brewing of beer.

YEAST ALLERGY

According to the Royal Prince Alfred Hospital Allergy Unit, yeast allergy is very rare and yeast is not one of the major eight allergens. However, yeast is rich in amines and glutamates, so may trigger food intolerance reactions.

YEAST-FREE DIET AND CANDIDA INFECTIONS

A yeast-free diet is often claimed to clear up vaginal infections, fatigue, digestive upsets, skin disorders and headaches—all supposedly due to the excessive growth of the micro-organism *Candida albicans* that takes over your digestive system. Once it spreads, it produces toxins that 'poison' your whole body.

This diet seeks to address this by avoiding yeast in any form, any food that may grow mould (for example certain cheeses), and sugar and refined carbohydrates found in cakes, biscuits and sweets. Yeast, sugar and mouldy foods supposedly 'feed' the growth of the candida. If you cut off its food supply, it should die off and your symptoms disappear, or so the theory goes.

Many people swear they feel better and have more energy on the diet, but this could be attributed to eating better quality of food and the exclusion of sugar, white flour and junk foods—people on this diet must cook proper meals and eat lots of vegetables, rice, beans, fruit, fish, lean meat and yoghurt. Scientifically, there have been no sound clinical trials to show whether a yeast-free diet has any beneficial effect. Allergy dietitians say that the same symptoms can often be a result of food sensitivity—an intolerance to various chemicals, both natural and artificial, in food.

DID YOU KNOW?

Sourdough bread is not free of yeast. While it contains no baker's yeast, the sourdough starter is teeming with live wild yeasts, which grow during proving, generating bubbles of gas that make the bread rise.

Yoghurt

Yoghurt is one of my must-eat, easy superfoods. It's packed with calcium, protein and B vitamins (especially riboflavin, a B vitamin needed for healthy skin and eyes). Yoghurt offers the nutrients of milk but in a more concentrated form. It is also more easily digested and absorbed than milk due to the partial predigestion by its bacteria. Studies show the protein, fat and lactose it contains are better absorbed and the calcium is more available.

The carbohydrate in yoghurt is also absorbed slowly, producing only a modest rise in blood-glucose levels making it a filling low-GI snack or dessert for anyone with diabetes.

NUMBER CRUNCH

A 200 gram carton of plain low-fat yoghurt supplies 10 grams of protein, 2 grams of fat, 14 grams of carbohydrate, 14 grams of sugar, no starch, no dietary fibre and 480 kilojoules.

A 200 gram carton of strawberry low-fat yoghurt supplies 10 grams of protein, 2 grams of fat, 24 grams of carbohydrate, 24 grams of sugar, no starch, no dietary fibre and 660 kilojoules.

LACTOSE INTOLERANCE

People with lactose intolerance are more likely to tolerate yoghurt than milk. During yoghurt-making, the bacteria partly break down the milk sugar lactose, turning it into lactic acid, creating yoghurt's sour taste.

WEIGHT LOSS

Research shows that when cutting kilojoules to lose weight, three servings of milk or yogurt each day actually help people burn more fat and lose more weight, rather than simply cutting down on kilojoules. The mix of nutrients found in dairy foods, especially calcium, may be responsible for helping the body break down and burn fat.

MY TAKE

I prefer the set types of yoghurt, which have a firmer jelly-like texture, rather than the stirred yoghurt that pours out of the container. That's just my tastebuds talking, though—nutritionally there's little difference. Sometimes yoghurt is also marketed as fromage frais, even though they're not strictly equivalent.

WHAT YOGHURT IS THAT?

DESSERT YOGHURTS

You'll find these in the dairy section next to the yoghurts, but they're a far cry from regular yoghurt. Yes they may contain a little yoghurt, but there's also added cream or chocolate, and flavouring like cheesecake, caramel or tiramisu. Think of these as an indulgent dessert, not a healthy snack.

DIET YOGHURTS

Diet yoghurts contain virtually no fat, no added sugar and the least kilojoules of all yoghurts—this is as low as you can get! They are artificially sweetened (usually with acesulfame K or sucralose). For the serious dieter, here's how they compare:

- Low-fat yoghurt, 200 gram tub (0–1 grams of fat; 6 grams of added sugar) = 800 kilojoules
- Diet yoghurt, 200 gram tub (0 grams of fat; 0 grams of added sugar) = 380 kilojoules.

DRINKING YOGHURT

Drinking yoghurt (like the Indian *lassi*) is refreshing and convenient. Most brands have the same or slightly less calcium than yoghurt, but are still nutritious. Think of them as a sweetened, low-fat yoghurt in drinkable form—good for hungry teens who need a snack on the run.

FROZEN YOGHURT

With its slightly tart flavour and healthy-sounding fruit flavours like pomegranate and raspberry, frozen yoghurt cashes in on the health image of yoghurt, but it's not a direct substitute for the real thing. Yes it's a healthier option than regular ice-cream with less sugar, fat and kilojoules and a low GI, but it's got roughly twice the kilojoules of low-fat yoghurt, so it's not entirely guiltless. I regard it as halfway between gelato and ice-cream. Enjoy it as a treat on a hot day.

FULL-FAT YOGHURT

At 4 per cent fat, full-fat plain or natural yoghurt reflects the fat content of its starter milk. It's suitable for families and growing children who need the fat and kilojoules for growth and energy.

GREEK YOGHURT

Greek yoghurt is considerably thicker than plain yoghurt. It generally has around 8–10 per cent fat, compared with 4 per cent for normal plain yoghurt. It is made by straining yoghurt through muslin, cloth, paper or some other sort of filter, which removes the liquid whey and leaves the final yoghurt thicker and more creamy. You get a consistency similar to sour cream or mascarpone, while retaining yoghurt's distinctive sour taste. In Greece, it's traditionally made from sheep's milk. Here in Australia, we use cow's milk instead. Some brands add extra cream or powdered milk (milk solids), or boil off some of the water content in the milk, both of which increase the richness of the yoghurt.

You can buy low-fat Greek yoghurt, which has less than 3 per cent fat (like all foods labelled low-fat). To get the best of both worlds I recommend buying this one, and adding your own stewed rhubarb or canned apricots for flavour.

Growing bodies
Low-fat, reduced-fat and light yoghurts are suitable for children over the age of 2.

LOW-FAT, REDUCED-FAT, LIGHT YOGHURT

Like low-fat milk, low-fat yoghurts have around half the fat (less than 2 per cent) of full-fat types and are often labelled 'light', so you save fat and kilojoules. They can be plain or sweetened with sugar and fruit or fruit flavours. Look for a brand with less than 20 per cent total sugars in the label (from fruit and added sugar). These yoghurts make a handy office snack or lunch box addition.

NON-FAT OR SKIM YOGHURT

Plain skim milk yoghurt has almost no fat but is often thin and watery in texture. You still get the calcium and protein though, as this stays with the watery portion and not the fat.

See also Probiotics.

Z

Zeaxanthin

This is a carotenoid and antioxidant that may protect against loss of vision in the elderly. Rich sources include broccoli, spinach, silverbeet, parsley and dark-green lettuces.

See also Eye Health and Diet.

Zinc

Zinc is an essential mineral for many enzyme systems, concentrated in the bones, prostate glands, sperm and hair. Zinc serves many purposes:

- ✔ Combines with vitamin A to maintain eyesight
- ✔ Aids the healing of wounds and cuts
- ✔ Facilitates normal taste, smell and sight

- ✔ Makes up many enzymes
- ✔ Provides the hard structure of the bones
- ✔ Assists in sexual maturation and reproduction
- ✔ Is believed to prevent or shorten the duration of the common cold, but results are inconclusive.

RECOMMENDED DAILY INTAKE	ZINC (mg)
Adult women	8
Adult men	14
Safe upper limit for supplements 40 mg	
Sources Lean meat, liver, kidney, chicken, seafood (especially oysters) and milk are the most reliable source. Nuts, wholegrain foods, wholemeal bread and legumes also contain zinc, but much of it is in a form not biologically available to humans.	

ZINC LOZENGES

The cure for the common cold remains elusive; however, that doesn't stop those claiming to have found it from marketing their wares each winter. There have been many magic bullets—tea with lemon and honey, garlic, chicken soup, megadoses of vitamin C, echinacea, and in the last few years, zinc. A review of all trials of zinc and colds concluded last year that positive evidence is still lacking, and so the benefits remain uncertain. While some swear by their zinc lozenges, others find they suffer its annoying side effects, which can include nausea, upset tummy and a bad taste in their mouth. You decide if it's worth it!

Appendix 1—Energy

RECOMMENDED DAILY INTAKE (RDI)

DAILY KILOJOULE REQUIREMENTS MEN				
MEN DOING LIGHT ACTIVITY*				
Weight (kg)	19–30 yrs	31–50 yrs	51–70 yrs	Over 70 yrs
56	10,300	10,200	9300	8300
63	11,000	10,700	9800	8900
71	11,800	11,300	10,400	9500
79	12,600	11,900	11,100	10,200
88	13,500	12,600	11,700	10,800

DAILY KILOJOULE REQUIREMENTS WOMEN				
WOMEN DOING LIGHT ACTIVITY*				
Weight (kg)	19–30 yrs	31–50 yrs	51–70 yrs	Over 70 yrs
49	8200	8400	7900	7400
56	8800	8700	8300	7800
63	9600	9100	8700	8300
71	10,300	9500	9100	8700
79	11,100	10,000	9600	9200

DAILY KILOJOULE REQUIREMENTS CHILDREN				
	GIRLS		BOYS	
Age	Light activities*	Heavy activities or strenuous sport**	Light activities*	Heavy activities or strenuous sport**
3	5300	6400	5600	6900
4	5500	6800	5900	7300
5	5700	7200	6200	7800
6	6100	7600	6600	8200
7	6500	8100	7000	8700
8	6900	8600	7300	9200
9	7300	9100	7800	9700
10	7600	9500	8300	10,400
11	8000	10,000	8800	11,000
12	8500	10,600	9300	11,600
13	8900	11,100	10,000	12,400
14	9200	11,500	10,600	13,200
15	9400	11,700	11,200	14,000
16	9500	11,900	11,800	14,700
17	9600	12,000	12,200	15,200
18	9700	12,100	12,500	15,600

Energy Requirements will differ depending on your weight, height and physical activity level.

These figures are provided as a guide only:

* Based on a Physical Activity Level (PAL) of 1.6, which is considered light activity.

** Based on a Physical Activity Level (PAL) of 2.0, which is considered heavy activity.

Source: NHMRC (2006) Nutrient Reference Values for Australia and New Zealand, *Executive Summary*. Department of Health and Ageing, Australian Government.

Appendix 2—Minerals

RECOMMENDED DAILY INTAKE

MINERAL	RECOMMENDED DIETARY INTAKE (RDI) FOR ADULTS	RECOMMENDED DIETARY INTAKE (RDI) FOR CHILDREN AND TEENS	SAFE MAXIMUM INTAKE OR UPPER LIMIT (UL) FOR ADULTS
Calcium	1000 mg women (19–50 yrs) 1300 mg women (over 50 yrs) 1000 mg men (19–70 yrs) 1300 mg men (over 70 yrs)	500 mg (1–3 yrs) 700 mg (4–8 yrs) 1000 mg (9–11 yrs) 1300 mg (12–13 yrs) 1300 mg (14–18 yrs)	2500 mg
Chromium	25 mcg women 35 mcg men	11 mcg (AI) (1–3 yrs) 15 mcg (AI) (4–8 yrs) 21 mcg girls (AI) (9–13 yrs) 25 mcg boys (AI) (9–13 yrs) 25 mcg girls (AI) (14–18 yrs) 35 mcg boys (AI) (14–18 yrs)	It is not possible to set an upper limit, but no adverse effects have been reported with doses ranging from 200 to 1000 mcg daily, mostly in the form of chromium picolinate for diabetes.
Copper	1.2 mg women 1.7 mg men	0.7 mg (AI) (1–3 yrs) 1.0 mg (AI) (4–8 yrs) 1.1 mg girls (AI) (9–13 yrs) 1.3 mg boys (AI) (9–13 yrs) 1.1 mg girls (AI) (14–18 yrs) 1.5 mg boys (AI) (14–18 yrs)	10 mg
Fluoride	3 mg women 4 mg men	0.7 mg (AI) (1–3 yrs) 1.0 mg (AI) (4–8 yrs) 2 mg (AI) (9–13 yrs) 3 mg (AI) (14–18 yrs)	10 mg
Iodine	150 mcg	90 mcg (1–3 yrs) 90 mcg (4–8 yrs) 120 mcg (9–13 yrs) 150 mcg (14–18 yrs)	1100 mcg
Iron	18 mg women (19–50 yrs) 8 mg women (over 50 yrs) 8 mg men	9 mg (1–3 yrs) 10 mg (4–8 yrs) 8 mg (9–13 yrs) 15 mg girls (14–18 yrs) 11 mg boys (14–18 yrs)	45 mg
Magnesium	310 mg women (19–30 yrs) 320 mg women (over 30 yrs) 400 mg men (19–30 yrs) 420 mg men (over 30 yrs)	80 mg (1–3 yrs) 130 mg (4–8 yrs) 240 mg (9–13 yrs) 360 mg girls (14–18 yrs) 410 mg boys (14–18 yrs)	350 mg (supplements only)
Manganese	5 mg women 5.5 mg men	2 mg (AI) (1–3 yrs) 2.5 mg (AI) (4–8 yrs) 2.5 mg girls (AI) (9–13 yrs) 3 mg boys (AI) (9–13 yrs) 3 mg girls (AI) (14–18 yrs) 3.5 mg boys (AI) (14–18 yrs)	No upper limit has been set, but up to 11 milligrams a day is considered safe.
Molybdenum	45 mcg men and women	17 mcg (1–3 yrs) 22 mcg (4–8 yrs) 34 mcg (9–13 yrs) 43 mcg (14–18 yrs)	2000 mcg

MINERAL	RECOMMENDED DIETARY INTAKE (RDI) FOR ADULTS	RECOMMENDED DIETARY INTAKE (RDI) FOR CHILDREN AND TEENS	SAFE MAXIMUM INTAKE OR UPPER LIMIT (UL) FOR ADULTS
Phosphorus	1000 mg men and women	460 mg (1–3 yrs) 500 mg (4–8 yrs) 1250 mg (9–13 yrs) 1250 mg (14–18 yrs)	4000 mg
Potassium	2800 mg women 3800 mg men	2000 mg (AI) (1–3 yrs) 2300 mg (AI) (4–8 yrs) 2500 mg girls (AI) (9–13 yrs) 3000 mg boys (AI) (9–13 yrs) 2600 mg girls (AI) (14–18 yrs) 3600 mg boys (AI) (14–18 yrs)	No firm data but more than 10,000 mg (10 g) in a single dose may cause cardiac arrest.
Selenium	60 mcg women 70 mcg men	25 mcg (1–3 yrs) 30 mcg (4–8 yrs) 50 mcg (9–13 yrs) 60 mcg girls (14–18 yrs) 70 mcg boys (14–18 yrs)	400 mcg
Sodium	460–920 mg	200–400 mg (AI) (1–3 yrs) 300–600 mg (AI) (4–8 yrs) 400–800 mg (AI) (9–13 yrs) 460–920 mg (AI) (14–18 yrs)	2300 mg 1600 mg for older, overweight hypertensives and those wishing to maintain low blood pressure over the lifespan.
Zinc	8 mg women 14 mg men	3 mg (1–3 yrs) 4 mg (4–8 yrs) 6 mg (9–13 yrs) 7 mg girls (14–18 yrs) 13 mg boys (14–18 yrs)	40 mg

Source: Nutrient Reference Values for Australia and New Zealand, NH&MRC 2006. Adult figures apply to adults over 18 yrs. Where no RDI has been established, an Adequate Intake (AI) figure is given instead.

RECOMMENDED DIETARY INTAKE (RDI)

The RDI is the average daily dietary intake level that is sufficient to meet the nutrient requirements of nearly all (97–8 per cent) healthy individuals in a particular life stage and gender group.

UPPER LIMIT (UL)

This is the highest average daily intake likely to pose *no* adverse health effects to almost all individuals in the general population.

Appendix 3—Vitamins

RECOMMENDED DIETARY INTAKE

NUTRIENT	RECOMMENDED DIETARY INTAKE (RDI) FOR ADULTS	RECOMMENDED DIETARY INTAKE (RDI) FOR CHILDREN AND TEENS	SAFE MAXIMUM INTAKE OR UPPER LIMIT (UL) FOR ADULTS
Vitamin A as retinol equivalents	700 mcg women 900 mcg men	300 mcg (1–3 yrs) 400 mcg (4–8 yrs) 600 mcg (9–13 yrs) 700 mcg girls (14–18 yrs) 900 mcg boys (14–18 yrs)	3000 mcg RE = 10,000 IU Note: 1 retinol IU = 0.3 mcg Retinol Equivalents
Thiamin (Vitamin B_1)	1.1 mg women 1.2 mg men	0.5 mg (1–3 yrs) 0.6 mg (4–8 yrs) 0.9 mg (9–13 yrs) 1.1 mg girls (14–18 yrs) 1.2 mg boys (14–18 yrs)	Not established but 50–100 mg a day is considered the maximum
Riboflavin (Vitamin B_2)	1.1 mg women (19–70 yrs) 1.3 mg women (>70 yrs) 1.3 mg men (19–70 yrs) 1.6 mg men (>70 yrs)	0.5 mg (1–3 yrs) 0.6 mg (4–8 yrs) 0.9 mg (9–13 yrs) 1.1 mg girls (14–18 yrs) 1.3 mg boys (14–18 yrs)	Not established but 200 mg a day is considered the maximum
Niacin (Vitamin B_3)	14 mg women 16 mg men	6 mg (1–3 yrs) 8 mg (4–8 yrs) 12 mg (9–13 yrs) 14 mg girls (14–18 yrs) 16 mg boys (14–18 yrs)	35 mg—can cause flushing reaction at doses over 1000 mg a day
Pyridoxine (Vitamin B_6)	1.3 mg women (19–50 yrs) 1.5 mg women (>50 yrs) 1.3 mg men (19–50 yrs) 1.7 mg men (>50 yrs)	0.5 mg (1–3 yrs) 0.6 mg (4–8 yrs) 1.0 mg (9–13 yrs) 1.2 mg girls (14–18 yrs) 1.3 mg boys (14–18 yrs)	50 mg—more than 2000 mg can lead to neuritis, a painful numbing in the hands and feet due to damage to the nerves
Cyanocobalamin (Vitamin B_{12})	2.4 mcg	0.9 mcg (1–3 yrs) 1.2 mcg (4–8 yrs) 1.8 mcg (9–13 yrs) 2.4 mcg (14–18 yrs)	Non-toxic even in large doses
Folic acid (Folate) (Folate equivalents)	400 mcg	150 mcg (1–3 yrs) 200 mcg (4–8 yrs) 300 mcg (9–13 yrs) 400 mcg (14–18 yrs)	1000 mcg
Biotin	25 mcg women (AI) 30 mcg men (AI)	8 mcg (AI) (1–3 yrs) 12 mcg (AI) (4–8 yrs) 20 mcg (AI) (9–13 yrs) 25 mg girls (AI) (14–18 yrs) 30 mcg boys (AI) (14–18 yrs)	Not established but 2500 mg a day is considered the maximum
Pantothenic acid (Vitamin B_5)	4 mg women (AI) 6 mg men (AI)	3.5 mg (AI) (1–3 yrs) 4 mg (AI) (4–8 yrs) 4 mg girls (AI) (9–13 yrs) 5 mg boys (AI) (9–13 yrs) 4 mg girls (AI) (14–18 yrs) 6 mg boys (AI) (14–18 yrs)	Not established but 1000 mg a day is considered the maximum

NUTRIENT	RECOMMENDED DIETARY INTAKE (RDI) FOR ADULTS	RECOMMENDED DIETARY INTAKE (RDI) FOR CHILDREN AND TEENS	SAFE MAXIMUM INTAKE OR UPPER LIMIT (UL) FOR ADULTS
Choline	425 mg women (AI) 550 mg men (AI)	200 mg (AI) (1–3 yrs) 250 mg (AI) (4–8 yrs) 375 mg (AI) (9–13 yrs) 400 mg girls (AI) (14–18 yrs) 550 mg boys (AI) (14–18 yrs)	3500 mg
Ascorbic Acid (Vitamin C)	45 mg women and men	35 mg (1–3 yrs) 35 mg (4–8 yrs) 40 mg (9–13 yrs) 40 mg (14–18 yrs)	1000 mg. It is not toxic, but doses greater than 2000 mg a day can cause upset stomach and diarrhoea, and increases the risk of iron overload
Cholecalciferol (Vitamin D)	5 mcg or 200 IU women and men (19–50 yrs) (AI) 10 mcg or 400 IU women and men (51–70 yrs) (AI) 15 mcg or 600 IU women and men (>70 yrs) (AI)	5 mcg or 200 IU (AI) (1–3 yrs) 5 mcg or 200 IU (AI) (4–8 yrs) 5 mcg or 200 IU (AI) (9–13 yrs) 5 mcg or 200 IU (AI) (14–18 yrs)	80 mcg or 3200 IU—if you're taking supplements or for those unable to get exposure to sunlight Note: 1 mcg = 40 IU
Tocopherols (Vitamin E)	7 mg women (AI) 10 mg men (AI)	5 mg (AI) (1–3 yrs) 6 mg (AI) (4–8 yrs) 8 mg girls (AI) (9–13 yrs) 9 mg boys (AI) (9–13 yrs) 8 mg girls (AI) (14–18 yrs) 10 mg boys (AI) (14–18 yrs)	300 mg or 450 IU as d-alpha tocopherol
Phylloquinone (Vitamin K)	60 mcg women (AI) 70 mcg men (AI)	25 mcg (AI) (1–3 yrs) 35 mcg (AI) (4–8 yrs) 45 mcg (AI) (9–13 yrs) 55 mcg (AI) (14–18 yrs)	Not established but it appears safe even at quite high intakes

Source: Nutrient Reference Values for Australia and New Zealand. NH&MRC 2006. Adult figures apply to adults over 18 years. Where no RDI has been established, an Adequate Intake (AI) figure is given instead.

RECOMMENDED DIETARY INTAKE (RDI)

The RDI is the average daily intake level that is sufficient to meet the nutrient needs of nearly all (97–8 per cent) healthy individuals in a particular life stage and gender group.

UPPER LIMIT (UL)

The UL is the highest average daily intake that is likely to pose *no* adverse health effects to almost all individuals in the general population.

INDEX

Note: page references for major entries are highlighted in **bold**.

foodwatch

Keep up to date and connect with Catherine in the following ways

Online	www.foodwatch.com.au
Twitter	Follow @foodwatch
Facebook	Like FoodwatchAustralia or www.facebook.com/FoodwatchAustralia
Pinterest	Follow Foodwatch at https://pinterest.com/foodwatch
Instagram	Check out Catherine's latest pics on Instagram at http://statigr.am/catherine_saxelby